AF606318

The Baby Under 1000 g

The Baby Under 1000 g

David Harvey MB FRCP DCH
Senior Lecturer in Paediatrics, Institute of Obstetrics and Gynaecology, London

Richard W. I. Cooke MD FRCP DCH
Professor in Neonatal Medicine, University of Liverpool

Gillian A. Levitt BSc DCH MRCP
Senior Paediatric Registrar, Hospital for Sick Children, Great Ormond Street, London

WRIGHT
London Boston Singapore Sydney Toronto Wellington

Wright
is an imprint of Butterworth Scientific

 PART OF REED INTERNATIONAL P.L.C.

First published 1989

British Library Cataloguing in Publication Data
The Baby under 1000 g.
1. Premature babies & newborn babies with low birth weight
I. Harvey, David II. Cooke, Richard W. I.
III. Levitt, Gillian A.
613.92'011
ISBN 0–7236–0952–7

Library of Congress Cataloging in Publication Data
Harvey, David (David Robert)
The baby under 1000 g.
Bibliography: p.
Includes index.
1. Infants (Premature) 2. Birth weight, Low.
I. Cooke, Richard W. I. II. Levitt, Gillian A.
III. Title. IV. Title: Baby under one thousand g.
RJ250.H29 1989 618.92'011 89–7276
ISBN 0–7236–0952–7

Typeset in Great Britain by Latimer Trend & Company Ltd, Plymouth
Printed and bound in Great Britain by Butler and Tanner, Frome, Somerset

Foreword

It has been a pleasure to produce this book on the care of extremely premature babies. As neonatal medicine has advanced over the last 15 years, we have seen the survival of more and more tiny babies. All neonatal intensive care units now look after babies that were considered unsalvagable only a few years ago. The problem is that the management of these babies is very much more complicated than that for babies who are only mildly pre-term or who are born at term. They usually require ventilation for long periods and have particular difficulties with water loss because of their very thin skin.

As a result of these changes in medical care, we held a symposium on the subject. Some of those who were at the meeting have been joined by other specialists in the field. We are extremely grateful for a very generous donation from Cow and Gate Limited which allowed us to hold the meeting and for a donation from Orange Medical Instruments. The public meeting held after the symposium was also supported by other instrument and pharmaceutical companies.

We believe that joint efforts like this between industry and the profession can contribute both to the advancement of science and to the improvement of care of premature babies.

We have one sadness at the time of the publication of this book. Our friend and colleague Jean Boxall died in the autumn of 1988. She, more than anyone else, raised the status of neonatal nursing. Not only did she care for babies beautifully but she also worried about their families and the problems that the birth of such small babies had in a wider social context. Her chapter in this book bubbles over with her enthusiasm and new ideas for us to use.

Glossary of abbreviations

ABR	Auditory brainstem response
AGA	Appropriate for gestational age
AIDS	Acquired immunodeficiency syndrome
AVP	Arginine vasopressin
BBB	Blood-brain barrier
BP	Blood pressure
BPD	Bronchopulmonary dysplasia
CMV	Cytomegalovirus
CNS	Central nervous system
CLP	Chronic lung disease of prematurity
CPD	Cephalopelvic disproportion
C/S	Caesarean section
CVP	Central venous pressure
DEHP	Diethylhexyl phthalate
ECF	Extracellular fluid
ECG	Electrocardiogram
EEG	Electroencephalogram
ELBW	Extremely low birth weight (less than 1000 g)
EMG	Electromyelogram
FDP	Fibrinogen degradation products
$F\text{io}_2$	Fraction of inspired oxygen concentration
FPF	Fibroblast-pneumocyte factor
FRC	Functional residual capacity
GA	Gestational age
GFR	Glomerular filtration rate
GVHD	Graft verus host disease
HDN	Haemolytic disease of the newborn
HFPPV	High frequency positive pressure ventilation (> 60 breaths/min)
HIV	Human immunodeficiency virus
HMWK	High molecular weight kininogen
ICP	Intracranial pressure
IPPV	Intermittent positive pressure ventilation

IQ	Intellectual quotient
IUGR	Intrauterine growth retardation
IVH	Intraventricular haemorrhage
LBW	Low birth weight (less than 2500 g)
L:S ratio	Lecithin:sphingomyelin ratio
MAP	Mean airways pressure
MRC	Medical Research Council
MRS	Magnetic resonance spectroscopy
NICU	Neonatal intensive care unit
NMR	Nuclear magnetic resonance
PAL	Pulmonary air leak
PCA	Post-conceptual age
PCV	Packed cell volume
PDA	Patent ductus arteriosus
PEEP	Positive end expiratory pressure
PET	Pre-eclamptic toxaemia
PG	Phosphatidyl glycerol
PGA	Post-gestational age
PI	Phosphatidyl inositol
PIA	Pulmonary interstitial air
PIP	Peak inspiratory pressure
PK	Prekallikrein
PMA	Post-menstrual age
PROM	Prolonged rupture of membranes
PTT	Partial thromboplastin time
PUFA	Polyunsaturated fatty acids
PVC	Polyvinyl chloride
PVH	Periventricular haemorrhage
PVL	Periventricular leucomalacia
RAAS	Renin-angiotensin-aldosterone system
RCM	Red cell mass
RDS	Respiratory distress syndrome
$S\text{ao}_2$	Oxygen saturation
SCBU	Special care baby unit
SGA	Small for gestational age
$T_{\frac{1}{2}}$	Half life
T_3	Tri-iodothyronine
TI	Inflation time
TLC	Total lung capacity
$\text{tc}P\text{co}_2$	Transcutaneous partial pressure for carbon dioxide
$\text{tc}P\text{o}_2$	Transcutaneous partial pressure for oxygen
TRH	Thyrotropin-releasing hormone
TTP	Thrombotic thrombocytopaenic purpura
VEP	Visual evoked potential
VLBW	Very low birth weight (less than 1500 g)

Contributors

Jean Boxall
Late Honorary Research Fellow,
Department of Child Health,
Royal Devon and Exeter Hospital,
Exeter, UK

Elizabeth M. Bryan
Honorary Consultant Paediatrician,
Queen Charlotte's Hospital for Women,
London, UK

Geoffrey Chamberlain
Professor of Obstetrics and Gynaecology,
St George's Hospital Medical School,
London, UK

Richard W. I. Cooke
Professor in Neonatal Medicine,
University of Liverpool, Liverpool, UK

Malcolm Coulthard
Consultant Paediatric Nephrologist,
The Children's Department,
Royal Victoria Infirmary,
Newcastle, UK

John de Louvois
Top Grade Microbiologist,
Queen Charlotte's Hospital for Women,
London, UK

Robert Dinwiddie
Consultant Paediatrician,
Hospital for Sick Children,
Great Ormond Street,
London, UK

Lilly M. S. Dubowitz
Research Lecturer,
Department of Child Health and Neonatal Medicine,
Hammersmith Hospital,
London, UK

Murdoch G. Elder
Professor of Obstetrics and Gynaecology,
Institute of Obstetrics and Gynaecology,
Hammersmith Hospital,
London, UK

Janet Eyre
First Assistant in Child Health,
Department of Child Health,
The Medical School,
University of Newcastle upon Tyne, UK

Anne Greenough
Senior Lecturer in Neonatology,
Department of Child Health,
King's College Hospital, London, UK

David Harvey
Senior Lecturer in Paediatrics,
Institute of Obstetrics and Gynecology,
London, UK

Jean W. Keeling
Consultant Paediatric Pathologist,
John Radcliffe Maternity Hospital, Oxford, UK

Richard F. Lamont
Consultant Obstetrician and Gynaecologist,
Northwick Park Hospital and
Clinical Research Centre, London, UK

Elizabeth Letsky
Consultant Haematologist,
Queen Charlotte's Hospital for Women,
London, UK

Gillian A. Levitt
Associate Specialist,
The Hospitals for Sick Children,
Great Ormond Street,
London, UK

Neil McIntosh
Senior Lecturer in Child Health,
St George's Hospital Medical School,
London, UK

Neena Modi
Consultant Paediatrician,
Queen Charlotte's Hospital for Women,
London, UK

Colin J. Morley
Consultant Paediatrician
University Department of Paediatrics,
Addenbrooke's Hospital,
Cambridge, UK

Clifford Roberton
Head of Paediatrics,
Riyadh Armed Forces Hospital,
Riyadh, Kingdom of Saudi Arabia

Martin Richards
Head of Child Care and Development Group,
University of Cambridge, UK

Naren Patel
Consultant Obstetrician and Gynaecologist,
Department of Reproductive Medicine,
Ninewells Hospital,
Dundee, UK

Kathrine L. Peters
Neonatal Research Laboratory,
Alexandra Children's Pavilion,
Edmonton, Canada

Peter Rolfe
Professor, Department of Biomedical Engineering and Physics,
University of Keele,
Stoke on Trent, UK

Nicholas Rutter
Senior Lecturer in Child Health and Honorary Consultant Paediatrician,
Department of Neonatal Medicine and Surgery,
City Hospital,
Nottingham, UK

Ann L. Stewart
Honorary Senior Lecturer in Perinatal Medicine,
Department of Paediatrics and Obstetrics,
University College and Middlesex School of Medicine,
Rayne Institute,
London, UK

William Tarnow-Mordi
Senior Lecturer,
Department of Child Health,
Ninewells Hospital and Medical School,
Dundee, UK

Ewan Walker
Consultant Obstetrician and Gynaecologist,
Ayrshire Central Hospital,
Irvine, Ayrshire, UK

Andrew Whitelaw
Consultant Neonatologist,
Department of Paediatrics and Neonatal Medicine,
Hammersmith Hospital, London, UK

James L. Wilkinson
Director of Cardiology,
Royal Children's Hospital,
Parkville, Victoria, Australia

Antony F. Williams
Senior Lecturer in Child Health,
St Georges Hospital Medical School, London, UK

Victor Y. H. Yu
Director of Neonatal Intensive Care,
Queen Victoria Medical Centre; Clinical Associate Professor,
Monash University,
Melbourne, Australia

Contents

Foreword v

Glossary of abbreviations vii

Contributors ix

1 **Aetiology and incidence** 1
Ewan Walker and Naren Patel
2 **Obstetrical management** 9
Geoffrey Chamberlain
3 **Mode of delivery** 16
Richard F. Lamont and Murdoch G. Elder
4 **Prevention of respiratory distress syndrome** 23
Colin J. Morley
5 **Resuscitation** 50
Clifford Roberton
6 **Ventilator care and respiratory audit** 65
William Tarnow-Mordi
7 **Pulmonary air leak** 78
Anne Greenough
8 **Chronic lung disease** 86
Robert Dinwiddie
9 **The hazards of an immature skin** 94
Nicholas Rutter
10 **Monitoring** 106
Peter Rolfe
11 **Jaundice** 120
Neena Modi
12 **Feeding** 134
Anthony F. Williams
13 **Intravenous nutrition** 141
Victor Y. H. Yu
14 **Calcium and phosphorus metabolism and rickets** 155
Neil McIntosh
15 **Haematology** 163
Elizabeth Letsky

16	**Infection** John de Louvois	190
17	**Cardiac disorders including ductus arteriosus** James L. Wilkinson	200
18	**Renal function** Malcolm Coulthard	211
19	**Neurological abnormalities** Richard W. I. Cooke, Lilly M. S. Dubowitz, Janet Eyre, Andrew Whitelaw	226
20	**Iatrogenic disease** Jean W. Keeling and Elizabeth M. Bryan	289
21	**Nursing procedures and chest physiotherapy** Kathrine L. Peters	304
22	**Preparation for home** Jean Boxall	316
23	**The social and emotional needs of the parents and baby** Martin Richards	325
24	**Outcome** Ann L. Stewart	331
25	**The cost of intensive care** Richard W. I. Cooke	340

Index 345

Chapter 1

Aetiology and incidence

Ewen Walker and Naren Patel

Any attempt to define the incidence of babies born weighing less than 1000 g is fraught with problems. The commonly quoted figure of just under 1% [1] only relates to live or stillbirths after 28 weeks of gestation, and is inherently biased to exclude stillbirths or babies born dead earlier than this gestation (late abortions). In an attempt to discover the obstetric factors leading to delivery of live births of less than 1000 g, one must look also at late abortions at less than 28 weeks gestation. The survivors at birth are only a minority of pregnancies that have come to grief. The factors that lead to the delivery of these extremely low birth weight (ELBW) infants are likely to be the same as those causing late abortions in mid-trimester.

The majority of ELBW infants are small because of extreme prematurity (less than 28 weeks gestation) but some are small for dates at a later gestation. Much of the published data deal with birth weight alone and it is understandable why this is so. Weight is easily established by placing the infant on scales. Length of gestation, however, is much more difficult to assess retrospectively. It has long been recognized that a woman's recall of the date of her last menstrual period is poor; about one-fifth of UK women surveyed in 1970 were unable to provide reliable enough dates to calculate length of gestation [2] and this has been confirmed by other workers [3]. Paediatric scoring systems for assessing gestational age are difficult to perform on these infants and are designed primarily for older gestations. Unless reliable ultrasound data are available from earlier in the pregnancy, it is not always possible to estimate gestational age. Since we cannot predict which women will produce a baby weighing less than 1000 g, all women in an obstetric population would have to have an ultrasound measurement of crown–rump length (between seven and 11 weeks gestation) or biparietal diameter (from 14 to 20 weeks gestation) in order to know the gestational age at birth. Few centres have such intensive use of ultrasound scanning.

In Dundee we have a policy of routine scanning at 19 weeks gestation which is primarily for confirmation of gestational age, exclusion of fetal abnormality and diagnosis of multiple pregnancy. We have recently conducted a retrospective review of all pregnancies ending between 20 and 28 weeks gestation to determine what antenatal factors resulted in these late abortions and extremely premature deliveries.

During the five years studied (1980–1984 inclusive), 144 mothers delivered 156 infants between 20 and 28 weeks (12 sets of twins). Only 137 of these women had an ultrasound scan performed before 20 weeks gestation and those who had not been scanned were excluded from the study. The case notes of the remaining 149 infants were reviewed. Terminations of pregnancy for fetal abnormality during this period are discussed separately later.

Table 1.1 The causes of delivery between 20 and 28 weeks gestation and the subsequent infant outcome in 149 infants (1980–1984)

Cause	*Stillborn or abortion*	*Live <7 days*	*Died 8–28 days*	*Died 1–18 months*	*Alive (handi-capped)*	*Alive (well)*	*Total*	*Percentage*
Premature labour	39	14	3	2	5[a]	8	71	47.7
Antepartum haemorrhage	15	5			3[b]	3	23	15.4
Preterm spontaneous rupture of membranes	15	1				2	21	14.1
Unexplained IUD	7						7	4.7
Intrauterine growth retardation	2						2	1.3
Intrauterine asphyxia	1						1	0.7
Fetal abnormality	3						3	2.0
Hypertension	4					3	7	4.7
Cervical incompetence	5	1					6	4.0
Maternal disease	1						1	0.7
Infection	7						7	4.7
Total no. (%)	99 (66.4)	21 (14.1)	3 (2.0)	2 (1.3)	8 (5.4)	16 (10.7)		

Type of disability:
[a] Right hemiplegia; right hemiplegia; blind; blind; osteogenesis imperfecta.
[b] Left hemiplegia; microcephaly; spastic dysplegia.

Of the 149 infants, 99 were registered as abortions. Of the 50 infants who were liveborn, 21 died within one week, another three died within one month, and a further two within 18 months. Mean birth weight between 25 and 26 weeks gestation was 681 g, between 26 and 27 weeks was 889 g and between 27 and 28 weeks was 978 g. Of the 24 surviving, eight have a major degree of handicap on follow-up to 18 months (although in one case the disability is congenital in origin).

Table 1.1 shows the causes of delivery between 20 and 28 weeks gestation. The most frequent precipitating cause of delivery was uncomplicated spontaneous preterm labour (47%). Spontaneous preterm labour complicated by antepartum haemorrhage (15%) and preterm rupture of membranes (14%) were other significant antenatal precedents. Only 4% could be attributed to cervical incompetence which therefore offers hope that medical intervention in a subsequent pregnancy could prevent a recurrence. It is worth looking in more detail at what is known about these antenatal factors which precipitated delivery of these very small infants.

Spontaneous preterm labour

Despite recent advances in knowledge about prostaglandins and other locally acting agents involved in parturition, we still do not know why the human uterus starts to contract at term, and even less about causes of preterm labour. Factors associated with birth at less than 37 weeks gestation have been studied in Oxford in 1973–

Table 1.2 The percentage of major causes of preterm delivery ($n = 393$) [4]

	Percentage
Spontaneous	
Twins	10
Singleton – known cause	24
– unknown cause	38
Total	72
Elective	28

1974 [4] and Aberdeen [5]. These studies divided deliveries into elective, uncomplicated preterm and preterm labour complicated by, for example, antepartum haemorrhage or preterm spontaneous rupture of membranes. About half of all preterm births occurred in the absence of any specific complications – so-called uncomplicated preterm labour (Table 1.2).

Uncomplicated preterm labour

Despite the fact that no definite complication such as antepartum haemorrhage or spontaneous rupture of membranes precedes the onset of labour in most cases, there must be a factor as yet unrecognized which precipitates delivery in these 'uncomplicated preterm labours'. Several possible causes have been investigated.

Psychosocial stress

A number of studies have been performed to determine the influence of psychological stress on the incidence of preterm delivery. Standardized questionnaires have been designed to measure perceived levels of anxiety and depression along with a record of recent life events. Some of these earlier studies were performed in retrospect – interviewers visited the women after a preterm delivery [6]. This was a major criticism of their method, since women who have had an adverse outcome tend to seek a cause and this tendency has been recognized in other retrospective studies [7]. Perhaps the best example of this is a study by Stott [8], which showed that mothers who had delivered a child with Down's syndrome had experienced more 'shocks' during that pregnancy than mothers with normal children. It was two years later that the first report linking Down's syndrome and chromosomal abnormality appeared!

A recent prospective study, however, has confirmed that there is a significant association between the experience of major life events in pregnancy such as divorce or bereavement, etc. and preterm delivery [9], but the mechanism by which psychosocial stress precipitates labour is not known. In the same study cigarette smoking was related to some extent to preterm delivery.

Complicated preterm delivery

Bleeding in pregnancy

Threatened abortion seems to predispose to an increased risk of preterm birth. In a study of threatened abortion where the bleeding settled and the pregnancy appeared to progress satisfactorily, the incidence of preterm labour was 16.5% compared with 6.5% in all booked cases [10]. Placenta praevia, placental abruption and non-specific antepartum haemorrhage are all associated with a high perinatal mortality rate mainly due to preterm delivery [11].

Premature rupture of membranes

Spontaneous rupture of the membranes precedes the onset of labour in a high percentage of preterm deliveries [12]. In our study of pregnancies ending spontaneously between 20 and 28 weeks, spontaneous preterm rupture of membranes was the principle precipitating obstetric factor in 14% of cases (Table 1.1). The mechanism whereby the amniotic membranes rupture prematurely in some women is not entirely clear although some interesting research has been performed. Tension in the intact membranes appears to increase as full term approaches, but there is a significant decrease in the elasticity of membranes which rupture spontaneously before the onset of labour [13]. The epithelial surfaces of amnion and chorion are hydrophobic and it has been demonstrated that in women with spontaneous premature rupture of membranes the surface energy is significantly higher than in controls. This probably results in impaired mechanical resistance. One interesting suggestion was that this phenomenon may be regulated by the deposition of surfactant from the amniotic fluid [14].

Infection

Several studies have attempted to identify a specific cervical infection which might weaken membranes and make preterm spontaneous rupture of membranes more likely. An association has been found between preterm spontaneous rupture of membranes and infection of amniotic fluid with bacteria which produce high phospholipase A_2 activity [15,16]. However, this association was also found in premature labour where the membranes were intact, so the mechanism may be increased uterine activity rather than weakening of the membranes. A prospective study of vaginal flora in early pregnancy has been carried out to try to predict preterm spontaneous rupture of membranes but no single microorganism proved to be either a highly specific or sensitive indicator of risk [17]. Women with group B streptococci in their *urine* seem to have a significantly increased risk of premature rupture of membranes and delivery [18]; it may be that screening and appropriate antibiotic treatment could reduce this cause of premature delivery.

Cervical incompetence

The incidence of true cervical incompetence is probably between 1 and 2% [19]. It is difficult to be sure since the condition is often overdiagnosed, and whilst the number of cerclage operations may well reflect the frequency of diagnosis, this is not necessarily the true incidence. Cervical incompetence has been estimated to be the principal precipitating cause in up to one-fifth of late miscarriages [19]. The classical picture is of late miscarriage resulting in the birth of a live fetus following a short painless labour not preceded by significant bleeding. Cervical incompetence is thus a loose term which describes the failure of the cervix to fulfil its role in the second

Table 1.3 Effect on subsequent pregnancies of conization with removal of small and large conus [21]

Cone volume	*Second trimester abortion (%)*	*Preterm birth (%)*
<4 ml	6.5	3.2
>4 ml	18.2	31.7

Table 1.4 The comparison of death, survival and handicap in singleton and twin infants delivered between 20 and 28 weeks gestation

	Abortion	*Deaths*			*Alive/ handicapped*	*Alive/ well*	*Total*
		< 1 week	*1 week–1 month*	*< 8 months*			
Singleton	88	20	1		6	10	125
Twin	11	1	2	2	2	6	24

trimester of pregnancy as a sphincter for the uterus. Much effort has been made to determine the causes.

The first report of abortion due to cervical incompetence was published by Gream [20] and he campaigned against the then fashionable practice of surgically dividing or forcefully dilating the cervix to treat adolescent dysmenorrhoea. It seems to have taken more than a century for this to be abandoned but iatrogenic damage still occurs.

Cone biopsy of the cervix has also been implicated; subsequent cervical incompetence is related to the volume of the tissue excised [21] (Table 1.3). This should become much less common now that the introduction of colposcopy has significantly reduced the need for cone biopsy in most centres. Uterine abnormalities [22] and *in utero* exposure to diethylstilboestrol [23] have also been implicated. It is interesting to note that whilst dilatating an unripened cervix with blunt Hegar dilators beyond 10 mm has been shown to cause rupture [24], the increased incidence of second trimester induced abortions in the last 15 years does not seem to have resulted in increased risk of spontaneous abortion in subsequent pregnancies [25]. This is almost certainly due to the improved techniques available.

Multiple pregnancy

It has long been recognized that multiple pregnancy is associated with a high risk of preterm labour and contributes significantly to ELBW babies admitted to special baby care units. In our recent review of pregnancies ending between 20 and 28 weeks gestation, 24 of 149 infants (16.1%) were twins (Table 1.4). Quite why multiple pregnancies should feature as such a significant underlying cause in this gestational age group is not entirely clear. While it may be true that many multiple pregnancies deliver before term because the uterus is very distended and simply cannot accommodate any more volume change, this cannot satisfactorily explain the high incidence of spontaneous labour at less than 28 weeks when a twin pregnancy does not yet distend the uterus as much as a 36-week singleton gestation. Some more subtle factor may be at work. In addition to increased total fetal weight there is also a much greater placental size and oestrogen levels are much higher. It may be that this alters myometrial activity and predisposes to earlier onset of spontaneous labour.

Fetal abnormality

Early detection of fetal abnormality is now an important part of antenatal care in the UK. Apart from specific investigations for groups at particular risk, e.g. amniocentesis for maternal age, many UK centres now perform whole population screening for specific abnormalities if there is a sufficiently high incidence of that defect in their area, e.g. serum alpha-fetoprotein to detect neural tube defects which is now routinely offered to pregnant women in areas with a high prevelance of this abnormality. In our hospital we rely on serum alpha-fetoprotein and the 19-week scan to detect neural tube defects. In addition, amniocentesis is available to all mothers over 36 years or younger women if indicated.

During 1980–84 there were 54 fetuses identified as abnormal and the pregnancies terminated (Table 1.5). Had these pregnancies, complicated by fetal abnormality, not been detected, many would have gone on to term but some may well have delivered at less than 28 weeks gestation, especially those abnormalities such as anencephaly which are often complicated by polyhydramnios. Only three fetuses which had slipped through the screening net delivered spontaneously between 20 and 28 weeks during 1980–84 and all were dead at birth. The abnormalities were chromosomal and could not have been detected by our screening techniques. As antenatal detection of fetal abnormalities becomes more effective, fetal abnormality should become a less common cause of birth weight under 1000 g.

Intrauterine growth retardation

Intrauterine growth retardation (IUGR) has been extensively investigated by many centres with access to good ultrasound facilities but most studies have concentrated on detection of poor fetal growth late in the third trimester. This is partly because some authors feel that IUGR only becomes manifest after 30 weeks gestation [26], i.e. that all fetuses grow at the same rate until then, and some fail to thrive thereafter. This hypothesis is not universally accepted [27]. Another reason why the emphasis has been placed on investigation later in pregnancy is the knowledge that intervention at

Table 1.5 Terminations for fetal abnormality (>20 weeks gestation) 1980–1984

Fetal abnormality	*No.*	*Percentage*
Anencephaly (+spina bifida)	31	57.4
Spina bifida (+hydrocephaly)	14	25.9
Encephalocoele	3	5.6
Hydrocephaly	1	1.9
Ophthalmocoele	1	1.9
Exophthalmos	1	1.9
Down's syndrome	1	1.9
Turner's syndrome	1	1.9
Other chromosomal	1	1.9

less than 30 weeks gestation is fraught with hazard for the fetus and the feeling that there is little point in detecting poor growth until the fetus is sufficiently mature to have a good chance of survival if delivered. Because of this there is a lack of data on ELBW babies and it is not possible to be certain what role IUGR plays in these deliveries.

References

1. *Health, United States* (1984) National Center for Health Statistics, Public Health Service, Washington D.C.
2. Chamberlain, G., Philipp, E., Howlett, B. and Masters, K. (1970) *British Births Survey*, Vol. **1**, pp. 8–54. Heinemann Medical, London
3. Hall, M. H., Carr-Hill, R. A., Fraser, C., Campbell, D. and Samphier, M. L. (1985) The extent and antecedents of uncertain gestation. *Br. J. Obstet. Gynaecol.*, **92**, 445–451
4. Rush, R., Keirse, M., Howard, P. *et al.* (1976) Contribution of preterm delivey to perinatal mortality. *Br. Med. J.*, **ii**, 956–968
5. Chng, P. K. (1981) An analysis of preterm singleton deliveries and associated deaths in a total population. *Br. J. Obstet. Gynaecol.* **88**, 814–824
6. Newton, R. W., Webster, P. A. C., Binu, P. S., Maskrey, N. and Philips, A. B. (1979) Psycho-social stress in pregnancy and its relation to the onset of premature labour. *Br. Med. J.*, **ii**, 411
7. Brown, G. W. and Harris, T. (1978) *Social Origins of Depression*, Tavistock, London
8. Stott, D. H. (1958) Some psycho-somatic aspects of casualty in reproduction. *J. Psychosom. Res.*, **3**, 42
9. Newton, R. W. and Hunt, L. P. (1984) Psychosocial stress in pregnancy and its relation to low birth weight. *Br. Med. J.*, **288**, 1191–1194
10. Turnbull, E. P. N. and Walker, J. (1956) The outcome of pregnancy complicated by threatened abortion. *J. Obstet. Gynaecol. Br. Emp.*, **63**, 553
11. Roberts, G. (1970) Unclassified antepartum haemorrhage incidence and perinatal mortality in a community. *J. Obstet. Gynaecol. Br. Emp.*, **77**, 492
12. Gillibrand, P. N. (1967) Premature rupture of membranes and prematurity. *J. Obstet. Gynaecol. Br. Commonw.*, **74**, 678
13. Parry-Jones, E. and Priya, S. (1976) A study of the elasticity and tension of fetal membranes and the relation of the area of the gestational sac to the area of the uterine cavity. *Br. J. Obstet. Gynaecol.*, **83**, 205
14. Hills, B. A. and Cotton, D. B. (1984) Premature rupture of membranes and surface energy. Possible role of surfactant. *Am. J. Obstet. Gynecol.*, **149**, 896
15. Bejar, R., Curbelo, V., Davis, C. and Gluck, L. (1981) Premature labour, II. Sources of phospholipase. *Obstet. Gynecol.*, **57**, 479
16. Curbelo, V., Bejar, R., Benirschke, K. and Gluck, L. (1981) Prostaglandin precursors in human placental membranes. *Obstet. Gynecol.*, **57**, 473
17. Minkoff, H., Grunebaum, A. N., Schwarz, R. H. *et al.* (1984) Risk factors for prematurity and premature rupture of the membranes: a prospective study of the vaginal flora in pregnancy. *Am. J. Obstet. Gynecol.*, **150**, 965
18. Moller, M., Thomson, A. C., Borch, K. *et al.*, (1984) Rupture of fetal membranes and prematurity associated with group B streptococci in urine of pregnant women. *Lancet*, **ii**, 69
19. McDonald, I. A. (1980) Cervical cerclage. *Clin. Obstet. Gynaecol.*, **7**, 461–479
20. Gream, G. T. (1865) Dilatation or division of the cervix uteri. *Lancet*, **i**, 381
21. Leiman, G., Harrison, N. A. and Rubin, A. (1980) Pregnancy following conisation of the cervix and complication related to cone size. *Am. J. Obstet. Gynecol.*, **136**, 14–18
22. Craig, C. J. T. (1974) Congenital abnormalities of the uterus and fetal wastage. *Obstet. Gynecol. Surv.*, **29**, 612–614
23. Quinlan, R. W. and Cruz, A. C. (1980) Reproductive failure and cervical incompetence in women exposed to diethyl stilbestrol. *S. Afr. Med. J.*, **73**, 89

24. Liu, D. T. Y., Black, M., Meldner, D. A., Melville, M. A. H. and Cameron, S. (1975) Dilatation of the parous non-pregnant cervix. *Br. J. Obstet. Gynaecol.*, **82**, 246–251
25. Chung, C. S., Smith, R. G., Steinhoff, P. G. and Ming-Pi, Mi (1982) Induced abortion and spontaneous fetal loss in subsequent pregnancies. *Am. J. Public Health*, **72**, 548–554
26. Beischer, N. A., Abell, D. A. and Drew, J. H. (1984) Intrauterine growth retardation. *Prog. Obstet. Gynaecol.*, **4**, 83
27. Geirsson, R. T. and Persson, P. (1984) Diagnosis of intrauterine growth retardation using ultrasound. *Clin. Obstet. Gynecol.*, **11**, 457–480

Chapter 2

Obstetrical management

Geoffrey Chamberlain

In the UK 0.3% of babies are born with a birth weight under 1000 g. In 1984 the stillbirth rate in this group was 207 per 1000 total births and the neonatal death rate 377 per 1000 live births [1]. Figure 2.1 shows how both these rates have been static until the mid 1970s but each has been reducing since then. Neonatal deaths have improved at a sharper rate than stillbirths since 1980, indicating the great improvement in neonatal care. There are many who allege that by saving very small babies we are providing problems for society later on. In general, this does not seem to be so.

By far the most common associated cause of death in babies with a birth weight under 1000 g is respiratory distress syndrome (about 40%), and the next largest is congenital abnormalities (about 15%).

Management

In all branches of medicine the best management of any condition is to prevent it,

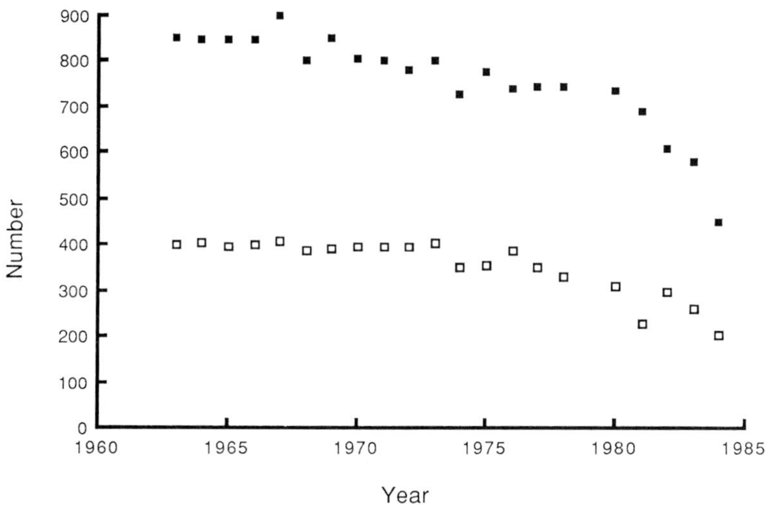

Figure 2.1 Neonatal deaths per 1000 live births (■) and stillbirths per 1000 total births (□) in babies under 1000 g birth weight in England and Wales

then no physician has to deal with the problems and the secondary problems that might arise. This may seem a counsel of perfection but it applies very much in the obstetric field of ELBW infants. Antenatal care as currently practised in the western world serves many functions but the one that particularly concerns this chapter is the prevention of very early preterm labour.

Background

During the course of antenatal care women at higher risk of such problems should be identified and special attention paid to them. For example, the woman who has had a previous preterm labour has at least twice the risk of another preterm delivery.

The three major components of perinatal epidemiology are shown in Figures 2.2, 2.3 and 2.4; in all these figures the percentage of babies born below 1000 g birth weight is so small that the effects are not easily seen. To facilitate visualization, the data on babies born under 2500 g are shown for this mirrors and exaggerates the changes seen in the under 1000 g group. The younger and older aged mothers have an increased risk with ELBW babies (Figure 2.2). A similar shaped curve is seen in Figure 2.3 which shows the effect of parity; the lowest incidence is with para 1 whilst those having their first or third baby or over have an increased incidence.

The socioeconomic class influence is shown in Figure 2.4. While those born under 2500 g follow the national trends of social deprivation, the babies under 1000 g do not do so. Any trends seen in this area seem to be a feature of the mother's body size rather than the simple categorization of their husband's occupation. Cigarette smokers have a much greater increased risk and women bearing multiple pregnancies are also at increased risk. Such women should be advised about their increased risks of preterm labour and warned of the signs of onset of such a labour. If their work is physically heavy they should be guided to try to reduce that effort, for fatiguing and boring jobs have been shown to double the risk of preterm labour [2]. Such advice is not always possible to follow in a society such as ours where employment is at a

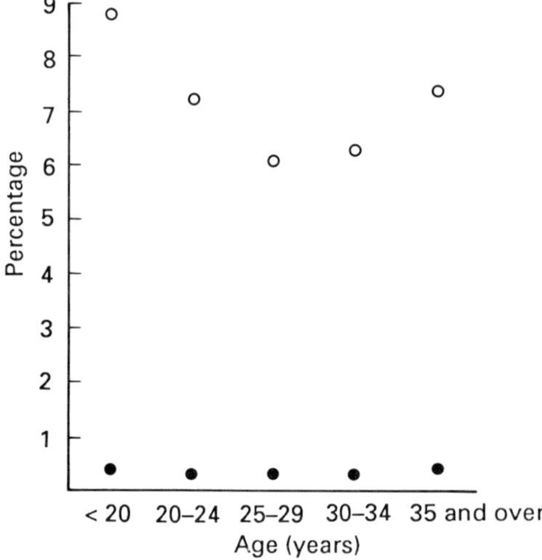

Figure 2.2 Relationship between birth weight and maternal age in England and Wales in 1985. ○ <2500 g; ● <1000 g

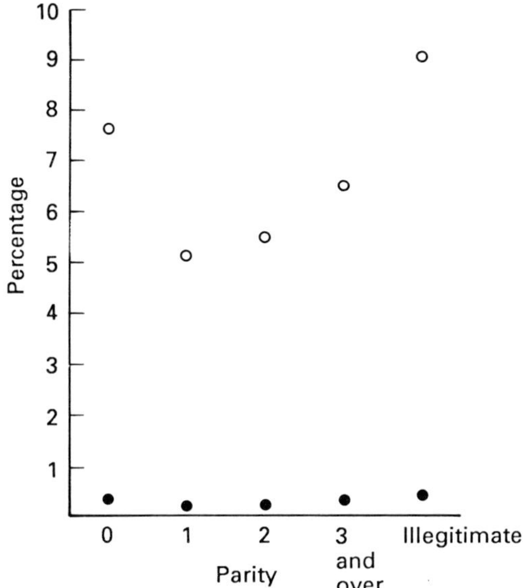

Figure 2.3 Effect of parity on birth weight in England and Wales in 1985. ○ <2500 g; ● <1000 g

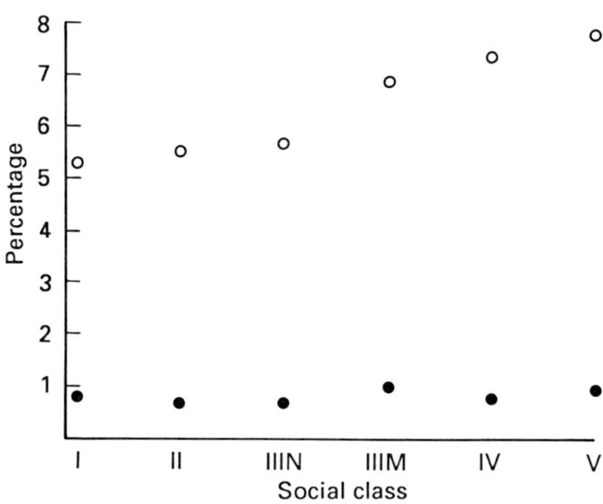

Figure 2.4 Effect of social class on birth weight in England and Wales in 1985. ○ <2500 g; ● <1000 g

premium, but if it could be arranged that a woman works less hard this may well postpone the onset of a very preterm labour. Work has many components, not the least of which is getting to work. Travelling to and from work in unpleasant circumstances for an hour each day can be as stressful as all the other features of work itself [3].

Growth of fetus

During the antenatal period most obstetricians try to estimate the growth of the fetus.

Clinical estimation is not good enough by itself; Paul, Koh and Monfared [4] showed that most clinicians underestimated babies weighing under 1500 g. In the UK almost 90% of women have an ultrasound reading of fetal size before the 20th week of pregnancy and some have a repeat of this later on. The first estimation confirms the dates of pregnancy assessed from the last menstrual period and enables a precise measure of fetal growth to be obtained by placing the baby on the correct part of the birth weight gestational age chart.

When a woman who has had early ultrasound runs into problems later in pregnancy, a repeat ultrasound estimation of the fetal head circumference and his abdominal circumference can give a precise measure of the estimated fetal weight. This is extremely useful in guiding obstetricians and neonatologists about delivery. Jeanty and Romero [5] have derived a series of charts from which the fetal weight can be calculated from the biparietal diameter and the abdominal circumference. These should be available in all labour wards where obstetricians at registrar and more senior level are capable of using an ultrasound machine to estimate fetal weight from such measurements. However, in the ELBW baby there is as yet a lack of data to make such valid charts of estimated birth weight and so errors of prediction are more likely. A fuller ultrasound scan should be performed by a more experienced obstetrician if time allows and labour does not follow.

Cervical incompetence

One of the major reasons for early preterm labour among ELBW babies is cervical incompetence. This is a concept which has grown up in the last 40 years; it owes acceptance in the obstetrical world to its simplistic nature. The diagnosis of this condition would ideally be made before pregnancy when a woman who has had previous mid-trimester abortions or early preterm labours should be investigated. She may be found to have a cervix which will accept an 8 mm dilator in the outpatients without any anaesthesia. She may require X-ray investigations to show the incompetence of the cervix. These are relatively crude but show up the worst cases.

In pregnancy, obviously investigations like these cannot be performed; one starts with the history of previous mid-trimester abortions or early preterm labours which gives rise to suspicion. Ultrasound investigation of the cervix in early and mid-pregnancy is rewarding provided a machine of sufficient resolution is used and the ultrasonographer is experienced. Varma, Patel and Pillai [6] found that accurate and reproducible readings could be made of the length of the canal and its diameter at the internal os; measurements provided an objective method of diagnosing an incompetent cervix and also helped to avoid unnecessary cerclage operations which might have been performed on history alone.

Treatment is simple and consists of putting in a non-absorbable suture at about the level of the internal cervical os to stop the cervix dilating. Shirodkar [7] was the pioneer in this although most people follow the technique of McDonald [8]. Unfortunately this simple operation has its complications. Stimulation of the myometrium to produce an abortion and septicaemia have been reported. Because of these doubts, the Medical Research Council and Royal College of Obstetrics and Gynaecology have performed a multicentre randomized controlled trial into cervical suture. The latest results indicate that there may be some assistance in preventing the very early preterm birth of babies to mothers who had a late mid-trimester abortion in a previous pregnancy. This applies also in women who have had previous deliveries at 24–28 weeks of gestation.

The cervical suture is best inserted before it is needed, usually at 14 weeks of gestation, allowing time for spontaneous abortions due to chromosomal abnormalities to have taken place. If the suture succeeds, pregnancy will proceed to the later weeks and the suture can be removed at about 37 weeks gestation. A full review of this subject is given by Chamberlain and Gibbings [9].

Tocolysis

The manipulation of uterine contractions has been the wish of many in obstetrics. For the last 20 years sympathomimetics have been the predominant drugs for the control of myometrial contractions. In the 1960s intravenous alcohol had a brief phase of popularity and spasmolytics such as isoxsuprine were tried. Whilst our knowledge of smooth muscle physiology of the uterus has increased greatly, the mechanisms responsible for starting the onset of contractions are still unknown and so the use of sympathomimetics is slightly illogical. They do not act against the factors that start preterm labour, only against the uterine contractions once started.

When very early preterm labour starts it is difficult for anyone – mother or doctor – to make the diagnosis. The differences between Braxton Hicks contractions of pregnancy and early labour contractions do not exist as well in practice as they seem to in the textbooks. It needs the passage of time with a competent observer watching and assessing the myometrial contractions. A tocograph helps and assessment of cervical dilatation finally allows the negative diagnosis of the Braxton Hicks contraction to be made. In consequence studies of tocolytic agents are bedevilled by the problems of deciding which women to enter into the study. The well-known placebo effect is important here. If one cares for a patient and looks after her properly, 25–50% of women will go out of labour even if given placebo tablets or infusions [10].

In essence there is little evidence that the use of betamimetics has improved fetal outcome. Certainly labour has been postponed by hours and days but the ultimate measurement of the fetus by perinatal mortality or morbidity has not been greatly improved. A *British Medical Journal* leading article [11] said: 'On balance and in terms of fetal outcome, the use of drugs to inhibit labour is usually unnecessary, frequently ineffective and occasionally harmful'. It is very hard to find truly randomized studies; to set these up is difficult for very few women present in the gestational stage who fulfil all the criteria and are willing to be randomized. There are a few valid studies, for example the work of Spellacy *et al.* [12] who could not find any neonatal beneficial effect of ritodrine in a truly randomized controlled study.

These agents have their side effects on the mother with an unpleasant tachycardia and, more seriously, pulmonary oedema. The use of such betamimetic agents has now decreased in the UK and they are used mostly to cover first aid situations such as the transfer of a woman to a unit where she should be delivered or to postpone labour to allow the use of steroids to help maturation of the fetal lungs.

In utero transfer

If the woman is at risk of going into very early preterm labour, she should be delivered at the place where the maximum paediatric care is available. If it is considered that the fetus is under 1000 g, this should be at a tertiary referral centre with expert neonatal help. The best incubator in which to transfer a baby of this size is the mother's uterus. This can be done after consultation between the peripheral and central units.

At the recipient unit the doctor concerned should be of senior registrar or consultant level. He should deal directly on the telephone with a consultant or registrar of the donor unit. It should be established that the woman is not likely to be delivered during the course of transfer. Hence it is unusual to accept women with a cervix over 4 cm dilated; another contraindication is vaginal bleeding which might imply the presence of placenta praevia. The senior registrar or consultant in the recipient unit should then check with his paediatric opposite number that there are staffed cots available and he should know whether there are any expected problems from his own unit that might need these cots. After this, acceptance is given and arrangements for escorted transport made. There is a further problem in the UK of transfer across regions. In the South West Thames region during 1986, of the women accepted for *in utero* transfer at the tertiary referral SCBU in St. George's Hospital, 30% came from out of the region implying some deficiency in the provision of care for the under 1000 g baby in the London area, as the different regions have insufficient facilities for modern neonatal care.

The major features in deciding whether to use *in utero* transfer are the condition of the fetus and his maturity. This should have been estimated by ultrasound in the peripheral unit. His presentation might sway transfer for, if he is a breech presentation, it is more than likely he will need help with operative delivery. The site of the placenta should be known.

It is very important to know about the family wishes of the potential transfer and to ensure that they are fully consulted before the woman leaves the donor centre. Much ill will has been engendered in the past when people have been transferred from one hospital to another without their family being fully informed of the reasons for this.

When the patient arrives at the recipient centre, the possibility of maturation of the lungs and postponement of labour must be considered again if both of these have not been fully worked out at the donor centre. At the stage of gestation appropriate for a 1000 g baby it is unlikely that the lecithin-sphingomyelin ratio will be used, as the results are not helpful at this very early stage of gestation and probably will not cause any change in the management of the case. If a test is not going to influence any clinical action taken there is no point in doing it. It may be performed in special cases and a phospholipid glycerol level may also be obtained by cross electrophoresis. Howie and Liggins [13] showed that betamethasone has a maximal effect in reducing respiratory distress syndrome when given for 48 h at a gestational age of between 32 and 34 weeks. Since then, Garite *et al.* [14] have shown that there are few advantages of corticosteroids compared with simple expectant management. It is probable that between 28 and 30 weeks a singleton baby (especially if female) would benefit from steroids given *in utero* to a greater extent than the disadvantages the therapy entails. This means the postponement of delivery for about 48 h, hence the use of betamimetics to aid this.

Conclusion

More babies of under 1000 g estimated birth weight are presenting in our labour wards. The obstetrician must consider in conjunction with the paediatrician the best way of coping with these. Background information or reported uterine contractions may warn of impending early preterm labour. The place of suturing of the cervix and of tocolytic drugs is at present less certain than it seemed ten years ago.

The features of the pregnancy should be reviewed and women at higher risk for delivery of very small babies should be offered accommodation in obstetrical units that can look after them. If a woman goes into labour with such a small baby, she should be transferred in labour to a unit where neonatal care will be of the highest standards.

References

1. OPCS (1987) *Infant and Perinatal Mortality*, HMSO, London
2. Mamelle, N. and Lauman, B. (1984) Occupational fatigue and preterm birth. In *Pregnant Women at Work* (ed. G. Chamberlain), Macmillan, London, pp. 105–116
3. Rodrigues-Escudero, R., Belanstegreguria, A. and Gutierrez-Martinez, S. (1980) Perinatal complications of work in pregnancy *An. Esp. Pediatr.*, **13**, 465–476
4. Paul, R., Koh, K. and Monfared, A. (1979) Obstetric factors influencing outcome in infants weighing from 1001 to 1500 g. *Am. J. Obstet. Gynecol.* **133**, 503–508
5. Jeanty, J. and Romero, R. (1984) Determining estimated fetal weight. In *Obstetrical Ultrasound*, McGraw Hill, New York, pp. 162–167
6. Varma, T., Patel, R. and Pillai, U. (1985) Ultrasonic assessment of the cervix in at-risk patients. *Acta Obstet. Gynecol. Scand.*, **65**, 147–152
7. Shirodkar, V. (1953) Observations on non-malignant conditions of the cervix. *J. Obstet. Gynaecol. India*, **3**, 287
8. McDonald, I. (1957) Suture of the cervix for inevitable miscarriage. *J. Obstet. Gynaecol. Br. Commonw.*, **64**, 346
9. Chamberlain, G. and Gibbings, C. (1983) Observations on non-malignant conditions of the cervix. In *Clinical and Diagnostic Procedures in Obstetrics and Gynaecology, Part A: Obstetrics* (eds M. Symmonds and F. Zuspan), Marcel Dekker Inc, New York pp. 34–47
10. Ingemarsson, I. (1984) Pharmacology of tocolytic agents. *Clin. Obstet. Gynaecol.*, **11**, 337–351
11. Leading article (1981) Drug treatment of premature labour. *Br. Med. J.*, **283**, 395–396
12. Spellacy, W., Cruz, A., Birk, S. and Burke, W. (1979) Treatment of premature labour with ritodrine. *Obstet. Gynecol.*, **54**, 220–223
13. Howie, R. and Liggins, G. C. (1977) Clinical trial of antepartum betamethasone therapy. In *Preterm Labour* (eds A. Anderson, R. Beard, J. M. Brudenell and P. M. Dunn), Royal College of Obstetricians and Gynaecologists, London, pp. 281–289
14. Garite, T. J., Freeman, R. K., Linzey, E. M., Braly, P. S. and Dorchester, W. L. (1981) Prospective randomized study of corticosteroids in the management of premature rupture of the membranes and the premature gestation. *Am. J. Obstet. Gynecol.*, **141**, 508–515

Chapter 3

Mode of delivery

Richard F. Lamont and Murdoch G. Elder

Introduction

The decision with respect to the route of delivery of the extremely low birthweight (ELBW) fetus estimated to weigh less than 1000 g will be influenced by a number of factors:

(1) Many women who present in early preterm labour have a past history of fetal or neonatal loss and this may persuade the obstetrician to choose the abdominal route.
(2) Those babies who are estimated to weigh less than 1000 g because of severe intrauterine growth retardation (IUGR) may be considered to have insufficient reserves to withstand a labour and vaginal delivery.
(3) Where elective delivery is planned at an early gestation for conditions such as severe IUGR, pregnancy-induced hypertension or antepartum haemorrhage, the state of the cervix may be so unfavourable that successful induction of labour and vaginal delivery would be improbable or impossible.
(4) Unless vaginal delivery is imminent, cardiotocographic evidence of intrapartum asphyxia will require delivery by caesarean section if the fetus is estimated to weigh more than 600 g and neonatal intensive care facilities are available.
(5) Most progressive spontaneous preterm labours are of relatively short duration but if it is felt that labour is becoming prolonged, or if there is evidence of intrapartum infection, most obstetricians would expedite delivery by caesarean section.

While these factors raise little controversy, the choice of a particular route of delivery continues to cause much argument.

Considerations for vaginal delivery

Cord complications such as compression or prolapse are more common with breech delivery. The lower limbs and trunk of the fetus presenting by the breech may be delivered through an incompletely dilated cervix and this may lead to entrapment of the head. Abdominal visceral injuries are more common when the soft abdomen of a breech rather than the bony pelvis has been compressed during manipulation at birth, and intracranial haemorrhage is more common after vaginal breech delivery. While these risks of vaginal breech delivery apply to breech presentations at all gestations, the lower the birth weight the higher the risk.

For vertex presentations, high intrauterine pressures during the expulsive phase of the second stage of labour may cause excessive head compression. With delivery of the tiny fetus, the increased ratio of the size of the maternal pelvis in relation to the size of the fetus may result in a compound presentation. It can be very worrying to see a scalp electrode disappear into the vagina with each maternal expulsive effort, as one realizes that the tiny fetus is gradually folding up in the vagina so that an arm or shoulder will soon appear at the introitus.

Considerations for caesarean section

Caesarean section carries a ten-fold increased risk of maternal mortality and morbidity over vaginal delivery. In the most recent triennium (1979–1981) of the Confidential Enquiry into Maternal Deaths there were 87 maternal deaths associated with caesarean section – a rate of 0.5 per 1000 operations.

Lethal congenital malformations, especially if associated with excess or deficiency of liquor volume, are associated with an increased incidence of preterm delivery. It is estimated that up to 13% preterm infants presenting by the breech have congenital malformations [1]. If appropriate steps are not taken to exclude such malformations where possible, many unnecessary caesarean sections may be performed because of cardiotocographic signs of intrapartum asphyxia in such infants.

Caesarean section below 30 weeks gestational age is a technically difficult procedure because of the poorly formed lower segment and, as with vaginal delivery, the fetus presenting by the breech may suffer head entrapment. This may require extension of the uterine incision into the upper segment.

Idiopathic respiratory distress syndrome (RDS) is more common after caesarean section, though this may only apply to elective caesarean sections where there has been no labour to stimulate release of endogenous fetal cortisol. It is less likely to occur in cases of IUGR where the fetus has been stressed for some time.

Delivery of the VLBW infant

Breech

From pooled data of 11 studies, Crowley and Hawkins [2] showed that preterm infants presenting by the breech and delivered vaginally suffered twice the mortality rate of comparable infants delivered by caesarean section. However, when the figures were presented as birth weight specific perinatal mortality rates, caesarean section only showed a reduction in mortality for those infants presenting by the breech who had a birth weight between 1000 and 1500 g. Since that time other review articles [3,4] have confirmed the findings of Crowley and Hawkins.

The results of a policy of caesarean section for infants presenting by the breech who were estimated to have a birth weight between 1000 and 1500 g were published by Lamont *et al.* [5]. Survival of such infants with a birth weight below 1500 g was 100% for those delivered by caesarean section compared to 63% for those delivered by the breech vaginally.

The rate of perventricular haemorrhage (PVH) in the same group of infants was 21% for breech presentations under 1500 g delivered by caesarean section compared with 59% for infants delivered vaginally.

Vertex

Studies which give recommendations for the best route to deliver the VLBW infant presenting by the vertex are far fewer than those for the preterm breech. For those vertex presentations above 34 weeks gestational age, in an otherwise uncomplicated labour, most obstetricians would agree that the vaginal route is the better mode of delivery.

For infants between 800 and 1350 g, Haesslein and Goodlin [6] showed an improvement in survival for infants delivered by caesarean section. Westgren *et al.* [7] recorded that for infants weighing less than 1500 g, delivery by caesarean section resulted in a reduced incidence of subsequent PVH over those infants delivered vaginally by the vertex. In a carefully matched study of infants weighing less than 2000 g Westgren *et al.* [8] showed that at follow-up 18 months to two years later, infants delivered vaginally had a higher incidence of psychomotor retardation over infants delivered by caesarean section.

In an observational study Lamont [9] recorded the outcome of 309 infants presenting by the vertex who delivered before 34 weeks gestation as a result of spontaneous preterm labour. Those infants who were delivered by caesarean section before 30 weeks (and who had a birth weight of less than 1500 g) had a higher survival rate and a lower rate of PVH compared to infants delivered vaginally. This was in spite of the fact that caesarean section was only performed for vertex presentations when there was some intrapartum complication such as haemorrhage, infection or cardiotocographic signs of intrapartum asphyxia.

Delivery of the infant weighing less than 1000 g (ELBW)

The data pertaining to the optimum mode of delivery for the ELBW infant are very difficult to obtain. A literature search for English language papers in the last ten years concerned with the mode of delivery of the VLBW revealed about 50 publications.

Breech

Only nine papers give adequate statistics from which conclusions can be drawn. The mortality of the infant weighing less than 1000 g presenting by the breech was calculated according to whether the delivery was vaginal or by caesarean section. These studies and their results are shown in Table 3.1.

Using the figures of Table 3.1 in combination, the mortality rate for infants presenting by the breech was 77% for vaginal deliveries compared to 49% for infants delivered by caesarean section. This difference is statistically significant (χ^2 with Yates correction = 26.4; $P < 0.001$).

Three studies of infants presenting by the breech quoted data for infants between 700 g (or 750 g) and 1000 g [10–12]. When only these infants were considered (Table 3.2), the overall mortality rate for these infants was 74% for infants delivered vaginally compared to 42% for infants delivered by caesarean section (χ^2 with Yates correction = 9.57; $P < 0.01$).

Table 3.1 Hospital mortality rates of infants presenting by the breech according to mode of delivery

Authors	*Birth weight range* (g)	*Caesarean section*		*Vaginal delivery*	
		Number	*Deaths*	*Number*	*Deaths*
Yu *et al.*[14]	501–1000	3	1	28	16
Doyle *et al.*[10]	500–999	10	3	49	33
Morales and Koerten[13]	500–1000	32	18	24	16
[a] Bowes *et al.*[15]	501–1000	5	3	34	29
[b] Effer *et al.*[16]	500–999	25	11	23	14
Worthington *et al.*[12]	500–999	10	2	18	13
Mann and Gallant[17]	500–1000	5	4	29	27
Main *et al.*[11]	750–999	15	9	52	45
Nissell *et al.*[1]	<1000	0	0	16	16
Total (%)		105	51 (49%)[c]	273	209 (77%)[c]

[a] Stillbirths plus neonatal deaths
[b] Neonatal mortality
[c] $P<0.001$

Table 3.2 Hospital mortality rates for infants between 750 and 1000 g according to presentation and mode of delivery

Authors	*Presentation*	*Caesarean section*		*Vaginal delivery*	
		Number	*Deaths*	*Number*	*Deaths*
[a] Doyle *et al.*[10]	Breech	8	2	40	26
Worthington *et al.*[12]	Breech	8	2	8	3
Main *et al.*[11]	Breech	15	9	52	45
Breech total (%)		31	13 (42%)[b]	100	74 (74%)[b]
Worthington *et al.*[12]	Vertex	12	4	36	12
Main *et al.*[11]	Vertex	9	5	132	73
Vertex total (%)		21	9 (43%)	168	85 (51%)

[a] 700–999 g
[b] $P<0.01$

In only two studies was it possible to quantify the rate of PVH among infants presenting by the breech. Morales and Koerten [13] detected PVH in 22 of 24 infants (92%) with birth weight between 500 g and 1000 g who delivered vaginally, compared to 26 of 32 infants (81%) for infants with similar birth weights delivered by caesarean section. Main, Main and Maurer [11] detected PVH in 17 of 34 infants (50%) weighing between 750 and 999 g delivered vaginally compared to six of ten infants (60%) delivered by caesarean section.

Vertex

Only four studies quoted adequate statistics for calculation of the mortality rate for infants weighing less than 1000 g and presenting by the vertex. These studies and their results are shown in Table 3.3.

For infants with a birth weight of 500–1000 g presenting by the vertex (Table 3.3), the trend was the same as for infants presenting by the breech (Table 3.1). Vaginal

Table 3.3 Hospital mortality rates of infants presenting by the vertex according to mode of delivery

Authors	*Birth weight range* (g)	*Caesarean section*		*Vaginal delivery*	
		Number	*Deaths*	*Number*	*Deaths*
Yu *et al.*[14]	501–1000	21	8	42	21
Main *et al.*[11]	500–1000	9	5	132	73
Morales and Koerten[13]	500–1000	26	9	88	32
Worthington *et al.*[12]	500–999	6	2	49	26
Total (%)		62	24 (39%)	311	152 (49%)

delivery was associated with a mortality rate of 49% compared to 39% for delivery by caesarean section (Table 3.3).

Two of these studies quoted mortality rates in the birth weight band 750–1000 g [11,12]. In this birth weight range the mortality rate for vertex presentations delivered vaginally was 51% compared to 43% for those infants delivered by caesarean section (Table 3.2).

The incidence of PVH among babies presenting by the vertex and weighing between 500 and 1000 g was 59 of 88 infants (67%) delivered vaginally compared to 16 of 26 infants (62%) delivered by caesarean section [13].

Long-term follow-up

There was only one report of survival at follow-up for infants weighing 501–1000 g depending on the presentation at birth and the mode of delivery. The survival at two years for vertex presentations with a birth weight of 501–1000 g was 11 of 13 (85%) delivered by caesarean section compared to 17 of 21 (81%) comparable infants delivered vaginally. The survival at two years for breech presentations with a birth weight of 501–1000 g was one of two (50%) delivered by caesarean section compared to eight of 12 (67%) of comparable infants delivered vaginally [14].

Data relating to handicap at long-term follow-up could not be found which quoted figures for the baby weighing less than 1000 g and which also broke down the data into presentation and mode of delivery.

Intrapartum management

The importance of ultrasound cannot be over-emphasized for a women admitted in preterm labour, when the birth weight is thought to be under 1000 g. The scan will give an estimate of birth weight, may detect congenital malformation, and will identify presentation, all of which are essential if the optimal mode of delivery is to be chosen.

To reduce the dangers of head compression for the infant presenting by the vertex, many advocate leaving the membranes intact. The membranes then act as the presenting part and spread the rise in intrauterine pressure that occurs during a contraction evenly over the liquor and fetus. This also reduces the incidence of cord prolapse. If external monitoring is unsatisfactory, it may be necessary to rupture the membranes and apply a fetal scalp electrode to monitor the fetal heart rate.

The transition of the fetus with its immature midbrain from intrauterine to extrauterine life will be helped if it is not depressed by central analgesics. Epidural analgesia is therefore the preferred method of analgesia rather than the use of narcotics.

The use of forceps for the delivery of the VLBW baby to protect the fetal head from compression at delivery has been advocated. Not only are forceps too big for the tiny baby but there is no evidence that the use of prophylactic forceps is beneficial [15]. Instead, we would advocate an adequate episiotomy to reduce perineal resistance to delivery of the fetal head.

The use of classical caesarean section has been advocated by Haesslein and Goodlin [6]. As a universal policy this seems unnecessary. Westgren *et al.* [7] found that a T-extension to the transverse lower segment uterine incision was needed in only three of 43 cases. The delivery of the preterm infant by caesarean section should be carried out by the most experienced member of the obstetric staff available and the decision about uterine incision should depend on the findings at the time of operation rather than making a policy in advance. Irrespective of the incision, some difficulty in delivering a tiny baby through thick myometrium may be encountered. In practice, the operation is not always as easy for the infant as one might expect.

Standardization

As increased attention is given to the infant weighing less than 1000 g, better standardization is required if data are to be compared and accumulated. The LBW baby and the VLBW baby are well defined birth weight groups. Nomenclature for the baby weighing less than 1000 g varies from 'tiny newborn' to 'extremely low birth weight' (ELBW). The latter would seem most appropriate and should be adopted for standardization.

There is a great difference in survival rates between babies weighing 500–749 g and babies of 750–1000 g. It would seem appropriate not to consider the group with birth weights less than 1000 g as a whole, but rather to group these babies into 250 g bands of 500–749 g and 750–999 g.

Many studies including those reviewed in this chapter quote birth weight ranges of 500–999 g or 501–1000 g or 500–1000 g. This may seem unimportant but in a busy regional referral centre the difference of 1 g can result in a number of infants each year being allocated to higher or lower birth weight bands which might adversely or favourably affect figures.

Conclusion

For the VLBW baby presenting by the vertex, there is evidence that caesarean section may result in a decrease in neonatal mortality and morbidity [9]. For the vertex presentation below 1000 g there also appears to be a trend towards improved survival following caesarean section (Table 3.3). The evidence, however, is not strong enough to recommend a policy of elective caesarean section for preterm infants presenting by the vertex.

Despite the limitations of the studies with regard to the VLBW infant presenting by the breech, a policy of caesarean section for infants estimated to weigh between 1000 and 1500 g appears to be vindicated [5].

From Table 3.2 mortality rates following caesarean section (42%) for infants between 750 and 1000 g presenting by the breech were significantly less than for such infants delivered vaginally (74%) ($P<0.01$). It would appear that with improved neonatal intensive care and hence improved survival for infants between 750 and 1000 g, the policy of caesarean section for infants presenting by the breech should be extended to cover infants with an estimated birth weight of 750–1500 g.

Finally, the views of the mother must not be ignored. Despite a poor prognosis, some women will request a caesarean section because they feel it gives their baby an increased chance of survival however tiny. Conversely, others may be totally against surgery for various reasons and these views must be respected, provided the patient has been fully informed of the situation.

References

1. Nissell, H., Bistoletti, P. and Palme, C. (1981) Preterm breech delivery: early and late complications. *Acta Obstet. Gynaecol. Scand.*, **60**, 363–366
2. Crowley, P. and Hawkins, D. F. (1980) Preterm breech delivery – the caesarean section debate. *J. Obstet. Gynaecol.*, **1**, 2–6
3. Howie, P. W. and Patel, N. B. (1984) Obstetric management of preterm labour. *Clin. Obstet. Gynaecol.*, **11**, 373–390
4. Steel, S. A. and Pearce, J. M. (1986) Delivery of the very low birth weight baby. *Br. J. Hosp. Med.*, **36**, 328–334
5. Lamont, R. F., Dunlop. P. D. M. D., Crowley, P. and Elder, M. G. (1983) Spontaneous preterm labour and delivery at under 34 weeks gestation. *Br. Med. J.*, **286**, 454–457
6. Haesslein, H. C. and Goodlin, R. C. (1979) Delivery of the tiny newborn. *Am. J. Obstet. Gynecol.*, **134**, 192–198
7. Westgren, M., Ingermarsson, I., Ahlstrom, H. Lindroth, M. and Svenningsen, M. W. (1982) Delivery and long term outcome of very low birth weight infants. *Acta Obstet. Gynaecol. Scand.*, **61**, 25–30
8. Westgren, M., Dolfin, T., Halperin, M. Milligan, J., Shennan, A., Svenningsen, M. W. and Ingermarsson, I. (1985) I. Mode of delivery in the low birth weight fetus. Delivery by caesarean section independent of fetal lie versus vaginal delivery in vertex presentation. *Acta Obstet. Gynaecol. Scand.*, **64**, 51–57
9. Lamont, R. F. (1985) Factors influencing the route of delivery of the preterm infant. In *Proceedings of the Thirteenth Study Group of the Royal College of Obstetricians and Gynaecologists* (eds R. W. Beard and F. Sharp), Royal College of Obstetrics and Gynaecology, London, pp. 263–271
10. Doyle, L. W., Rickards, A. L., Ford, G. W., Pepperell, R. J. and Kitchen, W. (1985) Outcome for the very low birth weight (500–1499 g) singleton breech: benefit of caesarean section. *Aust. NZ J. Obstet. Gynaecol.*, **25**, 259–265
11. Main, D. M., Main, E. K. and Maurer, M. M. (1983) Cesarean section versus vaginal delivery for the breech fetus weighing less than 1500 grams. *Am. J. Obstet. Gynecol.*, **146**, 580–584
12. Worthington, D., Davis, L. E., Grausz, J. P. and Sobocinski, K. (1983) Factors influencing survival and morbidity with very low birth weight delivery. *Obstet. Gynecol.*, **62**, 550–555
13. Morales, W. J. and Koerten, J. (1986) Obstetric management and intraventricular haemorrhage in very-low-birth-weight infants. *Obstet. Gynecol.*, **68**, 35–40
14. Yu, V. Y. H., Bajuk, B., Cutting, D., Orgill, A. A. and Astbury, J. (1984) Effect of mode of delivery on outcome of very low birth weight infants. *Br. J. Obstet. Gynaecol.*, **91**, 633–639
15. Liu, D. T. Y. and Fairweather, D. V. I. (1984) The management of preterm labour. In *Preterm Labour* (eds M. G. Elder and C. H. Hendricks), Butterworths, London, pp. 231–259
16. Effer, S. B., Saigal, S., Raud, C. *et al.* (1983) Effect of delivery method on outcomes in the very low birth weight breech infant: is the improved survival related to caesarean section or other perinatal case manoeuvres? *Am. J. Obstet. Gynecol.*, **145**, 123–128
17. Mann, L. I. and Gallant, J. M. (1979) Modern management of the breech delivery. *Am. J. Obstet. Gynecol.*, **134**, 611–614

Chapter 4

Prevention of respiratory distress syndrome

Colin J. Morley

This chapter outlines the different factors contributing to respiratory failure in very premature babies and suggests how they might be influenced to reduce its severity. Unfortunately there is very little information specifically concerned with the prevention of respiratory distress syndrome in babies under 1000 g. Therefore much of the information presented is extrapolated from basic physiology, biochemistry and studies on more mature babies.

Frequency of respiratory failure in very premature babies

Respiratory distress syndrome (RDS) is defined for the purpose of this chapter as the need by a premature baby for increased inspired oxygen requirements where the chest X-ray shows a fine granular pattern in the lung fields and there is no other obvious cause for the respiratory failure. This occurs in the majority of babies weighing less than 1000 g. In a recent Cambridge study [1] with 62 babies under 1000 g, 61 required resuscitation at birth and 58 subsequently needed artificial ventilation and increased inspired oxygen. Four were very small for dates; in those who were an appropriate size for dates 95% developed respiratory failure. A third of the babies died. The survivors required mechanical ventilation for an average of two weeks and additional oxygen for 35 days.

Respiratory failure in these small babies is the predisposing factor for most of the serious complications experienced in the neonatal period. The majority of these babies would die without meticulous management with carefully measured oxygen and ventilation therapy. It is therefore important that all the factors which might contribute to RDS are understood so that they can be controlled, prevented or manipulated to prevent or reduce the severity of RDS and its complications.

Factors affecting respiratory failure

The major problem facing the baby under 1000 g is immaturity of all the component parts of respiration. Since the work of Avery and Mead in 1959 [2], RDS in premature babies has been considered to be due to surfactant deficiency or abnormality. As a consequence pulmonary surfactant biochemistry and physiology and related factors have been extensively studied [3] with the idea that if the surfactant status of the babies could be enhanced either by endogenously improving synthesis and secretion, or by exogenously treating the babies with surfactant, their respiratory problems should improve considerably. However, surfactant is only one of the factors predisposing to RDS in very premature babies. The respiratory difficulties are due to many interrelated factors all of which would have to be removed or improved if RDS were to be prevented.

Gestational age

The factor which correlates best with the incidence and severity of neonatal respiratory disease is gestational age. The lower the gestational age the higher the incidence of RDS. As can be seen from Figure 4.1 most babies below 30 weeks gestation need respiratory support. This includes virtually all babies born weighing less than 1000 g.

Immature lung structure

Babies less than 28 weeks do not have mature alveoli. At about six months gestation lung structure is changing from the canalicular to the alveolar phase. The airways have developed a full complement of divisions but by 28 weeks gestation they end in small numbers of primitive saccules, the epithelium of which has just differentiated from a simple cuboidal epithelium to type I and II cells. The respiratory surface area of these saccules is small compared with the alveolar surface of a child. Although there is a full complement of pulmonary arteries at this stage the capillary network is comparatively sparse. Where the capillaries are closely adherent to the epithelial surface there is a satisfactory barrier for gas exchange but elsewhere the saccule walls are thicker due to a large connective tissue component. The structural development of the lung has been extensively reviewed by Hislop and Reid [4].

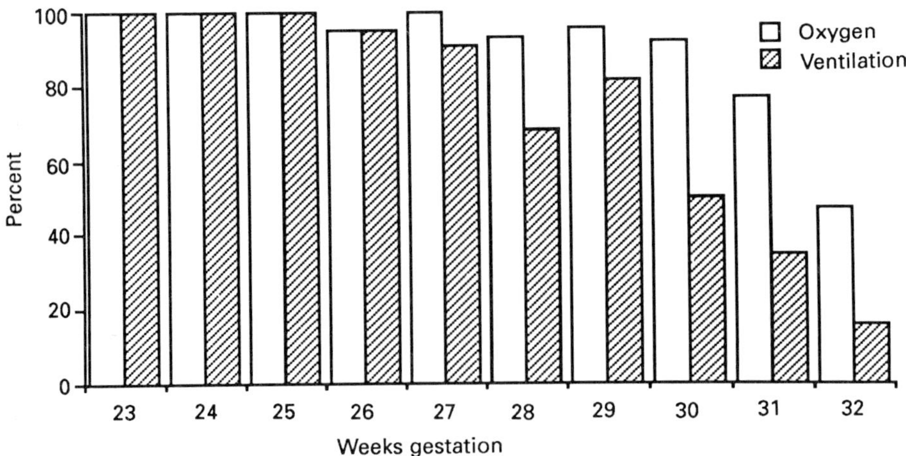

Figure 4.1 Requirements for ventilation and oxygen by very premature babies

Surfactant abnormality and deficiency

The role of surfactant on the surface of a normal, mature healthy alveolus is to split open the alveoli and terminal airways during expiration thus maintaining the functional residual capacity (FRC) and preventing atelectasis. It acts as a low surface tension lubricant during inspiration facilitating lung expansion and also helps keep the alveolar surface dry [5]. An excess of good surfactant at birth is vital for the rapid development and maintenance of lung volume.

Surfactant is a complex mixture of phospholipids, neutral lipids and proteolipids. The main phospholipid components are phosphatidyl choline and unsaturated phosphatidyl glycerol (PG). In very immature lungs the surfactant has low levels of phosphatidyl choline which is relatively unsaturated compared with surfactant from mature lungs [6,7]. It is therefore functionally poor at stabilizing the airways because it is less able to produce a high surface pressure on compression and thereby maintain the FRC during expiration [8]. This immature surfactant also has very low levels of PG [9], the role of which is unknown. It is probably one of the components which aid surface spreading. Immature surfactant which lacks PG does not function normally. The amount of surfactant produced by babies dying of RDS per 100 g lung tissue is about half that produced by full term babies [2,7,10,11]. This relative surfactant deficiency probably compounds the problem of immature surfactant composition and means that it is less able to maintain a patent airway.

The biochemical maturation of surfactant can be measured in the amniotic fluid using the lecithin:sphingomyelin (L:S) ratio. It has been shown that the lungs are functionally mature when this reaches 2:1, at about 34–35 weeks gestation [12]. However at 30–31 weeks the incidence of RDS is only about 50% [13] and many babies appear to have clinically good lung function. Therefore there is a discrepancy of about four weeks between studying the amniotic fluid of the fetus and the respiratory function of the baby. This may be due to the beneficial effect of labour and delivery on the lungs (see below).

Surfactant substrate deficiency

It has been suggested [14] that the variation in the incidence of RDS in various parts of the world may be due to different dietary intakes of palmitic acid. Palmitic acid is the 16-carbon saturated fatty acid which forms the major fatty acid component of phosphatidyl choline in mature surfactant. It has been shown in animals that mothers who have a diet high in palmitate have premature babies with a lower incidence of respiratory problems.

Hallman and his collegues have shown that the severity of RDS can be reduced by giving a baby inositol after birth. In a randomized trial in 74 babies weighing less than 2000 g who required ventilation for RDS, they showed that between the fourth and tenth day the inositol-treated infants tended to have a milder respiratory course than the controls. This effect was apparent in the babies under 28 weeks gestation [15]. Phosphatidyl inositol (PI) is one of the phospholipids which appears to be important to surfactant function in premature babies. The level of PI falls in premature babies not fed on milk. It can be increased and the L:S ratio improved by augmenting the plasma inositol level in these babies [16].

This suggests that dietary factors may be an important influence on the severity of RDS.

Protein exudation onto the airway surface

In the preterm baby there is often enough surfactant to sustain reasonable lung function if it is secreted properly, not inhibited and not lost prematurely. When the lungs of a very premature baby expand at birth in the presence of inadequate surfactant, the surface epithelium rapidly develops interstitial oedema, localized areas of necrosis, desquamation of the epithelium and hyaline membranes [17]. The hyaline membranes consist of both coagulated proteins which have exuded onto the lung surface and cell debris from the damaged and desquamated epithelial cells. Part of the coagulated protein appears to be polymerized fibrinogen.

Some, if not all, of the extruded proteins interfere with surfactant function. It has been shown that fibrinogen and fibrin monomers prevent surfactant generating high surface pressures under compression [18,19]. Ikegami, Jobe and Glatz [20] showed that when premature lambs were treated with natural surfactant they had an improvement in lung function which deteriorated after a few hours. This was due to the appearance of surfactant inhibitory proteins which interfered with the physical properties of the surfactant molecules in the surface monolayer.

The exudation of these inhibitory proteins may be a major factor in babies with marginal surfactant function developing severe RDS. This is probably the reason why asphyxiated and acidotic babies develop RDS when they might otherwise have reasonable neonatal lung function.

Labour and the clearance of lung fluid

Lung fluid which contains surfactant is secreted by the alveolar cells and prior to birth fills the lung. This secretion is controlled by epithelial cells which actively pump chloride ions into the alveolar fluid, passively carrying sodium ions and water with it. During labour, in mature animals, the secretion stops and fluid is absorbed from the lung so that at birth the lungs contain much less fluid. This effect is due to endogenous release of adrenaline by the fetus during labour and mediated by β-adrenergic receptors. It stimulates sodium transport from the lung lumen to the plasma and water passively follows. In the premature animals labour has much less effect on lung fluid secretion and reabsorption than in mature animals [21]. This means that very premature babies may not be able to clear their lung fluid from their airways and it is possible that secretion may continue for a while after birth. It is also possible that in the absence of satisfactory surfactant the rate of fluid absorption may be comparatively slow.

Extrapolating to the very premature baby, it is likely that at birth the lungs will contain fluid which is not rapidly absorbed. This will interfere with alveolar volume by it reducing the radius of curvature inside the air sac and thereby increasing its surface tension. This is another factor which reduces the ability of very premature babies to develop a stable aerated lung [22].

It has been known for a long time that babies born by elective caesarian section (C/S) are more at risk of RDS than babies born after normal labour. In term babies there is a catecholamine surge during labour [23] which is important for the enhancement of airway liquid absorption, increases cardiac performance, particularly during hypoxia, and mobilizes glucose and free fatty acids. There is a much smaller rise in endogenous catecholamines during elective C/S delivery than C/S during labour. C/S delivery without labour is common in premature babies. In a ten-centre surfactant trial [24] with babies between 25 and 29 weeks gestation 40% were delivered by C/S without labour. Rooney, Gobran and Wai-Lee [25] showed that neonatal rabbit lungs secreted more surfactant in the hours after birth if they were subjected to labour than if they were born after elective C/S. This effect was independent of gestational age. Although this is probably an important mechanism there is little evidence that it has much effect on the incidence of RDS below 33 weeks [23]. In premature lambs Lawson *et al.* [26] showed that infusion of adrenaline reduced the rate of pulmonary fluid secretion in term fetuses but had very little effect in premature fetuses. It is therefore possible that the premature human fetus may have a similar lack of response to adrenergic stimulation.

Immaturity of pulmonary blood pressure control and patent ductus arteriosus

In full term babies pulmonary vascular resistance falls after birth in association with air breathing and the ductus arteriosus closes within a few hours. This is delayed by acidosis or hypoxia [27]. In very premature babies it appears that the ductus arteriosus remains patent [28] partially under the influence of high levels of prostaglandins. The shunt of blood across the ductus is dependent on the difference between the pulmonary and systemic blood pressures. In the early stages of severe RDS the systemic blood pressure may be lower than the pulmonary arterial pressure so that a right-to-left shunt causes systemic hypoxia. Very premature babies appear to be less able to maintain a high level of pulmonary vasomotor tone after birth than more mature babies. As a result, the pulmonary vascular resistance drops causing a large left-to-right shunt which floods the lung capillaries with blood. This reduces the compliance of the lungs and contributes to pulmonary oedema and exacerbates the RDS.

Compliant chest wall

The chest wall in a baby under 1000 g is very soft and compliant. The muscles are hypotonic compared with a full term baby so that the intercostal muscles are not strong enough to stabilize the soft cartilaginous ribs. This means that the VLBW baby has difficulty stabilizing the chest wall against diaphragmatic contraction during inspiration particularly when the lung compliance is diminished by immature lung structure, surfactant deficiency, hyaline membranes or pulmonary fluid. The result is that as the baby inspires, the chest wall distorts along the insertion of the diaphragm and, rather than air entering the chest, the sternum and lower ribs are sucked in. This reduces the baby's ability to expand its lungs. The greater the inspiratory effort to inflate the lungs, the more the chest is indrawn and the lower the resulting tidal volume.

Apnoea

Apnoea is most common below 30 weeks of gestation and is inversely related to gestational age. An apnoeic pause of greater than 20 s is probably related to immaturity of the brainstem respiratory neurones [29]. In the VLBW baby, hypoxia and acidosis are the major factors leading to apnoea soon after birth [30]. It results in bradycardia, cyanosis and loss of lung volume. This contributes to the premature baby's difficulties in maintaining lung volume.

Acidosis

After gestational age, acidosis is the second major determinant of the severity of RDS. Worthington and Smith [31] in 1978 observed that, in 81 babies between 25 and 37 weeks gestation, of those with an L:S ratio less than 2.0 who were asphyxiated, 75% developed RDS compared with 40% of the unasphyxiated babies with a low L:S ratio. In those babies with an L:S ratio above 2.0, 33% of the asphyxiated and none of the unasphyxiated developed RDS. Jones *et al.* [32] found that the incidence of RDS was twice as high in babies with an Apgar score of 5 or less compared with those with a higher score. Omer, Robson and Neliger [33] showed that babies between 1000 and 2000 g who were pink on admission to the nursery were only one-quarter as likely to die of RDS as those who were blue. Robson and Hey [34] showed that resuscitation of premature babies at birth reduced the risk of their subsequently dying of hyaline membrane disease.

MacDonald *et al.* [35] reviewing 38 405 consecutive deliveries showed that asphyxia is more common in very premature babies. Using multiple regression analysis they showed that asphyxia occurred in 72% of babies weighing between 500 and 749 g and in 39% of babies weighing 750–999 g. They also showed that premature babies were more at risk of asphyxia if born by the breech or small for dates. The type of delivery was not associated with asphyxia, only the underlying conditions which determined the technique of delivery.

Acidosis probably compounds the respiratory problems because it increases pulmonary vascular resistance and reduces muscle tone, respiratory drive, surfactant synthesis and the integrity of the cell membranes. Asphyxia in premature babies may depress myocardial contractility resulting in heart failure which causes pulmonary oedema and compounds the respiratory failure [36].

Lung expansion

Part of the explanation for the beneficial effects of resuscitation of premature babies [33,34] may have been due to the early expansion of their lungs, surfactant secretion and early stabilization of lung volume. Lawson *et al.* [37] showed that expansion of the lungs of newborn rabbits was important for surfactant secretion. In those animals where the lungs did not expand despite active respiratory movements, there was no increase in surfactant in the airways.

Hypothermia

Very premature babies in a cold environment are more likely to drop their body temperature than full term babies because their surface area is greater, they have less fat and more immature temperature regulation. In an attempt to keep warm they consume more oxygen. If they are already having difficulties maintaining their arterial oxygen level this compounds their hypoxia.

Preterm infants who become cold at delivery have a greater chance of dying, particulary of RDS. Hypothermia is associated with acidosis and hypoxia. It is often difficult to separate the cause and effect but the poor outcome of cold babies justifies all attempts to keep them warm. Hypothermic babies are more likely to become hypoglycaemic which also compounds the acidosis. Cold babies commonly develop an expiratory grunt. This may be a sign that the hypothermia interferes with lung volume because grunting in expiration is a mechanism used by premature babies with lung disease to maintain their FRC.

Trauma

Very premature babies are much more likely to become bruised and oedematous during delivery than full term babies. This leads to a reduction in circulating blood volume and may contribute to the acidosis. The bruising consumes clotting factors and may predispose to pulmonary and intraventricular haemorrhage. Quirk *et al.* [38] in a review of mothers treated with antenatal steroids and their controls suggested that 'avoidence of a stressful labour coupled with an atraumatic delivery was as effective as glucocorticoids in reducing the incidence of RDS'.

Drugs causing respiratory depression

All drugs which are used during labour such as anaesthetics, sedatives or analgesics cross the placenta and depress the baby's respiration. This is particularly important for a very premature baby on the edge of respiratory failure because inadequate respiration leads to hypoxia, hypercarbia, acidosis and RDS.

Pre-eclamptic toxaemia

Evidence for the effect of pre-eclamptic toxaemia (PET) on the very premature baby is conflicting. In our experience the PET does not have any effect of its own on the baby's respiratory failure. Any apparent effects are due to associated factors such as caesarian section without labour and anaesthetic or sedative drugs. However, in a study of 678 consecutive babies weighing between 500 and 1000 g, Doyle *et al.* [39] showed by multiple regression analysis that PET had a significantly beneficial effect on survival.

In contrast, Szymonowicz *et al.* [40] showed that severe eclampsia in the mothers of babies under 1500 g was significantly associated with a higher incidence of RDS and worse severity than a matched group of babies born without PET. This may be because the babies whose mothers had severe PET were more likely to be subjected to depressant drugs and delivered by caesarian section without labour.

In the multicentre premature baby feeding trial [41] (A. Lucas and R. Morley, personal communication) which contained 99 babies under 1000 g, there was no significant effect of PET on days of ventilation.

Prolonged rupture of the membranes

It has been suggested that rupture of the membranes is beneficial to the very premature baby providing that intrauterine infection does not arise. The effect is again difficult to disentangle from associated factors. A mother with rupture of the membranes may be observed in hospital and treated with a number of drugs including steroids and tocolytics whereas a mother without ruptured membranes is more likely to deliver spontaneously and rapidly with little therapeutic intervention. However, in the study of Simpson and Harbert [42] where betamethasone was given to mothers threatening premature labour with ruptured membranes, the control group had a 31% incidence of RDS when the membranes had been ruptured for less than 48 h and

11% when the membranes had been ruptured for more than 48 h. However, in the study of Morales *et al.* [43] the length of time the membranes were ruptured did not affect the incidence of RDS, and in the study of Doyle *et al.* [39] rupture of the membranes was not shown to have a significant effect on mortality in babies between 500 and 1500 g. In 1975 Jones *et al.* [44] reviewed 16 458 consecutive live births of babies born weighing more than 500 g in Colorado from January 1956 to January 1968. When considering the whole group of babies and also the subgroup 25 to 29 weeks gestation there was no apparent effect of prolonged rupture of membranes (PROM) on the incidence of RDS or mortality. In the multicentre feeding trial [41] (A. Lucas and R. Morley, personal communication) which contained 99 babies under 1000 g, 79 had ruptured membranes for less than 24 h and 16 had ruptured membranes for more than 24 h. The ventilation time for the survivors was doubled in the babies with ruptured membranes for more than 24 h ($P=0.0025$). However, this effect was probably due to different gestations and modes of delivery because with regression analysis taking account of gestation, birth weight, delivery, PET, antenatal steroids and sex, the presence of ruptured membranes had no effect on days of ventilation.

In some premature deliveries there has been a chronic leakage of liquor for several weeks which has drained all the liquor. This is likely to lead to pulmonary hypoplasia, whereas it is possible that a small leak for a short time may stress the baby and stimulate lung maturation.

Maternal smoking

It has been known for some time that maternal smoking influences the growth of the fetus and reduces its ultimate size. In a study in Cambridge [1] (unpublished results) using multiple regression analysis it was shown that the mother's smoking significantly reduced the severity of neonatal RDS. This may be due to ill-understood stresses prematurely maturing the baby's lungs.

Infection

Infection of the very premature baby during labour and delivery usually presents with severe respiratory failure and circulatory collapse soon after birth. It is very difficult to distinguish the effects of infection from those associated with prematurity because some premature babies may have been delivered because of amnionitis. Infection is one of the factors that can tip the balance for a premature baby from mild to severe RDS. In consequence every very premature baby must be considered to be infected and treated with appropriate antibiotics.

Effect of mode of delivery

It is very difficult to disentangle the effect of the mode of delivery from the reasons for the delivery. In studies of larger premature babies there is good evidence that caesarian section delivery without previous labour predisposes to RDS. In the multicentre feeding trial [41] (A. Lucas and R. Morley, personal communication) involving 99 babies under 1000 g, 48 were delivered vaginally and 51 by C/S. The surviving babies born by C/S had significantly fewer days of ventilation (7 ± 9; mean $\pm$ SD) compared with the vaginal deliveries 17 ± 15 ($P=0.0003$). Using regression analysis to take account of the babies' gestation, birth weight, antenatal steroids, sex, ruptured membranes and toxaemia, C/S delivery still resulted in the surviving babies having significantly fewer days ventilation ($P=0.05$).

Antenatal steroid influence on lung maturation

Although there are a number of agents which have been used to stimulate the production of surfactant by the fetal lung, the greatest experience has been with glucocorticoids.

Liggins [45] in 1969 noticed that lambs delivered prematurely after intrafetal infusion of ACTH or glucocorticoids were viable and had better pulmonary aeration than untreated premature lambs.

Glucocorticoids act on the fetal lung fibroblasts to induce production of fibroblast-pneumocyte factor (FPF) which in turn stimulates surfactant synthesis in the alveolar type II cell. The induction of FPF in the fibroblast is relatively slow so that the clinical effect of antenatal steroids appears to be rather slow. Once formed, FPF quickly stimulates the rate-limiting enzyme in surfactant phospholipid synthesis. Males are less responsive to antenatal steroids than females. This is probably because the male lung fibroblast is less able to produce FPF than the female fibroblast [46].

Using lung cultures from 28 day fetal rabbits, there was a 12 h delay before an increase in phosphatidyl choline could be demonstrated after steroid stimulation, with the maximal effect detected at 24 h. This required mixed cell cultures containing fibroblasts and was much less apparent if the cultures were pure type II cells [47].

Administration of exogenous steroids increases and accelerates lung maturation in experimental animals as shown by improved pressure volume curves of lungs and surface tension properties of lung extracts, biochemical measurements of phospholipids, lung morphology, appearance and survival of the premature animal. Intrafetal injection is associated with fetal lung maturation [48]. Ablation of the fetal pituitary or adrenals delays lung maturation. The fetal lung contains specific glucocorticoid receptors. Glucocorticoids increase the activities of various enzymes which are important to surfactant synthesis. Also fetal plasma glucocorticoids rise prior to the increase in surfactant production.

Exogenous glucocorticoids have other effects on the lung than stimulating surfactant synthesis. They mature other tissues and structures in the lungs. Bunton and Plopper [49] showed that triamcinolone accelerated the maturation of the interstitial tissues. The septa became longer, thinner and less cellular with larger air spaces and increased numbers of alveolar divisions compared with controls. However, although steroids may mature the interstitial and epithelial components of the lungs, if they are given early they may retard growth. Glucocorticoids given antenatally may reduce the leak of protein onto the lung surface. Hemberger and Schanker [50] showed that antenatal steroids accelerate the development of adult permeability characteristics in the pulmonary epithelium.

It is important to stress that cortisol is not the sole physiological regulator of the enzymes which control surfactant formation and maturation. In experiments with ventilated premature rabbits Ikegami *et al.* [51] showed that maternal corticosteroid treatment did not appear to change surfactant-saturated phosphatidyl choline pool sizes or lung compliance but there were large improvements after the steroid-treated animals were treated with exogenous surfactant compared with surfactant-treated controls. They suggested that this was due to the corticosteroids making the preterm lung 'receptive' to surfactant, implying a maturational change in lung structure.

The human placenta is relatively permeable to the passage of glucocorticoids.

However, not all steroids cross the placenta. Cortisol is largely inactivated by the placenta although this degradation is resisted by the synthetic steroids such as betamethasone and dexamethasone. Betamethesone has a maternal:fetal gradient of 3:1 and dexamethasone a gradient of 1:1 [52,53].

After maternal steroids fetal cortisol synthesis is suppressed but returns to normal after five days.

Prevention of respiratory problems

Unfortunately, there are few data about specific therapeutic manoeuvres to prevent respiratory problems in babies under 1000 g. Most of the data available have been derived from studies on the management of slightly older premature babies.

Clinical trials of antenatal steroid therapy

There are no specific trials to study the effect of antenatal steroid administration to the mothers of babies under 1000 g. The available evidence from randomized trials will therefore be reviewed with an emphasis on the data for very premature babies.

In 1972 Liggins and Howie [54] undertook a randomized trial with 282 mothers threatening premature labour under 37 weeks gestation, comparing intramuscular betamethasone 12 mg with cortisone acetate 6 mg which has one-seventieth the potency. A second dose was given at 24 h if the baby had not delivered. There was a reduction in the incidence of RDS from 26% in the cortisone group to 9% in the betamethasone group ($P=0.003$) and the perinatal death rate was reduced from 18% to 7% ($P<0.02$). However, the benefit was restricted to infants born more than 24 h but less than seven days after treatment commenced. Unfortunately, the betamethasone-treated babies were slightly bigger which may have biased the effect. The incidence of RDS in the babies between 26 and 32 weeks gestation was reduced from 16/23 (70%) to 2/17 (12%) ($P=0.02$).

In 1976, Dluholucky, Babic and Taufer [55] used antenatal hydrocortisone 100 mg i.m. in a randomized trial with 120 treated babies and 40 control babies whose mothers were in premature labour at less than 37 weeks gestation. Fifty-five babies delivered at term with no perinatal complications and there were no stillbirths. The incidence of RDS was 5/31 (16%) in the treated babies, 11/34 (32%) in the partially treated and 18/40 (45%) in the controls. The mortality was 35% in the controls, 23% in the partially treated and 10% in the treated babies. From this trial it appears that a single injection of hydrocortisone may have the same effect as betamethasone although it does not provide data for very premature babies.

In 1977 Block, Kling and Crosby [56] undertook a blind trial of antenatal steroid treatment in mothers threatening premature delivery randomized between betamethasone 12 mg, methylprednisolone 125 mg and saline 1 ml i.m. with a second injection after one day if the baby had not delivered. The study enrolled 167 women, 14 delivered elsewhere, five were stillborn and six did not complete the protocol. Of the remainder there were 57 babies treated with betamethasone, 40 with methylprednisolone and 53 were controls. The incidence of RDS was 5/57 (9%) in the betamethasone group, 10/40 (25%) ($P=$ NS) in the methylprednisolone group and 12/53 (23%) of the control babies. In babies under 32 weeks gestation the incidence of RDS was: betamethasone-treated, 31%; methylprednisolone-treated, 53%; control, 47%. The incidence of RDS in babies with a low L:S ratio was betamethasone, 25%;

methylprednisolone, 71%; controls, 71%. There were no significant differences in the mortality. This study does not give the gestational age, sex or other factors which could have been imbalanced between the groups.

In 1979 Taeusch *et al.* [57] undertook a double blind trial involving 122 mothers. There were 56 infants whose mothers had received dexamethasone 4 mg intramuscularly every 8 h up to six doses and 71 infants whose mothers received a placebo. After exclusions there were 50 treated babies and 65 controls. The incidence of RDS was 14% in the treated group compared with 22% of the controls. In those babies where the mothers received the full course of injections the incidence was 2/30 (7%) of the treated babies compared with 14/65 (22%) of the controls. These are not significant differences using conventional statistics. There was no significant difference in mortality.

In 1979 Morrison *et al.* [58] undertook a randomized trial of intravenous hydrocortisone 100 mg 12-hourly for 48 h or placebo in 654 women threatening labour under 34 weeks gestation or with an amniotic fluid L:S ratio of less than 2:1, regardless of gestation. Only 136 remained in the study after delivery. They excluded babies if they had hypoxia or asphyxia or they were not delivered within 7 days. Ten were lost to follow-up and of the remaining 126, 77% were black. There were 67 treated and 59 controls. Because so many babies were excluded this study is difficult to interpret but it is one of the few that quotes data for very premature babies. The incidence of RDS for babies between 750 and 999 g was 2/3 of the treated and 2/2 of the controls; for the babies between 1000 and 1499 g it was 4/37 (10%) of the treated and 10/36 (27%) of the controls (P = NS) and for the babies weighing 1500–1999 g it was 0/27 (0%) of the treated and 2/21 (10%) of the controls (P = NS). Overall 6/67 (9%) of the treated babies had RDS compared with 14/59 (14%) of the controls ($P < 0.05$).

In the 1981 North American Collaborative study [59], five centres enrolled 696 mothers from an initial cohort of 7893 presenting in premature labour between 26 and 37 weeks. They were randomized to dexamethasone 5 mg or placebo given every 12 h up to four doses. Tocolysis was used to stop labour for 24 h if necessary. There were 720 babies available to be assessed, 359 had received placebo and 361 dexamethasone. The incidence of RDS was reduced in the dexamethasone group from 65/359 (18%) of the controls to 46/361 (13%) ($P = 0.04$) but there was no difference in the severity of RDS or mortality. There was no apparent effect on the incidence of RDS in males, twins and those delivered before they had received 24 h of therapy. About 17% delivered within 24 h. The only subgroup where antenatal steroids reduced the incidence of RDS was those babies born between 24 h and seven days after the treatment at 30–34 weeks gestation, 7/66 (11%) compared with 16/63 (25%) in the placebo group ($P = 0.03$) had RDS. This is the largest randomized trial of antenatal steroid treatment in premature labour and it demonstrates clearly the difficulty of antenatal steroid treatment where only 696 could be entered into the trial out of 7893 women whose babies were considered likely to benefit from steroid prophylaxis. Even in that group the effect was confined to female babies with a gestation between 30 and 34 weeks gestation who had not delivered for 24 h after the initiation of treatment. There is little evidence from this trial that antenatal steroids would greatly benefit babies under 1000 g mainly because there were only 36 single babies in this subgroup and these numbers are too small to show an effect. There is no evidence in this trial that antenatal steroids reduce periventricular haemorrhages (PVH), pneumothoraces or mortality, all of which are indicators that they only had a slightly beneficial effect on RDS.

In 1985 Simpson and Harbert [42] compared the use of betamethasone (12 mg i.m.

in two doses, 12–24 h apart, then repeated weekly until delivery) given to women in labour with ruptured membranes between 26 and 35 weeks gestation with matched controls. They excluded mothers with the usual contraindications to steroids and those who only received one dose of betamethasone; 42% of the mothers were black. The incidence of RDS *increased* from 42/112 (38%) in the controls to 47/105 (45%) of the treated babies. If the membranes were ruptured for less than 48 h the steroid treatment had no effect. In those babies whose membranes had been ruptured for more than 48 h the incidence of RDS was increased from 13/54 (24%) of the controls to 32/75 (43%) of the treated babies. There was no difference in the death rate between the treated and control babies. Sepsis occurred in 9% of the control babies and 19% of the treated ($P<0.05$). This paper suggests that antenatal steroids have little place in the management of preterm labour, particularly in the presence of ruptured membranes.

In 1986 Morales *et al.* [43] undertook a randomized study of antenatal dexamethasone (four i.m. 6 mg doses 12-hourly) in singleton pregnancies with ruptured membranes between 28 and 33 weeks gestation. Tocolysis was given to 36% of the treated group but to none of the controls and prolonged the pregnancy for 48 h in 70% of cases. Two mothers had acute pulmonary oedema. There were 121 steroid-treated and 124 control babies. RDS occurred in 53% of the controls and 25% of the steroid-treated babies ($P=0.001$). This effect was unaffected by the time the membranes were ruptured. The incidence of PVH was reduced from 27% to 11% but with no difference in parenchymal haemorrhages and no significant difference in mortality or infection. In the babies between 28 and 30 weeks gestation the incidence of RDS was reduced from 61% to 32% ($P=0.01$). In females it was reduced from 40% to 19% ($P=0.01$) and males 63% to 30%($P=0.01$).

In 1986 Doyle *et al.* [39] looked at the short and medium term outcome for 244 babies weighing between 500 and 1500 g at birth treated with at least one dose of antenatal steroids compared with 434 consecutively born babies who did not receive antenatal steroids. There were considerable antenatal differences in complications between the groups. The steroid group had a four-fold increase in the use of tocolytics, 50% less PET and 50% more multiple pregnancies. By multiple regression analysis tocolytic therapy, ruptured membranes for more than 24 h, increasing gestational age, electronic fetal heart rate monitoring and multiple pregnancy were significantly associated with antenatal steroid therapy. The results showed that 80% of the steroid-treated babies were more likely to be discharged home compared with 61% of the controls ($P<0.001$). The mortality in the steroid-treated group was almost halved after adjustment for birth weight, extreme immaturity, lethal malformations, confounding obstetric variables and the effect was similar for both boys and girls. From multiple regression analysis the most important association with survival was increasing birth weight followed by antenatal steroids and pre-eclampsia. Fatal cases of RDS were less common in the treated group ($P=0.04$). Of the hospital survivors the steroid-treated group required less ventilation ($P=0.003$) and fewer days in oxygen ($P=0.02$). The incidence of patent ductus arteriosus ($P=0.002$) and bronchopulmonary dysplasia ($P=0.003$) was lower. At two years the surviving treated babies were heavier ($P=0.016$) and had larger head circumferences ($P=0.03$) although all the children in this cohort were lighter and shorter than the standards for the population. There were no apparent adverse effects from antenatal steroids and no difference in the incidence of handicap among the survivors from each group. The treated group of babies born with weights between 700 and 1000 g had improved survival compared with controls. This is an important study because it looks at the effects in so many very small babies. Unfortunately the obvious differences in the antenatal complications and treatments of the two groups of babies may have influenced the results. Nevertheless, there is no evidence from this study that antenatal steroids are harmful to this group of babies.

The data about the influence of sex on the results of the steroid trials are inconclusive particularly in babies under 1000 g. From these trials it appears that although glucocorticoid treatment will reduce the incidence and severity of RDS in some groups of babies, the therapy is limited to those few women threatening premature labour who do not have any contraindications to the use of steroids and are able to complete a 36-hour course. This implies a stable, non-urgent situation with no evidence of fetal distress. This is rarely the case during very premature labour. There is no good evidence that antenatal steroids benefit babies under 1000 g.

Follow-up after antenatal steroid therapy

The most extensive follow-up of infants whose mothers received betamethasone for the prevention of RDS is MacArthur *et al.* [60]. They examined 86% of 305 infants in a New Zealand trial. They did not find any significant differences in neurological development, ophthalmological findings, immune status or post-neonatal deaths in the steroid-treated group compared with controls.

Tocolysis

Beta-adrenergic drugs have been used to prevent premature labour because they have a tocolytic betamimetic effect on the gravid uterus. They may also have potentially beneficial effects on the surfactant synthesis and fluid secretion of fetal lungs.

In animals β-receptor agonists given directly to the fetus or into the maternal bloodstream caused a release of surfactant into the fetal pulmonary fluid from the type II cells in relatively mature animals [61]. However, it appears that after the treatment the stores were depleted and there was relative surfactant deficiency until they were restored by the normal synthetic processes. The time this would take to occur in the human premature fetus is not known [62].

Even though there is widespread use of tocolysis in very premature infants there is considerable controversy about its effectiveness. In 1986 in a randomized trial involving 106 women between 24 and 33 weeks gestation in premature labour, Leveno *et al.* [63] assigned them to ritodrine or placebo. Ritodrine delayed labour and increased the number delivering after one day, 28% of the treated women delivering within 24 h compared with 48% of the controls ($P<0.02$). The numbers were too small to show any significant effect on neonatal outcome although the numbers of babies requiring ventilation was reduced from 31% to 23%. Merkatz, Peter and Barden [64] in a review of studies of tocolytic agents in babies under 33 weeks gestation suggested that their use resulted in less RDS and fewer deaths. In Sweden there has been a decline in births below 1500 g coincident with the increased use of β-receptor agonist drugs to prevent premature labour [65]. In contrast, a study from Ireland [66] showed that any apparent beneficial effect from β-adrenergic drugs was probably associated with a reduction in deaths and complications from preterm labour with time following many improvements in obstetric and neonatal care.

Tocolytics on average seem to prolong the pregnancy by about 24 h in 60% of mothers treated. However there is no satisfactory evidence that they are effective in pregnancies of babies under 1000 g.

Influences of hormones

Lung maturation is influenced by several hormones – insulin, prolactin, oestrogen, thyroxine and thyrotropin-releasing hormone (TRH). However, it must be borne in mind that the effect of premature labour is greater than the effect of any therapeutic effect of hormones.

Thyroid

During fetal life normal thyroid function is necessary for maturation of the lungs [67]. There are a number of studies which suggest from *in vitro* experiments that there are synergistic maturational effects of tri-iodothyronine (T_3) with glucocorticoids on phosphatidyl choline synthesis in the fetal type II cell and that the corticosteroids may also increase the fetal level of T_3 [68]. It appears that thyroid hormones act on the type II cell making it more responsive to FPF [46].

Recently there has been a growing interest in TRH because it crosses the placenta and stimulates the fetal thyroid and prolactin secretion. When TRH was given to pregnant rabbits it increased by 150% the amount of phosphatidyl choline in fetal lung lavage at 27 days [69]. Ikegami *et al.* [70] studied the effect on ventilated 27-day premature rabbits of maternal treatment with corticosteroids, TRH and T_3 in various combinations together with exogenous surfactant treatment at birth. T_3 and TRH did not increase the pool size of saturated phosphatidyl choline. TRH did not increase the fetal blood level of T_3 and therefore may work via mechanisms other than the thyroid gland. More T_3-treated fetuses died than in any other group. There were no fetal deaths in the animals treated with TRH. In the absence of surfactant treatment there was no benefit on lung function from corticosteroids or T_3 although TRH treatment caused a significant improvement. Although surfactant treatment improved lung function in all groups, the best effect after a single hormone treatment was with corticosteroids. The combined effect of corticosteroids, TRH and surfactant treatment resulted in the best response.

These animal experiments suggest that possibly the most effective antenatal therapy for RDS will be corticosteroids and TRH together with surfactant treatment at birth.

Ambroxol

Ambroxol, a bromhexine metabolite, has been used to reduce the severity of RDS. In a prospective controlled trial where mothers threatening premature labour were treated with 1000 mg per day intravenously, Wauer *et al.* [71] reported a reduction in the incidence of RDS from 41.7% of controls to 23.2% of treated babies. There were no data to suggest that it was useful in babies under 1000 g. No adverse effects on the babies were reported.

Inositol

Myo-inositol has been considered to be a regulator and augmentor of pulmonary surfactant synthesis and secretion in the fetal lung. Its role has been extensively reviewed by Hallman [72]. It increases surfactant phosphatidyl inositol (PI) and decreases phosphatidyl glycerol. It also potentiates the glucocorticoid and thyroid hormone-induced increase in surfactant phosphatidyl choline in the fetus. In a randomized double blind trial of myo-inositol supplementation for 10 days to babies with a birth weight of less than 2000 g and who needed ventilation for RDS, there was a reduction in the severity of RDS and 9/37 (24%) inositol-treated infants died or developed bronchopulmonary dysplasia compared with 19/37 (51%) of the controls ($P < 0.02$) [15]. These results support the concept that there are substrates which may aid the synthesis and secretion of mature surfactant by premature babies. The role of inositol needs to be clarified but it may provide an interesting clue to the development of future treatments to reduce the severity of RDS.

Exogenous surfactant therapy

Surfactant treatment to prevent or ameliorate neonatal RDS and its complications has been the dream of many paediatricians since the 1960s when it was shown that very premature babies were deficient in surfactant [2]. However, in the face of the factors presented above it is unlikely that surfactant therapy will prevent or cure RDS but animal experiments have shown that it is possible to reduce the severity of the respiratory disease.

In 1973 Enhorning and Robertson showed that premature, surfactant-deficient rabbit fetuses treated with concentrated natural surfactant at birth had improved lung expansion [73]. Similar effects were obtained in lambs [74] and monkeys [75,76]. In several recent studies babies have been treated with exogenous surfactant to prevent or ameliorate the problems of RDS [1,24,77–92,98]. They have used either artificial surfactants [1,24,78,81,82,98], extracted and purified animal pulmonary surfactants [77,79,84–86,88,89,90] or human amniotic fluid surfactants [80,83,87] which have been given either at birth [1,24,78,81,82,84–87,98] or several hours later to treat established RDS [77,79,80,82,83,88–90].

There have not been any trials specifically designed to look at the effect of surfactant treatment in premature babies under 1000 g. However, a number of the prophylactic trials have concentrated on babies under 30 weeks gestation [24,84–86,88–90] and one trial specifically stratified for babies of 25 and 26 weeks gestation [24]. There are now 14 reasonably well documented trials of surfactant therapy.

Japanese workers have extracted surfactant from minced bovine lungs, purified and sterilized it and then added phospholipids and fatty acids to improve its physical properties [91]. This has been called Surfactant TA. No controlled trials have been reported from Japan but it is now being tested in America.

Calf surfactant is extracted and purified from calf lung washings. This has been used by three groups all based round lake Ontario [84–86].

Surfactant extracted and purified from minced pig lungs has been produced in Stockholm and is under trial in various European centres [92].

Human amniotic fluid surfactant is being collected in San Diego and Helsinki and used in clinical trials [80,83,87]. Obstetricians collect litres of fluid from elective mature caesarian sections. About five collections of carefully extracted and purified amniotic fluid are required for each dose.

In Cambridge an artificial surfactant has been developed called ALEC, Artificial Lung Expanding Compound [1,24,95–98]. It is a simple mixture of two of the major surfactant phospholipids, dipalmitoylphosphatidyl choline and unsaturated phosphatidyl glycerol used as a powder or crystalline suspension in cold saline. This has been tested in Cambridge, Nottingham [1,98], Oxford [82] and in a ten-centre trial [24] involving Aberdeen, Edinburgh, Glasgow, Liverpool, Leeds, Newcastle, Birmingham, Cambridge, King's College Hospital, London and St George's Hospital, London.

Table 4.1 Randomized prophylactic trials

Authors	*Surfactant*	*Dose* (mg)	*Volume* (ml)	*Placebo*	*Number*	*Gestation* (weeks)	*Excluded*	*Intubated*
Enhorning *et al.*[84]	Calf	75–100	3–4	None	72	25–29	Acute delivery	All
Shapiro *et al.*[86]	Calf	90	3	NaCl	32	25–29	Acute delivery	All
Kwong *et al.*[85]	Calf	90	3	NaCl	27	24–28	Acute delivery	All
Merritt *et al.*[87]	Human AF	60	3	Air	60	24–29	L:S > 1.9	All
Halliday *et al.*[81]	DPPC/HDL	30	5	None	100	25–33	L:S > 1.9	All
Wilkinson *et al.*[82]	ALEC	25	Powder	None	24	< 32	L:S > 1.7	All
Morley *et al.*[78]	ALEC	25	Powder	None	129	25–35	None	All
Morley[1,98]	ALEC	50–100	1	NaCl	341	23–34	None	Some
10-centre[24]	ALEC	100	1	NaCl	328	25–29	None	Some

In Belfast, Professor Meban developed a surfactant composed of dipalmitoylphosphatidyl choline and human high density lipoprotein which was tested in clinical trials by Halliday *et al.* [81].

A satisfactory comparison of all the trials is impossible because of the great variation in the surfactant preparations, entry criteria to the trials, dosages, volumes and techniques of delivering the surfactant. Some trials have used a placebo and others not. Some only excluded babies with lethal malformations and others excluded babies who were delivered acutely, thereby excluding babies whose mothers had acute antepartum complications and enrolling a relatively high proportion treated with antenatal steroids. L:S ratios have been used as a criterion of entry to some trials but not others. In some of the trials the babies were intubated to deliver surfactant, in others the first dose was placed in the pharynx. The essential data from the controlled studies are summarized below.

Table 4.1 shows the basic data from the trials where surfactant was given at birth – the so-called prophylactic trials. The four at the top are trials with natural surfactants and the five at the bottom with artificial surfactant. The doses vary from 25 to 100 mg and the volume from 5 ml to just powder blown down the endotracheal tube. Some use a placebo and others do not. The numbers of babies in the trials vary from 24 to 341. The gestational age criterion for entry to the trials is one of the main differences. It varies from one trial entering all babies from 23 to 34 weeks, to another only entering babies of 25–29 weeks gestation. Some trials intubated the babies specifically for the trial to give either surfactant or placebo into the lungs. Others only recruited intubated babies and others entered all randomized babies putting the first dose into the pharynx and only giving the babies a dose into the lungs if they were intubated.

Table 4.2 shows the data from five 'rescue' trials where surfactant was not given until RDS was diagnosed and the baby fulfilled stringent entry criteria. In these trials the dosage varied from 25–200 mg with different volumes and varying use of placebo. The numbers of babies in each trial are all small. They all use birth weight limits which vary from one trial including babies between 700 and 2000 g to another with babies between 1000 and 1500 g. The trial entry criteria vary but all are based on a positive diagnosis of RDS with no obvious complications and various levels of inspired oxygen and ventilator pressure. The babies were treated at various times after birth. As can be appreciated, it is not posssible to compare satisfactorily the outcome of these trials. However, it is possible to postulate that the outcome in the trial by Gitlin *et al.* [88] should be better than in the trials by Hallman *et al.* [80] and Halliday *et al.* [90] because the babies entered the trial at a lower level of inspired oxygen and therefore were not so ill.

Obviously, the outcome between prophylactic and rescue trials is likely to be different when surfactant was given to babies at birth who may or may not develop RDS compared with treating babies with established RDS.

In each baby the severity of RDS can be reflected by the level of inspired oxygen required to maintain normal arterial oxygenation. Figure 4.2 shows the percentage improvement in inspired oxygen concentration in four prophylactic trials. The larger the percentage change the better the effect of surfactant. Two trials used calf surfactant [84,85], one human surfactant [87] and one artificial surfactant ALEC [1,98]. All the trials show some beneficial effect within an hour of birth which increases at 24 h, plateaus to 48 h and by 72 h the effect is waning except for the artificial surfactant.

Figure 4.3 shows the change in oxygenation for three rescue trials expressed as a change in the arterial–alveolar oxygen difference. The larger the percentage change

Table 4.2 Randomized rescue trials

Author	*Surfactant*	*Dose* (mg)	*Volume* (ml)	*Placebo*	*Number*	*Birth weight* (g)	*Inclusion*	*Time* (h)
Hallman *et al.*[80]	Human	60	3	None	45	<1500	RDS>60% O_2	<10
Wilkinson *et al.*[82]	ALEC	25	Powder	None	24	<31 weeks	RDS L:S<1.8	?
Gitlin *et al.*[88]	Bovine	100	3.3	NaCl	41	1000–1500	RDS>40% O_2	<8
Raju *et al.*[89]	Bovine	100	3.3	NaCl	30	751–1750	RDS>50% O_2	<6
Halliday *et al.*[90]	Pig	200	2.5	None	29	700–2000	RDS>60% O_2	1–15

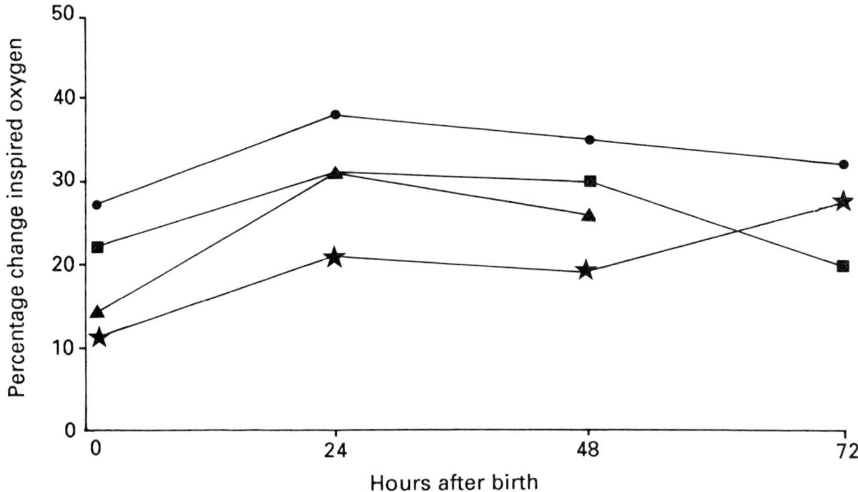

Figure 4.2 Percentage improvement in inspired oxygen concentration in four prophylactic trials: ★–★, Morley [1,98]; ■–■, Enhorning *et al.* [84]; ▲–▲, Kwong *et al* [88]; ●–●, Merritt *et al.* [87]

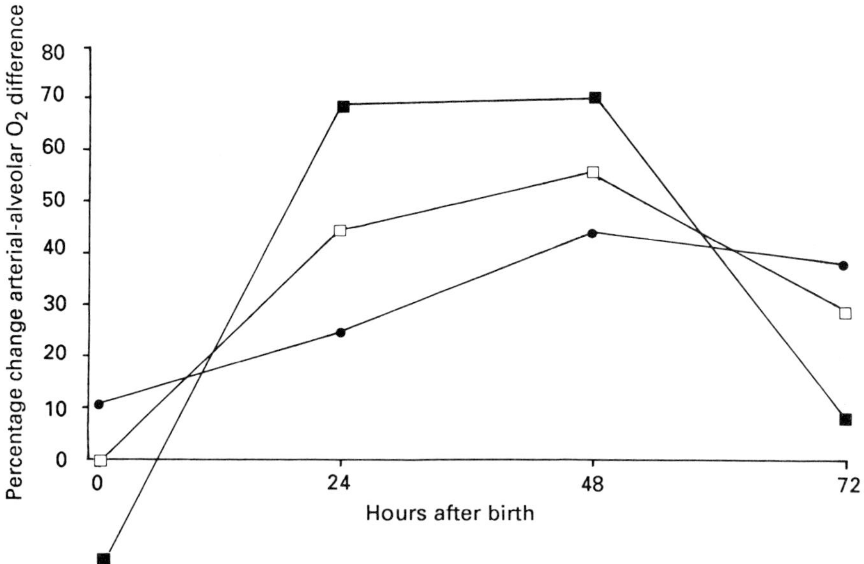

Figure 4.3 Percentage change in arterial-alveolar oxygen difference in three rescue trials: □–□, Hallman *et al.* [80]; ■–■ Gitlin *et al.* [88]; ●–● Raju *et al.* [89]

the better the effect of surfactant. Two are trials of the Japanese bovine Surfactant TA [88,89] and the other uses human surfactant [80]. All these trials show an acute improvement which diminished by 72 h. Note the difference in effect when Surfactant TA was used in different trials.

Figures 4.4–4.7 show the mean and 95% confidence intervals for the difference in

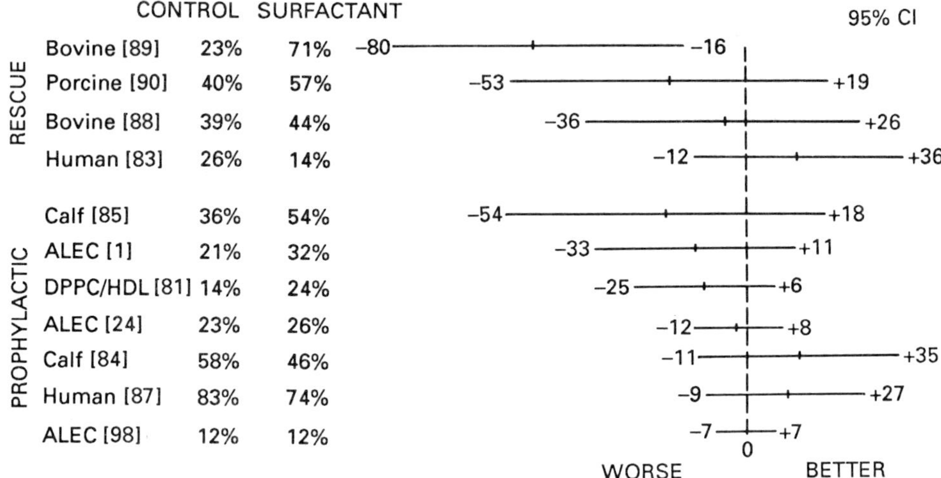

Figure 4.4 Mean and 95% confidence intervals for the effect of different surfactants on the incidence of patent ductus arteriosus

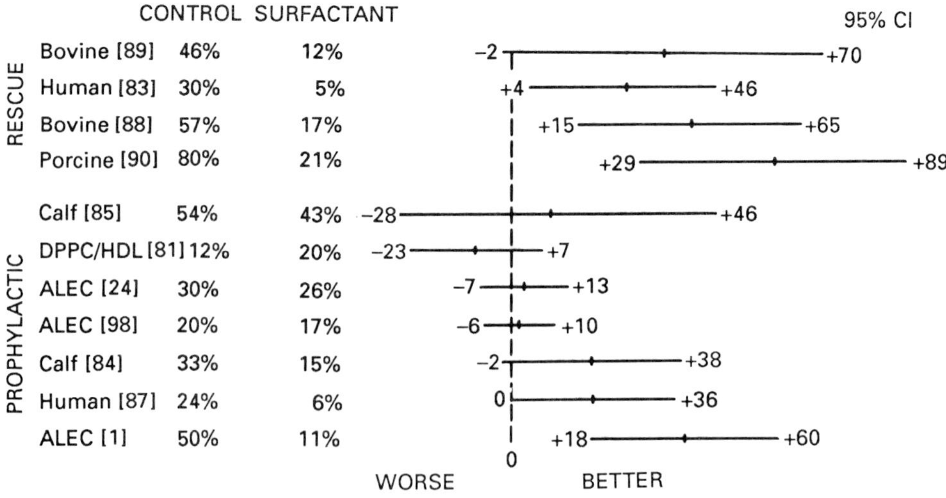

Figure 4.5 Mean and 95% confidence intervals for the effect of different surfactants on the incidence of pneumothorax.

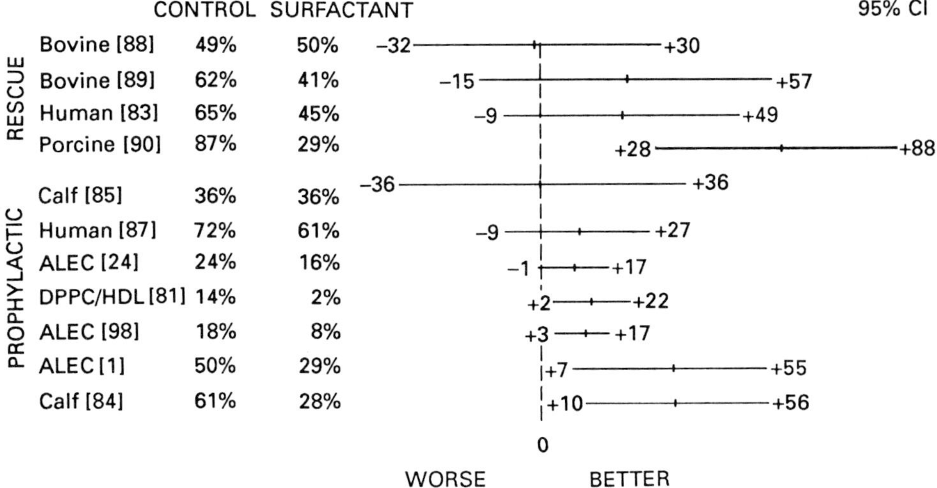

Figure 4.6 Mean and 95% confidence intervals for the effect of different surfactants on the incidence of PVH.

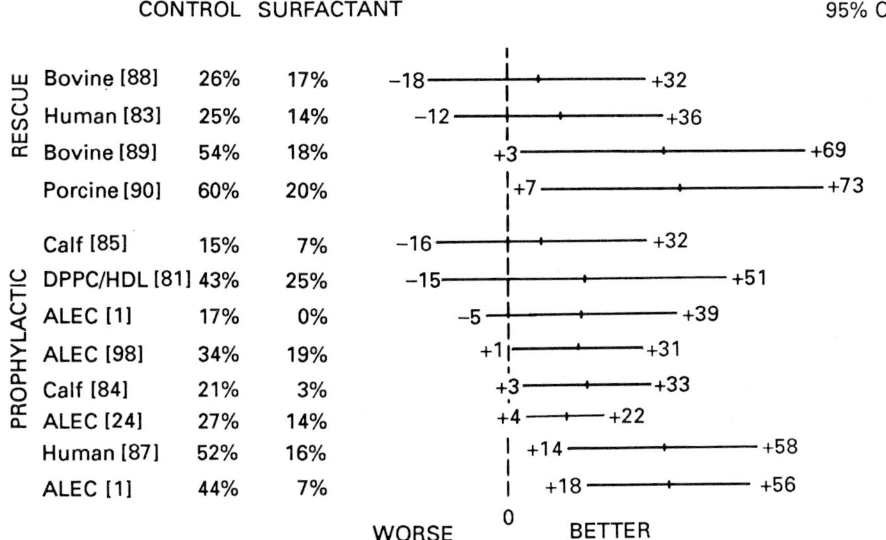

Figure 4.7 Mean and 95% confidence intervals for the effect of different surfactants on the mortality, calculated for babies under 30 weeks if possible.

incidence of various complications between the treated and control groups. This is easiest to think of in terms of the range of effect which might be achieved per 100 treated babies. The smaller the trial the wider the confidence intervals. You can tell whether there was a significant difference for any trial because the 5% level of significance is reached when one end of the horizontal line just touches the vertical zero line. The further the end of the confidence interval line is away from zero the more significant the difference. The data are presented in each figure so that the rescue trials are at the top and the prophylactic trials are at the bottom. They are ordered in each figure so that the trial with the best effect on that complication is at the bottom.

Figure 4.4 shows the effect of different surfactants on the incidence of patent ductus arteriosus (PDA). In the non-randomized trial of Fujiwara *et al.* [77] it occurred in nine out of ten babies and animal experiments have suggested that it might be a complication of surfactant therapy. This figure shows the rescue and prophylactic trials ranked for each group in increasing order of significance. It shows overall that surfactant therapy might increase the tendency to PDA although the lines and mid-points are more on the negative side. The only trial to show a significant effect was that of Raju *et al.* [89] of bovine surfactant TA with an increase in PDA from 23 to 71%, with a confidence interval from 12 to 80 more PDA. This is very significantly worse than the rescue and prophylactic trials with human surfactant, the two main ALEC trials [1,24,98] and Enhorning's calf surfactant trial [84]. No trial showed a significant reduction in PDA.

Figure 4.5 shows the effect on pneumothorax. When surfactant therapy was first used it was thought that a substance which improved lung expansion might increase the incidence of pneumothoraces. The overall trend is for surfactant treatment to produce fewer pneumothoraces. The chance of a deleterious effect with any surfactant is small. In the rescue trials the only surfactant not to produce a significant reduction in pneumothoraces was the bovine surfactant TA in the trial by Raja *et al.* [89], although the trend is similar to the other trials and with larger numbers it might well have shown a significant reduction. In the prophylactic trials the effect is smaller but this is because the incidence of pneumothoraces tends to be lower. Human surfactant [87] and ALEC powder [1,78] produced a significant reduction. ALEC crystalline suspension [1,24,98] appeared to have no effect.

Figure 4.6 shows the effect on all grades of PVH. Overall surfactant treatment appears to reduce the incidence. The only rescue trial with a significant effect is Halliday's trial with pig surfactant [90]. It is a significantly better effect than bovine surfactant in the trial by Gitlin *et al.* [88] but it is not different from the others. In the prophylactic trials significant reductions in PVH were shown by Halliday's trial with artificial surfactant [81], ALEC suspension [1,24,98], ALEC powder [1,78] and Enhorning's calf surfactant [84]. With wide confidence intervals and different trial designs it is difficult to say that one is better than another.

The length of time a baby is treated with oxygen or being ventilated is an important outcome. Few of the trials show this result. Those that do show little significant effect from surfactant treatment. However, ALEC suspension [24] showed a significant reduction in the number of babies in oxygen more than 28 days. In other trials surfactant therapy appears to be reducing the incidence of BPD [1]. The ten-centre artificial surfactant trial only collected data on the first ten days. This showed a significant reduction in the length of ventilation and time in more than 30% oxygen [24].

Mortality is a crude but important measure of the effect of surfactant treatment. The effect of surfactant is shown in Figure 4.7. Where possible the mortality has been calculated for babies under 30 weeks gestation because there are fewer deaths in the higher gestations. The overall trend is that surfactant treatment reduces mortality. In the rescue groups the confidence intervals are wide but the bovine and porcine surfactants produced significant reductions [89,90]. On average the mortality was halved by surfactant. In the prophylactic group there were significant reductions with Enhorning's calf surfactant [84], human surfactant [87] and ALEC powder [1,78] and suspension [1,24,98]. No surfactant increased the mortality and there is no significant difference between the effects of different preparations. On average there was a 65% reduction in mortality. This might be spuriously high because some of the trials were stopped when a significant difference in mortality was noted. Even at a lower level, surfactant therapy would be the best single therapy to improve neonatal mortality.

Few trials have yet published results on the long-term outcome for surfactant-treated babies. The 18-month follow-up of 235 surviving babies randomized to ALEC suspension in Cambridge shows that even though more small surfactant-treated babies survived, there were no differences between the two groups in Bayley mental and psychomotor scales, the IQ test, or the incidence of cerebral palsy, deafness, respiratory infections or hospital admissions.

Therefore it can be concluded that in the present state of knowledge surfactant therapy is effective but does not cure RDS. Apart from some concern about some natural surfactants causing an increased incidence of PDA, surfactant therapy appears to be harmless. Its most striking effect is the halving in mortality. It probably also reduces the incidence of PVH, pneumothoraces and BPD. Despite all the evidence accumulating and the speculation of some workers, it is not possible to show that one type of surfactant is more effective than others. The best dosage and treatment regime still needs to be elucidated.

From these results, with all their interpretation difficulties, it appears that surfactant therapy will be one of the most useful advances in neonatal care. If it truly halves the mortality in babies under 30 weeks gestation this would mean 500 fewer babies dying in the UK every year.

Conclusions

All babies under 1000 g are likely to suffer from RDS. It cannot be completely prevented because it is a consequence of their extreme immaturity. However, the severity can almost certainly be reduced by people being aware of those factors which are likely to make the disease worse and attending carefully to detail in the management of the baby from the onset of labour, through careful delivery to independent survival. Any technique should be used which could prevent or ameliorate the respiratory disease, without adding to the baby's complications. The best technique for preventing RDS would be the prevention of premature labour. At the moment, the treatment for RDS is supportive and symptomatic. In the near future surfactant therapy may be available as a specific therapy. The next few years will show whether antenatal steroids with or without TRH will be useful in this situation for the obstetricians.

References

1. Morley, C. J. (1987) The Cambridge experience of artificial surfactant. In *Physiology of the Fetal and Neonatal Lung* (eds D. V. Walters, L. B. Strang and F. Geubelle), MTP Press, Lancaster, pp. 255–272
2. Avery, M. E. and Mead, J. (1959) Surface properties in relation to atelectasis and hyaline membrane disease. *Am. J. Dis. Child.*, **97**, 517–523

3. Robertson, B., Van Golde, L. M. G. and Batenburg, J. J. (eds) (1984) *Pulmonary Surfactant*, Elsevier, Amsterdam
4. Hislop, A. and Reid, L. (1974) Growth and development of the respiratory system – anatomical development. In *The Scientific Foundations of Paediatrics* (eds J. A. Davis and J. Dobbing), Heinemann, London, pp. 214–270
5. Bangham, A. D. (1987) Lung surfactant: how it does and does not work. *Lung*, **165**, 17–25
6. Parkinson, C. E. and Harvey, D. R. (1977) Fatty acids of phospholipids in human neonatal lung surfactant. *Pediatr. Res.*, **11**, 723–727
7. Gluck, L., Kulovitch, M. V., Eidelman, A. I., Cordero, L. and Khazin, A. F. (1972) Biochemical development of surface activity in mammalian lung IV. Pulmonary lecithin synthesis in the fetus and newborn and etiology of the respiratory distress syndrome. *Pediatr. Res.*, **6**, 81–99
8. Boughton, K., Gandy, G. and Gairdner, D. (1970) Hyaline membrane disease. II: Lung lecithin. *Arch. Dis. Child.*, **45**, 311–320
9. Hallman, M., Feldman, B. H., Kirkpatrick, E. and Gluck, L. (1977) Absence of phosphatidyl glycerol (PG) in respiratory distress syndrome in the newborn: study of the minor surfactant phospholipids in newborns. *Pediatr. Res.*, **11**, 714–720
10. Brumley, G. W., Hodson, W. A. and Avery, M. E. (1967) Lung phospholipids and surface tension correlations in infants with and without hyaline membrane disease and in adults. *Pediatrics*, **40**, 13–19
11. Jobe, A., Ikegami, M., Jacobs, H. and Jones, S. (1983) Surfactant pool sizes and the severity of respiratory distress syndrome in prematurely delivered lambs. *Am. Rev. Resp. Dis.*, **127**, 751–755
12. Gluck, L., Kulovitch, M. V. and Borer, R. C. (1971) Diagnosis of respiratory distress syndrome by amniocentesis. *Am. J. Obstet. Gynecol.*, **109**, 440–445
13. Farrell, P. M. (1982) Overview of hyaline membrane disease. *Lung Development: Biological and Clinical Perspectives*, Volume II (ed. P. M. Farrell), Academic Press, New York, pp. 23–46
14. Nelson, G. H. and McPherson, J. C. (1985) Respiratory distress syndrome in various cultures and a possible role of diet. In *Pulmonary Development: Transition from Intrauterine to Extrauterine Life* (ed. G. H. Nelson), Marcel Dekker, New York, pp. 159–178
15. Hallman, M., Jarvenpaa, A-L. and Pohjavuori, M. (1986) Respiratory distress syndrome and inositol supplementation in preterm infants. *Arch. Dis. Child.*, **61**, 1076–1083
16. Hallman, M., Arjomaa, P. and Hoppu, K. (1987) Inositol supplementation in respiratory distress syndrome: relationship between serum concentration, renal excretion, and lung effluent phospholipids. *J. Pediatr.*, **110**, 604–610
17. Gandy, G., Jacobson, W. and Gairdner, D. (1970) Hyaline membrane disease. I: Cellular changes. *Arch. Dis. Child.*, **45**, 289–310
18. Taylor, F. B. and Abrams, M. E. (1966) Effect of surface active lipoprotein on clotting and fibrinolysis, and of fibrinogen on surface tension of surface active lipoprotein. *Am. J. Med.*, **40**, 346–350
19. Seeger, W., Stohr, G. and Neuhof, H. (1987) Surfactant inhibitory plasma derived proteins. In *Physiology of the Fetal and Neonatal Lung* (eds D. V. Walters, L. B. Strang and F. Geubelle), MTP Press, Lancaster, pp. 225–240
20. Ikegami, M., Jobe, A. and Glatz, T. (1981) Surface activity following natural surfactant treatment in premature lambs. *J. Appl. Physiol.*, **51**, 306–312
21. Walters, D. V. and Ramsden, C. A. (1987) The secretion and absorption of fetal lung liquid. In *Physiology of the Fetal and Neonatal Lung* (eds D. V. Walters, L. B. Strang and F. Geubelle), MTP Press, Lancaster, pp. 61–75
22. Guyton, A. C., Moffatt, D. S. and Adair, T. H. (1984) Role of alveolar surface tension in transepithelial movement of fluid. In *Pulmonary Surfactant* (eds B. Robertson, L. M. G. Van Golde and J. J. Batenburg), Elsevier, Amsterdam, pp. 171–186
23. Faxelius, G. (1983) Neonatal adaptation after vaginal delivery versus caesarian section with special regard to the sympatho-adrenal system. Thesis, Stockholm
24. Ten Centre Study Group (1987) Ten centre trial of artificial surfactant (artificial lung expanding compound) in very premature babies. *Br. Med. J.*, **294**, 991–996
25. Rooney, S. A., Gobran, L. I. and Wai-Lee, T. S. (1977) Stimulation of surfactant production by oxytocin-induced labor in the rabbit. *J. Clin. Invest.*, **60**, 754–759
26. Lawson, E. E., Brown, E. R., Torday, J. S., Madansky, D. L. and Taeusch, H. W. (1978) The effect of epinephrine on tracheal fluid flow and surfactant efflux in fetal sheep. *Am. Rev. Resp. Dis.*, **118**, 1023–1026

27. Rudolph, A. M. (1984) Regulation of pulmonary circulation in the fetus and newborn. In *Respiratory Distress Syndrome* (eds K. O. Raivio, N. Hallman, Kouvalainen and I. Valimaki), Academic Press, London, pp. 19–32
28. Rigby, M. L., Pickering, D. and Wilkinson, A. (1984) Cross-sectional echocardiography in determining persistent patency of the ductus arteriosus in preterm infants. *Arch. Dis. Child.*, **59**, 341–345
29. Henderson-Smart, D. (1986) Pulmonary disease of the newborn. I: Neonatal respiratory physiology. In *Textbook of Neonatology* (ed. N. R. C. Roberton) Churchill Livingstone, London, pp. 259–273
30. Rigatto, H. (1984) Control of ventilation in the newborn. *Ann. Rev. Physiol.*, **46**, 661–674
31. Worthington, D. and Smith, B. T. (1978) Relationship of amniotic lecithin/sphyngomyelin ratio and fetal asphyxia to respiratory distress syndrome in premature infants. *Can. Med. Assoc. J.*, **118**, 1384–1388
32. Jones, M. D., Burd, L. I., Bowes, W. A., Battaglia, F. C. and Lubchenco, L. O. (1975) Premature rupture of the membranes and respiratory distress syndrome. *N. Engl. J. Med.*, **292**, 1253–1257
33. Omer, M. I. A., Robson, E. and Neligan, G. A. (1974) Can initial resuscitation of preterm babies reduce the death rate from hyaline membrane disease? *Arch. Dis. Child.*, **49**, 219–221
34. Robson, E. and Hey, E. (1982) Resuscitation of preterm babies at birth reduces their risk of death from hyaline membrane disease. *Arch. Dis. Child.*, **57**, 184–187
35. MacDonald, H. M., Mulligan, J. C., Allen, A. C. and Taylor, P. M. (1980) Neonatal asphyxia. I. Relationship of obstetric and neonatal complications to neonatal mortality in 38405 consecutive deliveries. *J. Pediatr.*, **96**, 898–902
36. Cabel, L., Devaskar, U., Siassi, B., Hodgman, J. E. and Emmanouilides, G. (1980) Cardiogenic shock associated with perinatal asphyxia in preterm infants. *J. Pediatr.*, **96**, 705–710
37. Lawson, E. E., Birdwell, R. L., Huang, P. S. and Tausch, H. W. (1979) Augmentation of pulmonary surfactant secretion by lung expansion at birth. *Pediatr. Res.*, **13**, 611–617
38. Quirk, J. G., Raker, R. K., Petrie, R. H. and Williams, A. M. (1979) The role of glucocorticoids, unstressful labour and atraumatic delivery in the prevention of the respiratory distress syndrome. *Am. J. Obstet. Gynecol.*, **134**, 768–771
39. Doyle, L. W., Kitchen, W. H., Ford, G. W., Rickards, A. L., Lissenden, J. V. and Ryan, M. M. (1986) Effects of antenatal steroid therapy on mortality and morbidity in very low birth weight infants. *J. Pediatr.*, **108**, 287–292
40. Szymonowicz, W., Yu, V. Y. H., Astbury, J. and Bajuk, B. (1987) Severe pre-eclampsia and the very low birthweight infant. *Arch. Dis. Child.*, **62**, 712–716
41. Lucas, A., Gore, S. M., Cole, T. *et al.* (1984) Multicentre trial on feeding low birthweight infants: effects of diet on early growth. *Arch. Dis. Child.*, **59**, 722–730
42. Simpson, G. F. and Harbert, G. M. (1985) Use of betamethasone in management of preterm gestation with premature rupture of membranes. *Obstet. Gynecol.*, **66**, 168–175
43. Morales, W. J., Diebel, N. D., Lazar, A. J. and Zadrozny, D. (1986) The effect of antenatal dexamethasone administration on the prevention of respiratory distress syndrome in preterm gestations with premature rupture of membranes. *Am. J. Obstet. Gynecol.*, **154**, 591–595
44. Jones, M. D., Burd, L. I., Bowes, W. A., Battaglia, F. C. and Lubchencho, L. O. (1975) Failure of association of premature rupture of membranes with respiratory distress syndrome. *N. Engl. J. Med.*, **292**, 1253–1257
45. Liggins, G. C. (1969) Premature delivery of fetal lambs infused with glucocorticoids. *J. Endocrinol.*, **45**, 515–523
46. Smith, B. T., Post, M. and Floros, J. (1987) Differentiation of the pulmonary epithelium. In *Physiology of the Fetal and Neonatal Lung* (eds D. V. Walters, L. B. Strang and F. Geubelle), MTP Press, Lancaster, pp. 17–24
47. Smith, B. T. (1984) Prevention of hyaline membrane disease: an attempt to mimic a physiological process: hormonal control. In *Pulmonary Surfactants* (eds B. Robertson, L. M. G. van Golde and J. J. Batenburg), Elsevier, Amsterdam, pp. 357–381
48. Rooney, S. A., Gobran, L. I., Maniscalco, W. M., Marino, P. A. and Gross, I. (1979) Effects of betamethasone on phosphatidyl choline content, composition and biosynthesis in fetal rabbit lung. *Biochim. Biophys. Acta*, **572**, 64–76
49. Bunton, T. E. and Plopper, C. G. (1984) Triamcinolone induced structural alterations in the development of the lung of the fetal rhesus Macaque. *Am. J. Obstet. Gynecol.*, **148**, 203–215

50. Hemberger, J. A. and Schanker, L. S. (1981) Effect of cortisone on permeability of the neonatal rat lungs to drugs. *Biol. Neonate*, **40**, 99–104
51. Ikegami, M., Berry, D., Elkady, T., Pettenzanno, A., Seidner, S. and Jobe, A. (1987) Corticosteroids and surfactant change lung function and protein leaks in the lungs of ventilated premature rabbits. *J. Clin. Invest.*, **79**, 1371–1378
52. Ballard, P. I., Granberg, P. and Ballard, R. A. (1975) Glucocorticoid levels in maternal and cord serum after prenatal betamethasone therapy to prevent respiratory distress syndrome. *J. Clin. Invest.*, **56**, 1548–1554
53. Beitins, I. Z., Bayard, F., Ances, I. G., Kowarski, A. and Migeon, C. J. (1972) The transplacental passage of prednisone and prednisolone in pregnancies near term. *J. Pediatr.*, **81**, 936–945
54. Liggins, G. C. and Howie, R. N. (1972) A controlled trial of antepartum glucocorticoid treatment for prevention of respiratory distress syndrome in premature infants. *Pediatrics*, **50**, 515–525
55. Dluholucky, S., Babic, J. and Taufer, I. (1976) Reduction of incidence and mortality of respiratory distress syndrome by administration of hydrocortisone to mother. *Arch. Dis. Child.*, **51**, 420–423
56. Block, M. F., Kling, O. R. and Crosby, W. M. (1977) Antenatal glucocorticoid therapy for the prevention of respiratory distress syndrome in the premature infant. *Obstet. Gynecol.*, **50**, 186–190
57. Taeusch, H. W., Frigoletto, F., Kitzmiller, J. *et al.* (1979) Risk of respiratory distress syndrome after prenatal dexamethasone treatment. *Pediatrics*, **63**, 64–72
58. Morrison, J. C., Whybrew, W. D., Bucovaz, E. T. and Schneider, J. M. (1979) Injection of corticosteroids into mother to prevent neonatal respiratory distress syndrome. *Am. J. Obstet. Gynecol.*, **131**, 358–366
59. Collaborative Groups in Antenatal Steroid Therapy (1981) Effect of antenatal dexamethasone administration on the prevention of respiratory distress syndrome. *Am. J. Obstet. Gynecol.*, **141**, 276–287
60. MacArthur, B. A., Howie, R. N., Dozoete, J. A. and Elkins, J. (1982) School progress and cognitive development of 6 year old children whose mothers were treated antenatally with betamethasone. *Pediatrics*, **70**, 99–105
61. Enhorning, G., Chamberlain, D., Contreras, C., Burgoyne, R. and Robertson, B. (1977) Isoxsuprine release of pulmonary surfactant in the rabbit fetus. *Am. J. Obstet. Gynecol.*, **129**, 197–202
62. Eklund, L., Burgoyne, R. and Enhorning, G. (1983) Pulmonary surfactant release in fetal rabbits: immediate and delayed response to terbutaline. *Am. J. Obstet. Gynecol.*, **147**, 437–443
63. Leveno, K. J., Klein, V. R., Gusick, D. S., Hankins, G. V. D., Young, D. C. and Williams, M. L. (1986) Single-centre randomised trial of ritodrine hydrochloride for preterm labour. *Lancet* **i**, 1293–1295
64. Merkatz, I. R., Peter, J. B. and Barden, T. P. (1980) Ritodrine hydrochloride: a betamimetic agent for use in preterm labour. *Obstet. Gynecol.*, **56**, 7–12
65. Ingermasson, I. (1982) Use of β-receptor agonists in obstetrics. *Acta Obstet. Gynaecol. Scand.* (Suppl.) **108**, 29–34
66. Boylan, P. and O'Driscoll, K. (1983) Improvement in perinatal mortality rate attributed to spontaneous preterm labour without use of tocolytic agents. *Am. J. Obstet. Gynecol.*, **145**, 781–783
67. Erenberg, A., Rhodes, M. L., Weinstein, M. W. *et al.* (1979) The effect of fetal thyroidectomy on ovine fetal lung maturation. *Pediatr. Res.*, **13**, 230–235
68. Gross, I., Dynia, D. W., Wilson, C. M. *et al.* (1984) Glucocorticoid–thyroid hormone interaction in fetal rat lung. *Pediatr. Res.*, **18**, 191–196
69. Rooney, S. A., Morino, P. A., Gobran, L. *et al.* (1979) Thyrotrophin-releasing hormone increases the amount of surfactant in lung lavage from fetal rabbits. *Pediatr. Res.*, **13**, 623–625
70. Ikegami, M., Jobe, A. H., Pettanzano, A., Seidner, S. R., Berry, D. D. and Ruffini, L. (1987) Effects of maternal treatment with corticosteroids, T_3, TRH, and their combinations on lung function of ventilated preterm rabbits with and without surfactant treatments. *Am. Rev. Resp. Dis.*, **136**, 892–898
71. Wauer, R. R., Schmalisch, G., Menzal, K. *et al.* (1982) The antenatal use of Ambroxol (bromhexine metabolite VIII) to prevent hyaline membrane disease: a controlled double blind study. *Biol. Res. Pregnancy*, **3**, 84–91
72. Hallman, M. (1987) Myo-inositol and the perinatal development of surfactant. In *Physiology of the Fetal and Neonatal Lung* (eds D. V. Walters, L. B. Strang and F. Geubelle), MTP Press, Lancaster, pp. 197–208
73. Enhorning, G. and Robertson, B. (1973) Lung expansion in the premature rabbit fetus after tracheal deposition of surfactant. *Pediatrics*, **50**, 58–66

74. Adams, F. H., Tower, B., Osher, A., Ikegami, M., Fujiwara, T. and Nozaki, M. (1978) Effects of tracheal instillation of natural surfactant in premature lambs. *Pediatr. Res.* **12**, 841–848
75. Enhorning, G., Hill, D., Sherwood, G., Cutz, E., Robertson, B. and Bryan, C. (1978) Improved ventilation of prematurely delivered primates following tracheal deposition of surfactant. *Am. J. Obstet. Gynecol.*, **132**, 529–536
76. Cutz, E., Enhorning, G., Robertson, B., Sherwood, W. G. and Hill, D. E. (1978) Hyaline membrane disease. Effect of surfactant prophylaxis on lung morphology in premature primates. *Am. J. Pathol.*, **92**, 581–594
77. Fujiwara, T., Chida, S., Watabe, Y., Maeta, H., Morita, T. and Abe, T. (1980) Artificial surfactant therapy in hyaline membrane disease. *Lancet*, **i**, 55–59
78. Morley, C. J., Bangham, A. D., Miller, N. and Davis, J. A. (1981) Dry artificial surfactant and its effect on very premature babies. *Lancet*, **i**, 64–68
79. Smyth, J. A., Metcalfe, I. L., Duffty, P., Possmayer, F., Bryan, M. H. and Enhorning, G. (1983) Hyaline membrane disease treated with bovine surfactant. *Pediatrics*, **71**, 913–917
80. Hallman, M., Merritt, T. A., Schneider, H. *et al.* (1983) Isolation of human surfactant from amniotic fluid and a pilot study of its efficacy in respiratory distress syndrome. *Pediatrics*, **71**, 473–482
81. Halliday, H. L., McClure, G., Reid, M., Lappin, T. R. J., Meban, C. and Thomas, P. S. (1984) Controlled trial of artificial surfactant to prevent respiratory distress syndrome. *Lancet*, **i**, 476–478
82. Wilkinson, A., Jenkins, P. A. and Jeffrey, J. A. (1985) Two controlled trials of dry artificial surfactant: early effects and later outcome in babies with surfactant deficiency. *Lancet*, **ii**, 287–291
83. Hallman, M., Merritt, T. A., Jarvenpaa, A. L. *et al.* (1985) Exogenous human surfactant for treatment of severe respiratory distress syndrome: a randomized prospective clinical trial. *J. Pediatr.*, **106**, 963–969
84. Enhorning, G., Shennan, A., Possmayer, F., Dunn, M., Chen, C. P. and Milligan, J. (1985) Prevention of neonatal respiratory distress syndrome by tracheal instillation of surfactant. A randomized clinical trial. *Pediatrics*, **76**, 145–153
85. Kwong, S. M., Egan, E. A., Notter, R. H. and Shapiro, D. L. (1985) Double-blind clinical trial of calf lung surfactant extract for the prevention of hyaline membrane disease in extremely premature infants. *Pediatrics*, **76**, 585–592
86. Shapiro, D. L., Notter, R. H., Morin, F. C. *et al.* (1986) Double blind, randomized trial of calf lung surfactant extract administered at birth to very premature infants for prevention of respiratory distress syndrome. *Pediatrics*, **76**, 593–599
87. Merritt, T. A., Hallman, M., Bloom B. T. *et al.* (1986) Prophylactic treatment of very premature infants with human surfactant. *N. Engl. J. Med.*, **315**, 785–790
88. Gitlin, J. D., Soll, R. F., Parad, R. B. *et al.* (1987) Randomized controlled trial of exogenous surfactant for the treatment of hyaline membrane disease. *Pediatrics*, **79**, 31–37
89. Raju, T. N. K., Vidyasagar, D., Bhat, R. *et al.* (1987) Double-blind controlled trial of single-dose treatment with bovine surfactant in severe hyaline membrane disease. *Lancet*, **i**, 651–656
90. McCord, F. B., Cursted, T., Halliday, H., McClure, G., McCreid, M. and Robertson, B. (1988) surfactant treatment and incidence of intraventricular haemorrhage in severe respiratory distress syndrome. *Arch. Dis. Child.*, **63**, 10–16
91. Tanaka, Y., Takei, T., Kanazawa, Y. *et al.* (1982) Preparation of surfactant from minced bovine lung, chemical composition and surface tension properties. *J. Jap. Med. Soc. Biol. Interface*, **13**, 27–34
92. Robertson, B. (1983) Lung surfactant for replacement therapy. *Clin. Physiol.*, **3**, 97–110
93. Bangham, A. D. (1980) Breathing made easy. *New Scientist*, **85**, 408–410
94. Bangham, A. D., Morley, C. J. and Phillips, M. C. (1979) The physical properties of an effective lung surfactant. *Biochim. Biophys. Acta*, **573**, 552–556
95. Bangham, A. D., Miller, N. G. A., Davies, R. J., Greenough, A. and Morley, C. J. (1984) Introductory remarks about Artificial Lung Expanding Compounds (ALEC). *Colloid Surfaces*, **10**, 337–347
96. Morley, C. J., Bangham, A. D., Johnson, P., Thorburn, G. D. and Jenkin, G. (1978) Physical and physiological properties of dry lung surfactant. *Nature*, **271**, 162–163
97. Morley, C. J., Robertson, B., Lachmann, B. *et al.* (1980) Artificial surfactant and natural surfactant. Comparative study of the effects on premature rabbit lungs. *Arch. Dis. Child.*, **50**, 758–765
98. Morley, C., Greenough, A., Miller, N. G., Bangham, A., Pool, J., Wood, S., South, M., Davis, J. and Vyas, H. (1988) Randomized trial of artificial surfactant (ALEC) given at birth to babies from 23 to 34 weeks gestation. *Early Human Development*, **17**, 41–54

Chapter 5

Resuscitation

Clifford Roberton

Intubation and intermittent positive pressure ventilation (IPPV) should be used routinely to resuscitate all extremely low birth weight (ELBW) neonates and should be started as soon as the infant reaches the resuscitation trolley. The only possible exceptions to this rule are:

(1) Previable infants less than 400–500 g birth weight and less than 22–24 weeks gestation. This decision, an ethical one, should only be taken by an experienced neonatologist [1] and should only be done after weighing the baby (which can be done virtually instantaneously on modern electronic scales), and after pre-delivery discussion with the parents and their obstetrician about the problems and prognosis of a very immature infant. It is not fair to leave a junior paediatrician in the early stages of his neonatal training to make snap decisions of this nature in the middle of the night.
(2) A baby, usually small for gestational age, who by the time he arrives on the resuscitation trolley is pink, vigorous, howling, waving his arms and legs about and is clearly in excellent condition.

The justification for this aggressive management is based on five major lines of evidence:

(1) The high incidence of low Apgar scores in ELBW neonates which may not necessarily mean severe biochemical asphyxia, but undoubtedly identifies an at-risk infant who will rapidly develop the biochemical features of severe asphyxia if not resuscitated promptly.
(2) The literature suggesting that if an ELBW infant is spared hypoxia, hypercapnia, hypotension and acidaemia in the first few hours of life he is much less likely to develop complications of prematurity such as respiratory distress syndrome (RDS), periventricular haemorrhage (PVH), periventricular leucomalacia (PVL), and subsequent neurological handicap.
(3) The association between active resuscitation at birth and improved neonatal outcome.
(4) The deficiencies in methods of neonatal resuscitation other than intubation and IPPV.
(5) Practical advantages inherent in active resuscitation.

High incidence of low Apgar scores in ELBW infants

The traditional method for assessing the severity of asphyxia at birth is the Apgar score and it is well recognized that the score is often very low in ELBW babies [2]. Furthermore, it is clear that those with low Apgar scores are less likely to survive [2,3] (Figure 5.1), though the low Apgar score is a poor predictor of neurological outcome [4]. What is not clear, however, is whether the reduced survival is due to asphyxia, or whether the poor Apgar score is a measure of a more complex depression of vital functions caused by something other than the acid-base changes of asphyxia.

The most accurate and physiologically acceptable way of assessing the presence of asphyxia at birth is to measure the blood gases in a segment of umbilical artery double-clamped immediately after delivery [5]. Even this is less than perfect, since adequate interpretation of cord blood gas values requires some assessment of the mother's acid-base status [6]. Furthermore, cord blood gas analysis may give a falsely optimistic indication of the likely incidence of early neonatal problems. The neonate may have suffered severe asphyxia, for example early in the second stage of labour, from which he has recovered from the acid-base point of view by the time of delivery, but may nevertheless have suffered serious myocardial, pulmonary or neurological damage which will cause symptomatic disease in the 3–4 h after delivery. There are, unfortunately, very few studies measuring umbilical cord blood gases in preterm babies, and even fewer in those under 1000 g at birth. As with term babies [7] the data suggest that the Apgar score is a poor indicator of asphyxia, and correlates very much better with gestation [8–10]. One of the problems with recent studies of this sort is that with modern perinatal care, intrapartum acidaemia even in preterm infants is so rare that it is difficult to establish statistically significant correlates for the few babies with intrapartum asphyxia [11]. However, the data in this study do suggest that the incidence of cord pH levels below 7.20 increases with falling birth weight. Furthermore, Goldenberg, Huddleston and Nelson [8] showed that although many preterm

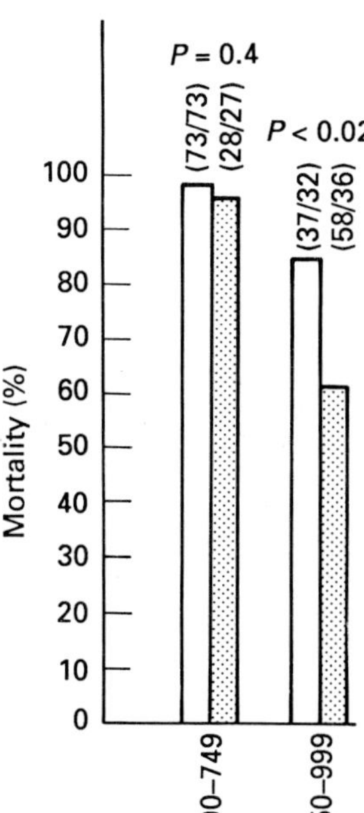

Figure 5.1 Neonatal mortality in asphyxiated infants (white bars) and unasphyxiated infants (shaded bars). Asphyxia is defined as those babies needing IPPV for >1 min after delivery. Figures in parentheses show absolute number of babies/number surviving. *P* values comparing outcome in asphyxiated and non-asphyxiated groups. From McDonald *et al.* [2], with permission

babies can have a low Apgar score without asphyxia, those that are asphyxiated ($pH < 7.25$) are much more likely to have a low Apgar score with its attendant risk of a higher neonatal mortality.

The low one-minute Apgar score in the ELBW infant does not, therefore, necessarily mean asphyxia in the strict biochemical sense of the term, but the neonate with a low score clearly has a problem whether or not it is asphyxia since he is more likely to die than the baby with a good Apgar score (Figure 5.1). Furthermore, if a baby with a 'non-asphyxial' low Apgar score is not promptly and adequately resuscitated, then hypoxia and asphyxia will be added rapidly to all his other pre-existing problems, and this should clearly be avoided at all costs.

Perinatal asphyxia and subsequent morbidity

Respiratory distress syndrome (RDS)

There is a large literature relating perinatal and intrapartum asphyxia, assessed either by Apgar score or cord blood gas analysis, to subsequent RDS [12–14].

In utero only 10% of the cardiac output goes to the lungs, but during fetal asphyxia lung perfusion may fall to even lower levels, which may cause ischaemic damage to pulmonary capillaries. Fetal resuscitation is then followed by pulmonary hyperperfusion [15] and pulmonary oedema [16]. If this type of prenatal damage has occurred, the infant's fate is sealed pre-delivery, and he is very likely to develop severe surfactant-deficient RDS. There is every reason, nevertheless, to try and minimize these prenatal effects, and to reverse any intrapartum asphyxia as quickly as possible after delivery by prompt and vigorous resuscitation.

However, the single most important justification for active resuscitation of ELBW babies is to prevent asphyxia developing in the first few minutes of life in small, puny, previously biochemically stable babies who even in the best of all possible worlds have great difficulty establishing adequate alveolar ventilation after birth. Common sense dictates, with any seriously ill patient, that it is important for the physician to establish control as soon as possible over such vital functions as ventilation, oxygenation and perfusion. More specifically in the ELBW infant at high risk from RDS, every effort must be made to avoid early neonatal events which are likely to increase the severity and complications of the disease. In theory at least there are five ways in which this can be done, all involving prompt vigorous resuscitation:

(1) Preventing postnatal hypoxic damage to lung capillaries leading to pulmonary oedema and RDS.
(2) Preventing decreased surfactant synthesis in the presence of acidaemia and hypoxia.
(3) Ensuring effective surfactant release from the type II pneumonocytes.
(4) Rapidly establishing normal blood gases and normal pulmonary perfusion.
(5) Avoiding and correcting systemic hypotension: postnatal hypotension is important in the aetiology not only of RDS but also of PVH and PVL.

Hypoxic capillary damage and RDS

In both fetal and neonatal animals hypoxaemia can cause pulmonary oedema. In part this is due to an increase in filtration pressure in the microcirculation and in part it is due to hypoxic ischaemic damage to the capillary and alveolar lining cells [16–18]. The resultant pulmonary oedema causes the surfactant-producing cells to slough off and die, and this is an early histological feature of fatal cases of RDS [19]. Even though the lung in the asphyxiated fetus does not appear to allow protein out of the capillaries [17], the early neonatal lung certainly does [20] and the presence of protein on the alveolar surface inhibits surfactant activity [21].

Every effort should therefore be made in the first 10–20 min after delivery to prevent hypoxia with its deleterious effects on the pulmonary vasculature and epithelium. This means using IPPV to establish immediate ventilation.

Surfactant synthesis and pH (see also Chapter 4)

Merritt and Farrell [22] in monkey lung tissue slices showed that dipalmitoyl phosphatidyl choline synthesis was pH sensitive and a fall in the pH of the tissue culture supernatant to just 7.20 was associated with reduced synthesis (Figure 5.2). This has a clear clinical message: the further the pH in a preterm neonate is below 7.20, the less likely he is to synthesize adequate amounts of surfactant. At resuscitation, therefore, every endeavour must be made to get his pH above 7.20 as quickly as possible, in part by ventilation and blowing off CO_2. Every effort should also be made to avert metabolic acidaemia (lactic acidaemia) by preventing hypoxia, anaemia, hypotension and hypoperfusion (Figure 5.3). Although asymptomatic term neonates who have suffered intrapartum asphyxia may be left safely postnatally to correct spontaneously a metabolic acidaemia of 10–20 mmol/l, there is no point in speculatively leaving an ELBW infant with a base deficit of more than 10 mmol/l in the hope that he might spontaneously correct it. The ability of sick low birth weight babies to correct metabolic acidaemia is reduced [23] and the data relating infusions of base to neonatal PVH are extremely unimpressive since they deal with inappropriate rates and volumes of bicarbonate given to infants many of whose cerebral haemorrhages were not of the periventricular variety [24,25].

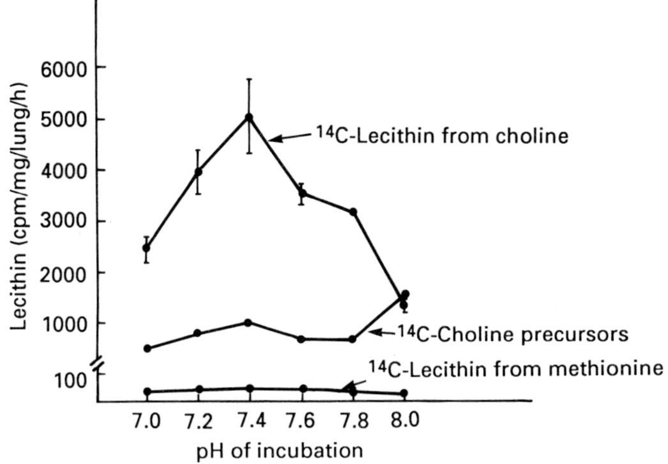

Figure 5.2 Rate of incorporation of ^{14}C into lecithin in monkey lung slices. From Merritt and Farrell [22] with permission

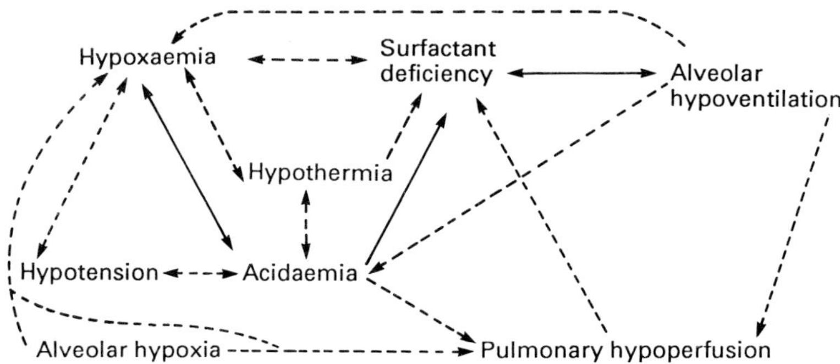

Figure 5.3 Inter-relationships of factors affecting surfactant production in ill neonates. From Roberton [68] with permission

Clearly in neonatal resuscitation the priority must be to prevent those conditions which predispose to acidaemia; however if the base deficit is more than 10 mmol/l in an ELBW infant in the first 30–60 min of life, it should be corrected with infusions of base given no faster than 0.5–1.0 mmol/kg/min [26].

Surfactant release

Surfactant release at birth is a complex combination of mobilization of intracellular reserves, pharmacologically mediated release of surfactant, in particular by beta-adrenergic mechanisms, and adequate physical expansion of the neonate's lungs [27–31]. Infants of less than 1000 g have a very compliant chest wall [32] which may cave in, even during the feeble respiratory efforts generated by their weak muscles [33]. Furthermore, these muscles fatigue easily [34] and their activity is often compromised by hypoxia and acidaemia [35]. The result is that the ELBW infant has considerable difficulty in expanding his fluid-filled surfactant-deficient lungs at birth [36], and has even greater problems maintaining a functional residual capacity [37].

There is, therefore, a potential vicious circle being created (Figure 5.3). Poor ventilation leads to poor surfactant release, resulting in hypoxia, hypercapnia, acidaemia and thus weaker muscles further compromising surfactant release. The most effective way of preventing this cycle is to ventilate the baby from birth, maximizing the release of whatever surfactant stores he possesses and reversing all the adverse changes (Figure 5.3).

An important factor to remember when ventilating such babies is that *over*-ventilation does reduce surfactant levels unless a small amount of positive end expiratory pressure (PEEP) is added [38].

Pulmonary perfusion and ventilation

The major cause of hypoxia in RDS is ventilation-perfusion imbalance in the diseased lungs [39,40]. There is also some right-to-left shunting through the patent ductus [41] and foramen ovale [42]. These true shunts are bigger in the presence of pulmonary hypertension which may be present in many neonates with severe RDS [43].

The classical studies of Cassin *et al.* [44] showed that during resuscitation lowering

$Pa\text{CO}_2$, increasing $Pa\text{O}_2$, even ventilation itself all had an important role in maximizing pulmonary perfusion and lowering pulmonary artery pressure. Therefore, to keep pulmonary hypertension and true shunting to a minimum, it is important to establish adequate ventilation and normal blood gases as soon after delivery of an ELBW infant as possible.

Hypotension

Hypotension, one of the cardinal features of terminal apnoea [45], is well recognized in asphyxiated babies, particularly those with myocardial injury [46]. It is also likely to develop in neonates who are hypoxic and acidaemic, and is virtually inevitable in neonates who have bled or have become anaemic for some other reason. Hypotension can damage many body systems in the neonate causing renal failure and necrotizing enterocolitis. In preterm neonates hypotension at birth has been reported to be associated with an increased incidence of RDS, and in particular an increased mortality from it [13,47]. It is also of crucial importance in the aetiology of PVH and PVL.

Prompt resuscitation by preventing hypoxia and acidaemia is likely to minimize the incidence of hypotension. In addition it is essential to measure the blood pressure in all ELBW infants within the first 30–60 min after birth, and if the blood pressure is low (systolic $BP < 40$ mmHg: mean $BP < 30$ mmHg) to correct it promptly by plasma expanders or blood, using dopamine if necessary.

Periventricular haemorrhage (PVH) and leucomalacia (PVL)

The current view is that a most important factor in the aetiology of PVL and the severe forms of PVH which carry a grave prognosis, is a period of periventricular hypoperfusion. This may cause a purely ischaemic lesion as in periventricular leucomalacia or may weaken the periventricular blood vessels so that they rupture easily causing haemorrhage either into the lateral ventricle (IVH) or into the pre-existing periventricular leucomalacia (PVH) [48]. This type of haemorrhage, secondary to vessel rupture, is more likely to occur during a period of raised cerebral blood flow. The factors influencing cerebral blood flow and thus the incidence of PVL and PVH are shown in Figure 5.4.

Periventricular damage of this type can be initiated by ischaemia occurring before and during delivery so that perinatal asphyxia can not only be an important antecedent of PVH, but as with RDS the fate of some babies as regards developing a PVH may be more or less sealed before they are delivered. The fact that careful cranial ultrasound studies do show that many periventricular haemorrhages appear shortly after delivery [49,50] supports this view, as does the fact that some epidemiological studies do show an association between prenatal asphyxia and an increased incidence of PVH [11,51–53]; however, these data are not consistent [54,55]. Nevertheless, in such babies, prompt resuscitation will prevent any further damage to the periventricular vasculature that might be caused by postnatal asphyxia.

Once the baby is delivered, however, there is a clear association between the development of a PVH and RDS in the neonate [56], and in particular the incidence of RDS complicated by a pneumothorax [57]. This association probably explains many cases of late onset (> 12–24 h of age) PVH, and the extension of haemorrhages which may have originally developed because of perinatal problems. Therefore, minimizing RDS in the ways outlined above, and in particular prompt resuscitation and early

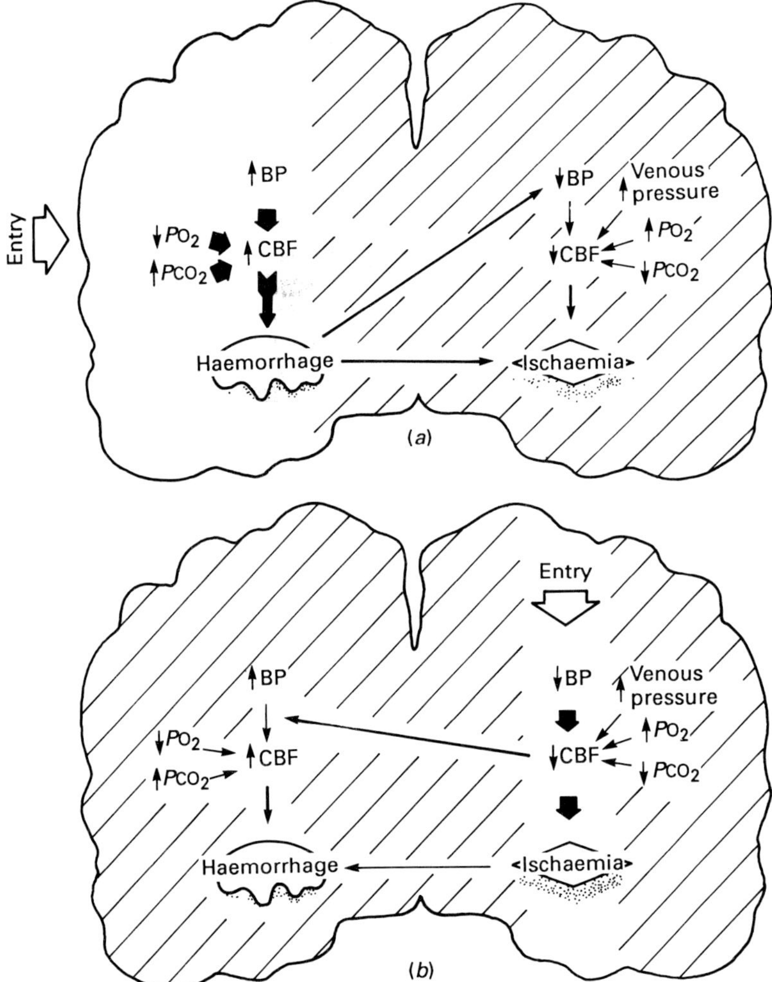

Figure 5.4 Factors influencing the development of PVH and PVL. In (*a*) the emphasis is placed on increased cerebral blood flow (CBF) and thus on PVH; in (*b*) the emphasis is on reduced flow and thus on PVL. From Wigglesworth and Pape [71] with permission

correction of hypotension to avoid cerebral hypoperfusion and ischaemia, is likely to decrease the incidence of PVH.

Although the current view is that, in order to prevent PVL and large PVH, cerebral *hypo*perfusion rather than *hyper*perfusion is to be avoided at all costs, some studies claim to show that early control (and reduction) of $Pa\text{CO}_2$ (thereby reducing cerebral blood flow and preventing hyperperfusion) reduces the incidence of PVH [58,59]. However, it is difficult to unravel the beneficial effects of the reduction in $Pa\text{CO}_2$ from all the other benefits alluded to in this chapter which are likely to result if there is active early resuscitation in ELBW babies. There are also theoretical hazards from overdoing the low $Pa\text{CO}_2$ approach, in particular *over*-ventilation causing lung damage, and hypocapnia reducing cerebral blood flow and predisposing to the very conditions (PVL) which prompt resuscitation is aiming to prevent.

Other acute neonatal illness

Birth asphyxia in term babies can damage many other body systems, causing renal failure, necrotizing enterocolitis, bleeding disorders, especially disseminated intravascular coagulation, and adrenal haemorrhage [60]. It is not unreasonable to assume that these illnesses may also be sequelae of intrapartum asphyxia in ELBW neonates and their incidence in such infants can be minimized by preventing postnatal asphyxia and hypotension.

Long-term neurological sequelae

Prevention of postnatal asphyxia and reduction in the incidence of RDS, PVL and PVH is likely to reduce the incidence of neurological sequelae causing handicap.

Studies on the effect of early intervention

Two attempts have been made to evaluate active resuscitation methods. Robson and Hey [61] compared consecutive periods in Newcastle when the resuscitation of infants weighing 1000–2000 g was passive or active. In the period with active resuscitation the babies were in better condition when admitted to the neonatal unit, and there was a statistically significant decrease of 20% in the mortality from RDS. Drew [62] prospectively randomized infants weighing 500–1500 g to electively resuscitation by intubation and ventilation or resuscitation by bag and mask and IPPV only when clinically indicated. He showed a very clear reduction in the morbidity and mortality in actively resuscitated infants. The overall mortality fell from 49% in the control group to 23% in the actively treated group ($P<0.01$) and from 86% to 59% when the analysis was limited to ELBW babies ($P<0.05$).

Why intubation?

It is hoped that the reader is now convinced that active resuscitation is indicated immediately after delivery in all ELBW infants. The next step is to justify why resuscitation should be carried out by intubation and positive pressure ventilation. This is based on studies on term infants since no comparable studies have, as yet, been done on preterm ones.

When using a bag and mask to resuscitate a term baby who has never breathed after delivery, it is a common clinical experience to find that, despite dramatic hissing and squelching noises as the gas escapes over the baby's face from under the mask, the chest does not move and air cannot be heard to enter the lungs.

Milner, Vyas and Hopkin [63] and Field, Milner and Hopkin [64] have confirmed that unless the physical assault on the baby is sufficient to provoke him to gasp or breathe on his own, useful tidal exchange does not take place during bag and mask ventilation. In the ELBW infant who has surfactant-deficient lungs with their inherent inability to establish a functional residual capacity (FRC), these data suggest that bag and mask ventilation is unlikely to be of any benefit.

Even with endotracheal intubation and IPPV in term babies, the tidal volume achieved for a given inflation pressure is much smaller than that which occurs with an identical pressure change during a spontaneous inhalation. The FRC is also slow to form during IPPV even down an endotracheal tube unless the inspiratory time is 3–5 s during the first few inflations [65–67].

Practical advantages

There are certain basic technical advantages which accrue when resuscitation is carried out by intubation and positive pressure ventilation down an endotracheal tube:

(1) Laryngoscopy is required and this allows the paediatrician to clear extraneous material out of the airway in a precise and accurate way, rather than blindly thrusting a suction catheter down the back of the baby's throat.
(2) The period between resuscitation in the labour ward and stabilizing the ELBW neonate in an incubator in the neonatal intensive care unit (NICU) is often one of the most hazardous 20–30 min of the ELBW neonate's existence [68]. Control of his care during this period and the transportation involved does become considerably easier if he is intubated. The incidence of the hypoxia, hypercapnia, acidaemia and hypotension which is so damaging to ELBW neonates in the first 60–90 min of life can thus be reduced to the absolute minimum.
(3) A previous study in which the decision to intubate ELBW infants at birth was left to clinical judgement has shown that the majority are intubated in any case (Figure 5.1), and since virtually all ELBW infants require a period of IPPV in the first few days, they might as well be intubated at birth to establish immediate control of their respiratory function.

The fact that laryngoscoping and intubating ELBW infants does require considerable skill should not be used as an excuse for relying on bag and mask ventilation which is a dangerously inadequate form of resuscitation. Rather it should motivate those responsible for the care of such fragile patients and their mothers to ensure that the birth takes place in a unit with adequate neonatal facilities.

Technique of resuscitation

Much of what goes on when resuscitating newborn babies is common to those of all birth weights, for example taking the perinatal history, providing appropriate equipment and drugs, and many of the techniques which are used [60]. In this section only those aspects of resuscitation which are specific to the ELBW baby will be considered.

Location and personnel

Infants weighing less than 1000 g should all be delivered in a level 3 NICU, but if in an emergency one needs to be delivered elsewhere, the most experienced paediatrician available must be present for resuscitation. Ideally a second person should be in the labour ward or immediately available should any complication arise.

Temperature control

In a conventional labour ward at 21°C(70 °F) the naked, wet ELBW infant loses heat about ten times faster than he can generate it, and as a result his body temperature may fall by 0.25–0.3 °C/min. The room in which the resuscitation takes place should, therefore, be as hot as possible, windows and doors should be shut and air conditioning turned off in an attempt to minimize convective and evaporative heat loss. To minimize radiant and conductive heat loss the radiant heater on the resuscitation trolley should be full on and warm towels should be available in which the baby can be wrapped as soon as he is delivered, and with which he can be dried.

Laryngoscope and endotracheal tubes (ETT)

In general straight-bladed laryngoscopes should be used. A common mistake is to use those with a ⊂ or L shape on cross-section. Particularly in the small mouth of the ELBW infant the cross-section of the laryngoscope blade should be C-shaped and large enough to pass the ETT through it and still visualize the laryngeal entrance. Although 2.5 mm ETTs have a much higher internal resistance than 3.0 mm ones, in most circumstances they will have to be used since the 3.0 mm tube will not pass through the vocal cords. For routine purposes a shouldered Cole's oral ETT should be used. Compared with nasal ETTs these are much easier to insert. Pushing the ETT too far into one or other division of the bronchial tree resulting in poor ventilation and increasing the risk of pneumothorax is also much less likely to occur with a shouldered tube. Furthermore, since they are quicker and easier to insert the adverse cardiorespiratory changes which take place during intubation [69] are likely to be minimized.

Although it is often suggested that nasal ETTs cause fewer complications when used for long-term IPPV and they are extensively used in neonates, the evidence on which this belief is based is far from convincing [70] and it is certainly absent where short-term intubation is concerned.

Inflation pressures and gas composition

Inflation pressures of 30 cmH_2O are likely to expand the lungs of most newborn babies [66,67]. Ideally the inflation time should be at least 1 s, and initially nearer 3 s, in an endeavour to establish an FRC as soon as possible; the ventilation rate will therefore be slow, no more than 30–40/min.

Self-inflating bags are frequently used for ventilation during neonatal resuscitation, but there is much to be said for using a simple Y connector attached to a blow-off valve since this allows for greater control of the duration of each inflation.

The practical and financial realities are such that, although 40–60% oxygen is theoretically preferable to pure oxygen for resuscitation, it is rarely used.

Drug administration

It is doubtful if drug therapy should ever be given to an ELBW infant in the labour ward. Those drugs that might be considered include:

(1) *Naloxone*. If the mother received an opiate during the 6 h before delivery and the baby makes no spontaneous respiratory effort, naloxone can be given. However, from what has been said it will be clear that the intention is to artificially ventilate the baby in any case, and there is therefore no urgency about giving an opiate antagonist to reverse apnoea.

(2) *Sodium bicarbonate*. Given the impossibility of assessing the severity of acidaemia clinically, this drug should not be used in the labour ward without measuring the neonate's blood gases. If a cord blood gas analysis has not been done, this can usually wait until the baby is transferred to the NICU. Bicarbonate should only be considered if there is persisting bradycardia (< 60/min) in the absence of some technical errors in the resuscitation, or in the case of a stillbirth when 5–10 mEq may be given intravenously over 1–2 min.

(3) *Glucose*. This should never be given unless hypoglycaemia is confirmed by Dextrostix.

(4) *Other drugs*. No other drugs should be considered for the neonate during routine resuscitation. In the event of a cardiac arrest appropriate dosages of calcium

Table 5.1 The causes of poor response to resuscitation at birth

Malformations
Upper respiratory tract:
- Choanal atresia
- Pierre-Robin syndrome
- Laryngeal and tracheal malformations
  - atresia
  - webs
  - luminal tumours
  - clefts

Lung:
- Pulmonary hypoplasia
  - Potter's syndrome
  - prolonged membrane rupture
  - idiopathic
- Pleural effusions; hydrops
- Congenital cystic adenomatoid malformation
- Congenital lobar emphysema
- Pulmonary lymphangiectasia

Extrapulmonary:
- Diaphragmatic hernia
- Diaphragmatic eventration
- Intrathoracic space-occupying tumours
- Gross abdominal distension splinting the diaphragm
  - tumours
  - hepatosplenomegaly
  - ascites ± hydrops
  - dilated renal tract
- Small chest
  - asphyxiating thoracic dystrophy
  - thanatophoric dwarfism

Pulmonary disease
Severe RDS
Congenital pneumonia (esp. Group B streptococcus)
Pneumothorax

gluconate, atropine and sympathomimetic drugs may be given in addition to bicarbonate.

The ELBW infant who does not respond to resuscitation

Despite carrying out the procedures outlined above the baby may remain cyanosed and often bradycardic at 5 min of age. The commonest cause for this is some technical error in the resuscitation procedure, and it is therefore essential to check as quickly as possible whether:

(a) the endotracheal tube is in the wrong place, either in the oesophagus, or down one main stem bronchus, or even in some more distant part of the bronchial tree;
(b) an adequate inflation pressure (usually set to 30 cmH_2O) is being applied. The blow-off valve on the resuscitation trolley may become inadvertently set at a low pressure;
(c) the oxygen has been disconnected.

As soon as these errors are recognized and remedied, the infant will rapidly pink up and become vigorous and active. The other causes of poor response to resuscitation are listed in Table 5.1 and are usually easy to diagnose clinically or by chest X-ray.

References

1. Campbell, A. G. M. (1986). Ethical problems in neonatal care. In *Textbook of Neonatology* (ed. N. R. C. Roberton), Churchill Livingstone, London and Edinburgh, pp. 35–41
2. McDonald, H. M., Mulligan, J. C., Allen, A. C. and Taylor, P. M. (1980) Neonatal asphyxia. I. Relationship of obstetric and neonatal complications to neonatal mortality in 28,405 consecutive deliveries. *J. Pediatr.*, **96**, 898–902
3. Rehnke, M., Carter R. L., Hardt, N. S., Eyler, F. D., Cruz, A. C. and Resnick, M. B. (1987) The relationship of Apgar scores, gestational age and birthweight to survival of low-birthweight infants. *Am. J. Perinatol*, **4**, 121–124
4. Nelson, K. B. and Ellenberg, J. H. (1981) Apgar scores as predictors of chronic neurologic disability. *Pediatrics*, **68**, 36–44
5. Wible, J. L., Petrie, B. H., Koons, A. and Perez, A. (1982) The clinical use of umbilical cord acid base determinations in perinatal surveillance and management. *Clin. Perinatol.*, **9**, 387–397
6. Dijxhoorn, M. J., Visser, G. H. A., Huisjes, H. J., Fidler, V. and Touwen B. C. L. (1985) The relation between umbilical pH values and neonatal neurological morbidity in full-term appropriate for dates infants. *Early Hum. Dev.*, **11**, 32–42
7. Sykes, G. S., Molloy, P. M., Johnson, P. *et al.* (1982). Do Apgar scores indicate asphyxia? *Lancet*, **i**, 494–497
8. Goldenberg, R. L., Huddleston, J. F. and Nelson, K. G. (1984) Apgar scores and umbilical arterial pH in preterm newborn infants. *Am. J. Obstet. Gynecol.*, **149**, 651–654
9. Perkins, R. P. and Papile, L. A. (1985) The very low birthweight infant: incidence and significance of low Apgar scores, "asphyxia" and morbidity. *Am. J. Perinatol.*, **2**, 108–113
10. Catlin, E. A., Carpenter, M. W., Brann, B. S. *et al.* (1986) The Apgar score revisited: influence of gestational age. *J. Pediatr.*, **109**, 865–868
11. Luthy, D. A., Shy, K. K., Strickland, D. *et al.* (1987) State of infants at birth and risk for adverse neonatal events and long term sequelae. A study in low birthweight infants. *Am. J. Obstet. Gynecol.*, **157**, 676–679
12. Jones, M. D., Burd, L. J., Bowes, W. A., Battaglia, F. C. and Lubchenko, L. O. (1975) Failure of association of premature rupture of membranes with respiratory distress syndrome. *N. Engl. J. Med.*, **292**, 1253–1257

13. Linderkamp, O., Versmold, H. T., Fendel, H. Riegel, K. P. and Betke, K. (1978) Association of neonatal respiratory distress with birth asphyxia and deficiency of red cell mass in premature infants. *Eur. J. Pediatr.*, **129**, 167–173
14. Thibeault, D. W., Hall, F. K., Sheehan, M. B. and Hall, R. T. (1984) Postasphyxial lung disease in newborn infants with severe perinatal acidosis. *Am. J. Obstet. Gynecol.*, **150**, 393–399
15. Dawes, G. S. and Mott, J. C. (1962) The vascular tone of the fetal lung. *J. Physiol.*, **164**, 465–477
16. Davis, J. A. and Stafford, A. (1964) Respiratory distress in newborn rabbits. *Biol. Neonate*, **7**, 129–140
17. Adamson, T. M. Boyd, R. D. H., Hill, J. R., Normand, I. C. S., Reynolds, E. O. R. and Strang, L. B. (1970) Effect of asphyxia due to umbilical cord occlusion in the foetal lamb on leakage of liquid from the circulation and permeability of lung capillaries to albumin. *J. Physiol.*, **207**, 493–505
18. Hansen, T. I., Hazinski, T. A. and Bland, R. D. (1984) Effects of asphyxia on lung fluid balance in fetal lambs. *J. Clin. Invest.*, **74**, 370–376
19. Gandy, G. M., Jacobson, W. and Gairdner, D. (1970) Hyaline membrane disease, I. Cellular changes. *Arch. Dis. Child.*, **45**, 289–310
20. Jeffries, A. L., Coates, G. and O'Brodovich H. (1984) Pulmonary epithelial permeability in hyaline membrane disease. *N. Engl. J. Med.*, **311**, 1075–1080
21. Ikegami, M., Jacobs, H. and Jobe, A. (1983) Surfactant function in respiratory distress syndrome. *J. Pediatr.*, **102**, 443–447
22. Merritt, T. A. and Farrell, P. M. (1976) Diminished pulmonary synthesis in acidosis. Experimental findings as related to respiratory distress syndrome. *Pediatrics*, **57**, 32–40
23. Allen, A. C. and Usher, R. H. (1971) Renal acid excretion in infants with respiratory distress syndrome. *Pediatr. Res.*, **5**, 345–355
24. Simmons, M. A. Adcock, E. Q., Bard, H. and Battaglia, F. C. (1974) Hypernatremia and intracranial hemorrhage in neonates. *N. Engl. J. Med.*, **291**, 6–10
25. Wigglesworth, J. S., Keith, J. H. Girling, D. J. and Slade, S. A. (1975) Hyaline membrane disease, alkali and intraventricular haemorrhage. *Arch. Dis. Child.*, **51**, 755–762
26. Baum, J. D. and Roberton, N. R. C. (1975) Immediate effects of alkaline infusion in infants with respiratory distress syndrome. *J. Pediatr.*, **87**, 255–261
27. Oyarzun, M. J. and Clements, J. A. (1978) Control of lung surfactant by ventilation, adrenergic mediators and prostaglandins in the rabbit. *Am. Rev. Resp. Dis.*, **117**, 879–891
28. Walters, D. W. and Olver, R. E. (1978) The role of catecholamines in lung liquid absorption at birth. *Pediatr. Res.*, **12**, 239–242
29. Oyarzun, M. J. and Clements, J. A. (1977) Ventilatory and cholinergic control of surfactant in the rabbit. *J. Appl. Physiol.*, **43**, 39–45
30. Lawson, E. E., Birdwell, R. L., Huang, P. S. and Taeusch, H. W. (1979) Augmentation of pulmonary surfactant secretion by lung expansion at birth. *Pediatr. Res.*, **13**, 611–614
31. Massaro, G. D. and Massaro, D. (1983) Morphological evidence that large inflations of the lung stimulate secretion of surfactant. *Am. Rev. Resp. Dis.*, **127**, 235–236
32. Stocks, J. (1977) The functional growth and development of the lung during the first year of life. *Early Hum. Dev.*, **1**, 285–309
33. Keens, T. G., Bryan, A. C., Levison, H. and Ianuzzo, C. D. (1978) Developmental pattern of muscle fibre types in human ventilatory muscles. *J. Appl. Physiol.*, **44**, 909–913
34. Muller, N., Gulston, G.,Cade, D., Witton, J., Froese, A. B. and Bryan, M. H. (1979) Diaphragmatic muscle fatigue in the newborn. *J. Appl. Physiol.*, **46**, 688–695
35. Watchko, J. F., LaFramboise, W. A., Standaert, T. A. and Woodrum, D. E. (1986) Diaphragmatic function during hypoxemia: neonatal and developmental aspects. *J. Appl. Physiol.*, **60**, 1599–1604
36. Scarpelli, E. M., Clutario, B. C. and Traver, D. (1979) Failure of immature lungs to produce foam and retain air at birth. *Pediatr. Res.*, **13**, 1285–1289
37. Scarpelli, E. M. (1984) Perinatal lung mechanics and the first breath. *Lung*, **162**, 61–71
38. Wyszogrodski I., Kyei-Aboagye, K., Taeusch, H. W. and Avery, M. E. (1975) Surfactant inactivation by hyperventilation, conservation by end-expiratory pressure. *J. Appl. Physiol.*, **38**, 461–466
39. Strang, L. B. and McLeish, M. H. (1961) Ventilatory failure and right to left shunt in newborn infants with respiratory distress. *Pediatrics*, **28**, 17–27
40. Warley, M. A. and Gairdner, D. (1962) Respiratory distress syndrome of the newborn – principles of treatment. *Arch. Dis. Child*, **37**, 455–465

41. Roberton, N. R. C. and Dahlenburg, G. W. (1969) Ductus arteriosus shunts in respiratory distress syndrome. *Pediatr. Res.*, **3**, 149–159
42. Stahlman, M. (1964) Treatment of cardiovascular disorders of the newborn. *Pediatr. Clin. North Am.*, **11**, 363–400
43. Emmanouilides, G. C. (1979) Persistence of fetal circulation. In *Neonatal Pulmonary Care* (eds D. W. Thibault and G. A. Gregory), Addison Wesley, Menlo Park, California, pp. 277–295
44. Cassin, S., Dawes, G. S. Mott, J. C., Ross, B. B. and Strang, L. B. (1964) The vascular resistance of the foetal and newly ventilated lungs of the lamb. *J. Physiol.*, **171**, 61–79
45. Dawes, G. S., Hibbard, E. and Windle, W. F. (1964) The effect of alkali and glucose infusion on permanent brain damage in rhesus monkeys asphyxiated at birth. *J. Pediatr.*, **65**, 801–806
46. Cabal, L. A., Devaskar, U. Siassi, B., Hodgman, J. E. and Emmanouilides, G. (1980) Cardiogenic shock associated with perinatal asphyxia in preterm infants. *J. Pediatr.*, **961**, 705–710
47. Phibbs, R. H., Clements, J. A., Creary, R. G. *et al.* (1976) Lung maturity, intrauterine growth, neonatal asphyxia and shock and the risk of hyaline membrane disease. *Pediatr. Res.*, **10**, 466 (Abstract)
48. Ment, L. R., Duncan, C. C. and Ehrencranz, R. A. (1987) Intraventricular hemorrhage of the preterm neonate. *Sem. Perinatol.*, **11**, 132–141
49. Ment, L. P., Duncan, C. C., Ehrencranz, R. A. *et al.* (1984) Intraventricular haemorrhage in the preterm neonate: timing and cerebral blood flow changes. *J. Pediatr.*, **104**, 410–425
50. McDonald, M. M., Koops, B. L., Johnson, M. L. *et al.* (1984) Timing and antecedents of intracranial hemorrhage in the newborn. *Pediatrics*, **74**, 32–36
51. Bada, H. S., Korones, S. B., Anderson, G. D., Magill, H. L. and Wong, S. P. (1984) Obstetric factors and relative risk of neonatal germinal layer intraventricular haemorrhage. *Am. J. Obstet. Gynecol.*, **148**, 798–804
52. Meidell, R. Martinelli, P. and Pettet, G. (1985) Perinatal factors associated with early onset intracranial haemorrhage in premature infants. *Am. J. Dis. Child.*, **139**, 160–163
53. Westgren, L. M., Malcus, P. and Svenningsen, N. W. (1986) Intrauterine asphyxia and long term outcome in preterm fetuses. *Obstet. Gynecol.*, **67**, 512–516
54. Szymonowicz, W., Yu., V. Y. H. and Wilson, F. E. (1984) Antecedents of periventricular haemorrhage in infants weighing 1250 g or less at birth. *Arch. Dis. Child.*, **59**, 13–17
55. Low, J. A. Galbraith, R. S., Sauerbrei, F. E. *et al.* (1986) Maternal, fetal and newborn complications associated with newborn intracranial haemorrhage. *Am. J. Obstet. Gynecol.*, **154**, 345–351
56. Dykes, F. D., Lazzara, A. Ahmann, P., Blumenstein, B., Schwartz, J. and Brann, A. W. (1980) Intraventricular haemorrhage. A prospective evaluation of etiopathogenesis. *Pediatrics*, **66**, 42–49
57. Lipscombe, A. P., Thorburn, R. J., Reynolds, E. O. R. *et al.* (1981) Pneumothorax and cerebral haemorrhage in preterm infants. *Lancet*, **i**, 414–416
58. Kenny, J. D., Garcia-Prats, J. A., Hilliard, J. L, Corbet, A. J. S. and Rudolph, A. J. (1978) Hypercarbia at birth – the possible role in the pathogenesis of intraventicular hemorrhage. *Pediatrics*, **62**, 465–467
59. Lou, H. C., Phibbs, R. H., Wilson, S. L. and Gregory, G. A. (1982) Hyperventilation at birth may prevent early periventricular haemorrhage. *Lancet*, **i**, 1047
60. Roberton, N. R. C. (1986) Resuscitation. In *Textbook of Neonatology* (ed N. R. C. Roberton), Churchill Livingstone, Edinburgh and London, pp. 244–245
61. Robson, E. and Hey, E. (1982) Resuscitation of preterm babies at birth reduces the risk of death from hyaline membrane disease. *Arch. Dis. Child.*, **57**, 184–186
62. Drew, J. H. (1982) Immediate intubation at birth for very-low-birthweight infants. *Am. J. Dis. Child.*, **136**, 207–210
63. Milner, A. D., Vyas, H. and Hopkin, I. E. (1984) Efficacy of face mask resuscitation at birth. *Br. Med. J.*, **289**, 1563–1565
64. Field, D., Milner, A. D. and Hopkin, I. E. (1986) Efficiency of manual resuscitation at birth. *Arch. Dis. Child.*, **61**, 300–302
65. Boon, A. W., Milner, A. D. and Hopkin, I. E. (1979a) Physiological responses of the newborn infant to resuscitation. *Arch. Dis. Child.*, **54**, 492–498
66. Boon, A. W., Milner, A. D. and Hopkin, I. E. (1979b) Lung expansion, tidal exchange and formation of the functional residual capacity during resuscitation of asphyxiated neonates. *J. Pediatr.*, **95**, 1031–1036

67. Milner, A. D. and Vyas, H. (1985) Resuscitation of the newborn. In *Neonatal and Paediatric Respiratory Medicine* (eds A. D. Milner and R. J. Martin), Butterworths, London, pp. 1–16
68. Roberton, N. R. C. (1986) *A Manual of Neonatal Intensive Care*, 2nd edn., Edward Arnold, London, Chapter 8
69. Kelly, M. A. and Finer, N. N. (1984) Nasotracheal intubation in the neonate: physiologic responses and affects of atropine and pancuronium. *J. Pediatr.*, **105**, 303–309
70. McMillan, D. D. Rademaker, A. W. Buchan, K. A., Reid, A., Machin, G. and Sauve, R. S. (1986) Benefits of oral tracheal and nasotracheal intubation in neonates requiring ventilatory assistance. *Pediatrics*, **77**, 39–44
71. Wigglesworth, J. S. and Pape, K. E. (1978). An integrated model for haemorrhage and ischaemic lesions in the newborn brain. *Early Hum. Dev.*, **2**, 179–199

Chapter 6

Ventilator care and respiratory audit

William O. Tarnow-Mordi

The substantial increase in the survival of ELBW infants over the last decade is largely due to improvements in ventilator care and respiratory support [1–6]. Nevertheless, respiratory complications are still common, and often lethal. Currently, about 35–60% of ELBW infants treated with artificial ventilation die, up to a third get pneumothoraces and 20–40% develop chronic lung disease (Table 6.1). Hyaline membrane disease, the commonest respiratory illness, occurs in 55–79% of ELBW infants [3–5] and is closely associated with intraventricular haemorrhage and its consequences [3,4,6]. Because of this, many still question whether it is ethical to persist with intensive respiratory treatment in every case. Effective surfactants [7–9] should bring a welcome reduction in the severity of hyaline membrane disease in ELBW infants, but artificial ventilation and its complications are still likely to remain important. If we are to improve outcome further, rigorous evaluation ought to become a standard part of our management [10]. Few units treat more than 50 ELBW

Table 6.1 Outcome and respiratory complications for ELBW infants 1977–85

Source		*No. infants*	*No. deaths*	*Infants receiving artificial ventilation*				
				No.	*Hyaline membrane disease (%)*	*Pneumo-thorax (%)*	*Chronic lung disease (%)*	*Deaths (%)*
Scotland (SMR 11)[48]	1981–85	719	465 (65%)	414	—	15	—	57
Queen Victoria Medical Centre, Melbourne[3]	1977–84	249	—	230	55	20	20	48
John Radcliffe Hospital, Oxford[b]	1981–85	120	52 (43%)	100	70	29	43	37
Addenbrooke's Hospital, Cambridge[6]	1980–83	—	—	59[a]	100	36	—	37

[a]Only artificially ventilated ELBW infants with hyaline membrane disease were reported. [b]unpublished data

infants each year, so multicentre cooperation will become increasingly helpful, both to identify useful therapies and to test and monitor their widespread use.

Because of the difficulties of obtaining detailed information on adequate numbers of ELBW infants, published reports on their respiratory management are sparse. This chapter will review current practice and outline the scope for cooperative respiratory audit in this vulnerable population.

Equipment

A blood gas analyser should be constantly available in the neonatal unit, with 24 h technical support. Most neonatologists now use pressure-limited, time-cycled ventilators which deliver positive end expiratory pressure (PEEP) with continuous gas flow. These are preferable to earlier intermittent flow ventilators which stopped gas flow during their expiratory phase so preventing a significant contribution to gas exchange by the baby's own respiratory effort. Volume preset ventilators like the Servo 900B also provide no gas flow during their expiratory phase, and are rarely used for ELBW infants in the UK. Accurate measurements and careful records of gas flow rate, peak inspiratory pressure (PIP), PEEP, mean airway pressure (MAP), ventilator rate, inspiratory and expiratory time or inspiratory:expiratory ratio, and inspired gas temperature are important aspects of artificial ventilation. Most neonatal ventilators are fitted with cheap needle gauge manometers designed for measurement of static pressure, which are often inaccurate, particularly at ventilator respiratory rates $\geqslant$60/min. Electronic airway pressure monitors are considerably more reliable and therefore safer, but more expensive.

Heated respiratory humidifiers are essential. To minimize the risk of thermal injury they must have a thermal cut-out device complying with BS 5724 [11]. The range of gas flow rates used should be tailored to the performance and operating temperature of the type of humidifier in use. Increasing the gas flow rate increases the humidity of inspired gas in some makes of humidifier, but tends to decrease it in others [12]. Disposable neonatal hygroscopic condensers are heat and moisture exchangers which are attached to the endotracheal tube where they trap exhaled heat and moisture, then give it back to freshly inspired gas [13]. Their benefits and risks, particularly at high flow rates, have not yet been assessed in ELBW infants so they cannot be recommended.

Blood pressure transducer systems connected to an umbilical artery catheter or peripheral artery cannula provide the most accurate measurements of arterial blood pressure, a very important adjunct to respiratory care. A cold light source is an important aid to prompt diagnosis of pneumothorax by transillumination of the chest.

Transcutaneous oxygen monitors use oxygen-sensitive electrodes which heat the skin to 'arterialize' the capillary circulation. They are a useful supplement to arterial or capillary blood gas analysis, and provide continuous data. They are unreliable when compressed over a rib or in severe shock, when capillary blood flow is severely reduced (and the risk of severe skin burns correspondingly increased). Oxygen saturation monitors provide continuous non-invasive data on haemoglobin saturation without heating the skin. Transcutaneous carbon dioxide electrodes and indwelling umbilical arterial oxygen electrodes are also available and indwelling fibreoptic umbilical artery catheters can also continuously monitor haemoglobin saturation.

Ventilator management

ELBW infants face several problems in achieving successful respiratory adaptation. These include low total respiratory system compliance [14] and poor respiratory drive [15], leading to stiff, easily collapsable lungs and recurrent apnoea. Nevertheless there is significant variation in the range and severity of respiratory illness. Up to 45% of ELBW infants receiving artificial ventilation do not have hyaline membrane disease (HMD) (Table 6.2) which itself varies considerably in severity. In 19 artificially ventilated ELBW infants in whom single breath lung mechanics were measured using a passive expiratory flow technique [14,16], values for total respiratory system compliance ranged widely from 0.5–1.6 ml/cmH_2O/m in those with HMD and from 1.7–3.6 ml/cmH_2O/m in those without lung disease (R. A. Wilkie and M. H. Bryan, unpublished data). Some of the controversy about ventilator management stems from the fact that appropriate settings for any baby depend on both the respiratory diagnosis and severity of illness [17].

Table 6.2 Primary respiratory diagnoses in 55 ELBW infants

Diagnosis	*Percentage*
Hyaline membrane disease	55
Apnoea of prematurity	30
Pneumonia	9
Respiratory depression due to birth asphyxia	6

Data from Queen Victoria Medical Centre, Melbourne [3]

The aim of intermittent positive pressure ventilation (IPPV) is to achieve sufficient lung volume and alveolar ventilation to maintain adequate gas exchange, minimizing the risk of:

(1) overdistension of parts of the lung, leading to rupture and air leak;
(2) damage to lung parenchyma and peripheral airways, causing chronic lung disease; and
(3) compression of the pulmonary vessels, causing increased pulmonary vascular resistance with extrapulmonary right-to-left shunting, hypoxia and acidosis.

Ventilator settings should be adjusted to take account of this, guided by the clinical signs (especially the movement of the chest wall), frequent blood gas estimations (supplemented if possible by continuous monitoring of $P\text{O}_2$, $P\text{CO}_2$ or oxygen saturation), the chest X-ray appearances and accurate measurements of systemic blood pressure.

Indications for artificial ventilation

These vary considerably. Most ELBW infants are resuscitated at birth by endotracheal intubation with manual inflation of the lungs. In many, IPPV is begun during transport and continued on admission to the neonatal unit, before blood gas data are available. In Melbourne between 1977 and 1984, 92% of ELBW infants received artificial ventilation [3]. Specific indications [2] were:

(1) Continuous positive airway pressure (CPAP) by single nasal prong or naso-

tracheal tube: increasing severity of HMD with $Pa\text{o}_2 < 60$ mmHg (8 kPa) in $F\text{io}_2 > 60\%$, or apnoea despite theophylline treatment.

(2) IPPV by nasotracheal tube: increasing respiratory distress with $Pa\text{o}_2 < 50$ mmHg (6.7 kPa) in $F\text{io}_2$ 90%, or $Pa\text{co}_2 > 70$ mmHg, or apnoea, gasping and bradycardia. (IPPV was given by nasal prong if peak and end expiratory pressures did not exceed 12/5 cmH_2O.)

Many clinicians would start IPPV or CPAP earlier at lower values of $F\text{io}_2$ and $Pa\text{co}_2$ than these to prevent further deterioration. Of the 55 infants reported by Yu and Hollingsworth [2], CPAP was the sole form of respiratory support in only 1/31 infants with HMD and 2/10 infants with preterm apnoea. Most ELBW infants therefore receive IPPV, whatever their diagnosis.

Recommended blood gas values during artificial ventilation

There are no definitive criteria for optimum blood gas values in ELBW infants. It seems sensible to aim for arterial oxygen tensions of 50–80 mmHg (6.7–10.7 kPa) to avoid the dual risks of hypoxic damage and retrolental fibroplasia. Acidosis and hypercapnia increase cerebral blood flow, which may lead to cerebral haemorrhage in the first three days. Conversely alkalosis and hypocapnia carry a potent risk of cerebral ischaemia [18,19]. In view of this, a reasonable policy is to aim for an arterial pH of 7.25–7.45 and $P\text{co}_2$ between 40 and 55 mmHg (5.3–7.3 kPa). When lung disease is severe and it seems best to avoid very high peak pressures, higher values of $P\text{co}_2$ must be accepted.

A prospective audit to relate blood gas values during the first 72 h to neurological outcome in ELBW infants would be a valuable undertaking [19].

Mild to moderate lung disease

This is seen in the majority of ELBW infants [2] and is also encountered in the recovery phase of severe hyaline membrane disease (see below). Priorities in management are to avoid obstruction of the pulmonary circulation and overinflation or gas trapping while maintaining adequate lung volume. Alterations in blood gases can be made with the same manoeuvres as those outlined below for severe lung disease, but generally lower pressures and gas flow rates of 4–8 l/min are needed.

Severe lung disease with low compliance

This is usually seen in severe hyaline membrane disease. The chest wall expands little despite a peak inspiratory pressure of >25 cmH_2O, mean airway pressure >12 cmH_2O and an inspiratory:expiratory ratio of 1:1 at ventilator rates <40/min. The chest deflates very quickly during expiration. Gas exchange is poor with an oxygen requirement of 80–100% and the chest X-ray shows low volume lung fields with increased density of the lung parenchyma, air bronchograms and partial or complete loss of the cardiac silhouette. The priority in management is to expand the lungs. Mean blood pressure is often <25–30 mmHg, suggesting hypovolaemia with poor systemic and pulmonary perfusion. Correcting this with blood or plasma frequently improves pulmonary perfusion and gas exchange, independently of any changes in ventilator settings.

Manipulations of ventilator settings to alter gas exchange were studied in a group of infants of more than 1000 g birth weight with severe HMD by Reynolds [20,21] using the Bennett PR2 intermittent flow ventilator at 30 breaths/min and an inspiratory:expiratory ratio of 1:1. Nearly all of his findings are applicable to ELBW infants managed on continuous flow ventilators.

Oxygenation

Three manoeuvres each depend on increasing the mean airway pressure (and therefore lung volume). They are to increase:

(a) peak inspiratory pressure;
(b) inspiratory:expiratory ratio; and
(c) positive end expiratory pressure.

Reynolds emphasized that increases in inspiratory:expiratory ratio from 1:1 to 2:1 could often improve oxygenation without the need for increasing peak inspiratory pressure. He also noted that oxygenation deteriorated at ventilator rates of 60–80/min and an inspiratory:expiratory ratio of 1:2. This is because mean airway pressure and lung volume fell markedly with the Bennet PR2 ventilator at those settings. Modern ventilators maintain mean airway pressure at rates of ≥60/min much better than the Bennett PR2, although some require substantial increases in gas flow to do it. Greenough *et al.* [22] showed an *increase* in oxygenation, keeping inspiratory:expiratory ratio at 1:1 or 1:1.2 and maintaining mean airway pressure by adjusting gas flow rate, at a rate of 120/min compared with rates of 30–60/min. This improvement in oxygenation was only seen in non-paralysed babies and was attributed to their synchronous breathing with the ventilator at a rate which approximates to their own intrinsic breathing frequency. This study used Bourns BP 200 and Sechrist IV 100B ventilators in infants of 25–33 weeks gestation with varying severities of hyaline membrane disease [22]. No study has compared slow versus rapid rates solely in ELBW infants with hyaline membrane disease of defined severity.

Carbon dioxide tension

Reynolds showed that arterial $P\text{CO}_2$ was reduced by:

(a) increasing the peak/end expiratory pressure difference; and
(b) increasing the respiratory rate up to 40/min.

These manoeuvres increase alveolar ventilation and are effective with modern ventilators in ELBW infants. An advantage of using respiratory rates ≥60/min is that hypercapnia is often controlled without the need to increase peak pressure, provided tidal volume is adequate.

Synchronous ventilation

Achieving a ventilator frequency which is synchronous with the baby's own breathing pattern may have several advantages. It may obviate the need for paralysis, thus preserving the baby's own contribution to gas exchange and avoiding the risk of hypotension. It may also reduce variability in cerebral blood flow velocity, possibly reducing the risk of adverse cerebrovascular events [23]. Several authors have reported improvements in gas exchange using various techniques for achieving synchrony [24–26], but more systematic studies are needed of both the indications and outcome in comparison with conventional techniques.

Specific recommendations have recently been advanced for management of babies of less than 31 weeks gestation with hyaline membrane disease using synchronous ventilation at rates of 60–120/min and inspiratory:expiratory ratios of 1:1 or 1:1.2 [27].

Weaning

There are few data on which to base recommendations for weaning ELBW infants from artificial ventilation. In larger infants with hyaline membrane disease a spontaneous diuresis begins between 24 and 36 h of age and is followed by a rapid increase in functional residual capacity and lung compliance between 36 and 72 h of age [28]. As lung function improves, the expiratory time constant of the lung increases [17] so a longer fraction of the respiratory cycle is needed for deflation. Hyaline membrane disease is likely to follow a similar course in ELBW infants so weaning should reflect these changes. Initially ventilator pressures and rates are decreased, then the inspiratory:expiratory ratio and gas flow rate are reduced, if they were increased during the acute phase. Greenough *et al.* have recently demonstrated a significantly shortened weaning period in babies of 24–32 weeks gestation randomized to a short inspiratory time of 0.5 s versus those treated with a long inspiratory time of 1.0 s [29].

Resistance to expiratory flow is inversely related to the size of endotracheal tube. Infants with a 3.0 mm internal diameter tube have a 15% reduction in respiratory system resistance compared to those with a 2.5 mm tube (R. A. Wilkie and M. H. Bryan, unpublished data). A larger tube may therefore help weaning. Deciding when to extubate the baby is essentially guesswork, based on the baby's respiratory effort and changes in blood gases during a period of slow rate IPPV, or endotracheal CPAP. Drugs such as theophylline and aminophylline are used to assist weaning (although evidence of their efficacy is confined to babies of more than 1000 g birth weight [30]). The risk of chronic lung disease in ELBW infants who remain intubated is high, even if they had no initial lung disease, so it is wise to attempt weaning early. After extubation, additional support with IPPV by mask (limiting PEEP to 12/5 cmH_2O [ref. 2]), or by CPAP with mask or nasopharyngeal tube is probably very useful, but has not been examined critically in ELBW infants.

Humidification, tracheal lavage, suction and physiotherapy

Although of great importance, these have been little studied. During normal breathing air attains a humidity of $\geqslant 32\ mgH_2O/l$ in the adult trachea. Figure 6.1 shows that this can only be achieved above 31°C (unless the gas is supersaturated). During endotracheal intubation the nasopharyngeal mucosa is bypassed. Grossly inadequate humidity causes depression of mucociliary clearance [31], with increased viscidity of secretions [32]. In larger babies, inspired gas humidity below 31 mgH_2O/l is associated with a ten-fold increase in the risk of blocked endotracheal tubes, from 1/600 to 1/60 ventilator hours [33]. Because their airways are narrower, ELBW infants are probably at even greater risk. The British Standard recommends a minimum of 33 mgH_2O/l inspired gas humidity for adults [34], but many babies receive less than this [12,35].

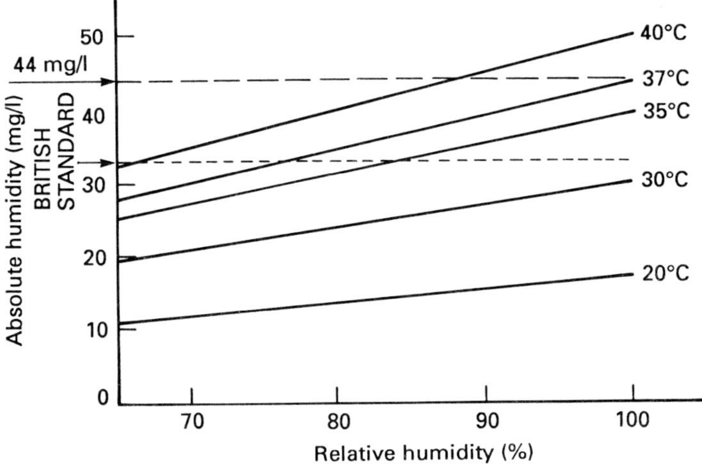

Figure 6.1 Relationship between absolute and relative humidity in water vapour at 760 mmHg

Table 6.3 Inspired gas temperature and ventilator settings in the first 96 hours and respiratory complications in ELBW infants who received artificial ventilation at the John Radcliffe Hospital, 1983–86[49]

	Inspired gas temperature in first 96 h		*Statistical significance*
	<36.5°C	*>36.5°C*	
Number of readings	456	875	
Average value for each patient[a]			
range (°C)	31.2–36.5	36.5–37.6	
mean (°C)	34.9 (1.6)	36.8 (0.4)	
Number of patients	19	27	
Birth weight (g)	788 (150)	814 (142)	NS (unpaired *t* test)
Gestation (weeks)	26.8 (1.9)	27.0 (2.2)	NS
Ventilator rate/min	44 (12)	48 (15)	NS
Peak pressure (cmH_2O)	20.3 (5.7)	20.4 (6.3)	NS
End expiratory pressure (cmH_2O)	3.7 (0.6)	3.8 (0.5)	NS
Flow rate (l/min)	6.5 (1.4)	6.3 (1.2)	NS
Air leak[b] (%)	8 (42%)	2 (7%)	
No air leak	11 (58%)	25 (93%)	$P=0.014$, $\chi^2=5.98$
Fio_2 at 29 days in survivors (%)	53 (28)	34 (11)	$P<0.001$ (t test)

[a] For each patient the average value was calculated of all readings of inspired gas temperature in the first 96 h. The range and mean of these average values was then expressed for each group.
[b] Pneumothorax and pneumomediastinum.
Figures in parentheses give standard deviations.

Among 46 ELBW infants artificially ventilated at the John Radcliffe Hospital, there was a six-fold increase in the relative risk of air leak for those managed with a mean inspired gas temperature of <36.5 °C versus >36.5 °C ($P<0.015$) and an increase in the severity of chronic oxygen dependency at 29 days ($P<0.001$) (Table 6.3). The slightly cooler gas with lower humidity might have caused depression of mucociliary clearance, leading to increased peripheral airway obstruction gas trapping with air leak and chronic lung disease. Pneumothorax and chronic lung disease may therefore be associated with inadequate inspired gas humidity. Pneumothorax is also strongly associated with two patterns of spontaneous breathing:

EXTREMELY LOW BIRTHWEIGHT INFANT: RESPIRATORY AUDIT FORM

1. BABY SURNAME/S ______________________ 2. HOSPITAL: ______________________

3. HOSPITAL NO. __________________ (or enter a study number if anonymity preferred)

4. DATE OF BIRTH: ________ 5. TIME OF BIRTH (24 h clock): ________________

6. INBORN [ ] or OUTBORN [ ] 7. MALE [ ] or FEMALE [ ] 8. BWT__________ G

9. GESTATION (completed weeks): _______________10. PRESENTATION: VERTEX [ ] or BREECH [ ] or OTHER [ ] 11. DELIVERY: VAGINAL [ ] or CAESAREAN [ ]

11. APGAR AT 5 MINS: _______________12. AGE WHEN FIRST HAD CPAP/IPPV/IMV BY ET TUBE WITH MECHANICAL VENTILATOR: DAYS____________ HRS_____________
(if never had ET Tube CPAP/IPPV/IMV by ventilator, write N)

13. PLEASE ENTER ALL BLOOD GASES TAKEN DURING FIRST 12 HOURS OF LIFE:

Time (24 h)												
Age (h)												
PIP (cmH_2O)												
PEEP (cmH_2O)												
MAP* (cmH_2O)												
Rate/min												
I:E ratio												
Flow l/min												
Airway temp												
Site A = Art V = Ven C = Cap												
$F\text{iO}_2$												
pH												
$P\text{co}_2$ (kPa/mmHg)**												
$P\text{o}_2^{\dagger}$ (kPa/mmHg)**												
Base excess												

* Mean Airway Pressure – if measured. ** Delete as appropriate PLEASE TURN OVER

† Only arterial or transcutaneous values, please

14. PRIOR TO IPPV OR IMV BY ET TUBE, WAS ANY OF THESE TREATMENTS GIVEN:

ET BY CPAP [ ] MASK CPAP/IMV/IPPV [ ] NASAL PRONG/S [ ] ?

15. MANAGEMENT DURING THE FIRST 72 HOURS OF LIFE:

TYPE OF VENTILATOR __________ TYPE OF HUMIDIFIER ______________________________

	MAXIMUM	MINIMUM
PIP (cmH_2O)		
PEEP (cmH_2O)		
MAP (cmH_2O)		
Rate/min		
I:E ratio		
Flow l/min		
Airway temp		
$F\text{IO}_2$		
pH		
$P\text{CO}_2$		
$P\text{O}_2$		

16. REASONS FOR MECHANICAL VENTILATION: TICK MORE THAN ONE IF NECESSARY

HMD [ ] Birth Asphyxia [ ] Apnoea [ ] Spontaneous Air Leak [ ]
Pneumonia [ ] Septicaemia [ ] Persistent fetal circulation [ ]
Meconium Aspiration [ ] Other (please specify):

17. DRUGS: MARK BOXES IF GIVEN PANCURONIUM [ ]
SURFACTANT [ ] or METHYLXANTHINE [ ] or DEXAMETHASONE [ ]

18. WEANING: AGE IN DAYS AND HOURS WHEN WEANING FIRST ATTEMPTED BY:

ET TUBE CPAP_____ _____ MASK _____ _____ NASAL PRONG/S_____ _____
(Complete more than one if necessary. If none of these were given for weaning write N):

19. OUTCOMES: WRITE AGE IN COMPLETED DAYS AT EACH OUTCOME
(If outcome never occurred, write N):

First Pn'thorax [ ]; Pn'mediastinum [ ]; Pulm Int Emphysema* [ ]
Final extubation [ ]; Finally O_2 independent [ ]; Death [ ]
*(Campbell R, *AJR*, 1970; 110:447)

PERSON COMPLETING AUDIT: Time Taken ______________ mins.

Figure 6.2 Respiratory audit form for ELBW babies

(a) active expiration during ventilator inflation with cessation or reversal of gas flow [36]; and
(b) summation of inspiration within ± 0.2 s of ventilator inflation [37].

Further studies are needed to show whether these breathing patterns and the risk of air leak are reduced in ELBW infants when inspired gas humidity remains in a certain range. Inspired gas temperature should be part of respiratory audit.

Tracheal lavage and suction is usually performed at 2–4-hourly intervals in intubated ELBW infants, with instillations of 0.2–0.5 ml of normal saline and is often preceded by chest physiotherapy [38]. Chest physiotherapy is usually started after 48 h of life and repeated 4–8-hourly [2]. In two ELBW infants studied by Etches and Scott, chest physiotherapy consistently increased the weight of secretions obtained on suction by 10–1600 mg [38]. Significant reductions in total respiratory system resistance have been shown after removal of tracheal secretions by suction and lavage [39]. However, these benefits of tracheal lavage, suction and physiotherapy must be balanced against the risks of hypoxia [40], bradycardia [41], bacteraemia [42] and even fatal bronchopleural fistula following perforation of the lung [43]. The need to perform these procedures routinely has been questioned [38–40], particularly during the first 48 h of life when secretions are scant. More work is needed to define the place of these routine practices in the care of ELBW infants.

Current respiratory humidifiers are of widely varying efficacy [12,35]. Until the safest levels of inspired gas humidity have been defined, it seems reasonable to recommend that temperatures and gas flow rates which produce inspired gas humidity of 30 mgH_2O/l or less should never be used [33].

Respiratory audit in ELBW infants

Cooperative study seems a promising source of further advances in the care of ELBW infants. Associations between treatment variables and outcomes could be tested on a large scale, as part of routine management. This chapter has outlined a number of hypotheses which could be examined by prospective audit or randomized controlled trials. Doctors and nurses who care for the newborn are busy people! If respiratory audit is to be feasible, the information recorded should be reasonably brief and easy to extract from clinical records.

Figure 6.2 illustrates an audit form for ELBW infants which can be completed in 15–30 min from suitably kept records. It is designed to investigate in a large population of ELBW infants receiving ventilatory assistance the relative association of:

(1) Air leak.
(2) Chronic lung disease, and
(3) Death
with:

(a) intrinsic severity of disease: e.g. mean pressure–shunt product in first 12 h [44];
(b) ventilator variables: rate, pressure, I:E ratio, flow rate;
(c) early nasal CPAP [45];
(d) type of ventilator [22];

(e) type of humidifier;
(f) mean inspired gas temperature;
(g) type of surfactant treatment [8,9];
(h) pancuronium treatment [45];
(i) methylxanthine treatment [30].

Once completed the audit form is sent to a coordinating centre for data entry and analysis. The relationship between the three outcome measures and the management variables can be analysed with multiple regression techniques using logistic interactive modelling [46]. Agreed definitions for audit purposes are:

Disease severity: the pressure–shunt product is a quantitative measure of disease severity, obtained by multiplying the mean airway pressure by the calculated right-to-left shunt (MAP × QS/QT) for each blood gas determination during the first 12 h [44]. The pressure–shunt product is automatically calculated by computer for all respiratory illnesses from the audit form.

Hyaline membrane disease: this has been defined by Yu and Hollingsworth [2] in ELBW infants as respiratory distress not due to other causes with:

(a) chest wall retractions;
(b) diffuse granular infiltrates on chest X-ray lasting at least 48 h;
(c) $F\text{io}_2 \geqslant 30\%$ to keep $P\text{ao}_2 > 60$ mmHg (8 kPa) before 12 h and for at least 72 h; and
(d) maximum $F\text{io}_2$ requirement $\geqslant 40\%$ [2].

Birth asphyxia: an Apgar score of 6 or less at 5 min of age, or an arterial or capillary blood gas showing a base deficit of >4.5 mmol/l within the first hour of birth.

Pneumonia: suggestive shadowing on chest X-ray, persisting at least 48 h, with an organism cultured from tracheal secretions or blood which needed antibiotics.

Pulmonary interstitial emphysema: defined according to Campbell [47].

References

1. Stewart, A. L., Reynolds, E. O. R. and Lipscomb, A. P. (1981) Outcome for infants of very low birthweight: survey of the world literature. *Lancet*, **i**, 1038–1041
2. Yu, V. Y. H. and Hollingsworth, E. (1979) Respiratory failure in infants weighing 1000 g or less at birth. *Aust. Paediatr. J.*, **15**, 152–159
3. Yu, V. Y. H., Wong, P. Y., Bajuk, B. and Szymonowicz, W. (1986) Pulmonary air leak in extremely low birthweight infants. *Arch. Dis. Child.*, **61**, 239–241
4. Yu, V. Y. H., Downe, L., Astbury, J. and Bajuk, B. (1986) Perinatal factors and adverse outcome in extremely low birthweight infants. *Arch. Dis. Child.*, **61**, 554–558
5. Kraybill, E. N., Kennedy, C. A., Teplin, S. W. and Campbell, S. K. (1984) Infants with birthweight less than 1001 grams. *Am. J. Dis. Child.*, **138**, 837–842
6. Greenough, A. and Roberton, N. R. C. (1985) Morbidity and survival in neonates ventilated for the respiratory distress syndrome. *Br. Med. J.*, **290**, 597–600
7. Hallman, M., Merritt, T. A., Jarvenpaa, A-L. *et al.* (1985) Exogenous human surfactant for treatment of severe respiratory distress syndrome: a randomized prospective clinical trial. *J. Pediatr.*, **71**, 473–482
8. Raju, T. N. K., Vidyasagar, D., Bhat, R. *et al.* (1987) Double-blind controlled trial of single-dose treatment with bovine surfactant in severe hyaline membrane disease. *Lancet*, **i**, 651–656
9. Ten Centre Study Group (1987) Ten centre trial of artificial surfactant (artificial lung expanding compound) in very premature babies. *Br. Med. J.*, **294**, 991–996

10. Tarnow-Mordi, W. O. and Wilkinson, A. R. (1986) Mechanical ventilation of the newborn. *Br. Med. J.*, **292**, 575–576
11. British Standards Institution. Specifications for safety of medical electrical equipment. Part 1. General requirements (BS 5724), London, British Standards Institution
12. Tarnow-Mordi, W. O., Sutton, P. and Wilkinson, A. R. (1986) Inadequate humidification of respiratory gases during mechanical ventilation of the newborn. *Arch. Dis. Child.*, **61**, 698–700
13. Gedeon, A., Mebius, C. and Palmer, K. (1987) Neonatal hygroscopic condenser humidifier. *Crit. Care Med.*, **15**, 51–54
14. Wilkie, R. A., and Bryan, M. H. (1987) The effect of nebulised bronchodilators on compliance in ventilated infants with chronic lung disease. *J. Pediatr.*, **111**, 278–282
15. Henderson-Smart, D. J., Pettigrew, A. G. and Campbell, D. J. (1983) Clinical apnea and brainstem neural function in preterm infants. *N. Engl. J. Med.*, **308**, 353–357
16. Le Souef, P. N., England, S. J. and Bryan, A. C. (1984) Passive respiratory mechanics in newborns and children. *Am. Rev. Resp. Dis.*, **129**, 552–556
17. Ramsden, C. A., Reynolds, E. O. R., Morley, C., South, M. and Milner, A. D. (1987) Ventilator settings for newborn infants. *Arch. Dis. Child.*, **62**, 529–538
18. Tarnow–Mordi, W. O. (1982) Hyperventilation at birth may prevent early periventricular haemorrhage. *Lancet*, **ii**, 212
19. Greisen, G., Munck, H. and Lou, H. (1986) May hypocarbia cause ischaemic brain damage in the preterm infant? *Lancet*, **ii**, 460
20. Herman, S. and Reynolds, E. O. R. (1973) Methods for improving oxygenation in infants mechanically ventilated for severe hyaline membrane disease. *Arch. Dis. Child.*, **46**, 612–617
21. Reynolds, E. O. R. (1979) Ventilator therapy. In *Neonatal Pulmonary Care* (eds D. W. Thibeault and G. A. Gregory), Addison Wesley, Menlo Park, California, pp. 217–236
22. Greenough, A., Greenall, F., Pool, J., Morley, C. and Gamsu, H. (1987) Comparison of different rates of artificial ventilation in preterm infants with respiratory distress syndrome. *Acta Paediatr. Scand.*, **76**, 706–712
23. Rennie, J. M., South, M. and Morley, C. J. (1987) Cerebral blood flow velocity variability in infants receiving assisted ventilation. *Arch. Dis. Child.*, **62**, 1247–1251
24. Greenough, A. and Greenall, F. (1988) Observation of spontaneous respiratory interaction with artificial ventilation. *Arch. Dis. Child.*, **63**, 168–171
25. Mehta, A., Wright, B. M., Callan, K. and Stacey, T. E. (1986) Patient-triggered ventilation in the newborn. *Lancet*, **i**, 17–19
26. South, M. and Morley, C. J. (1986) Synchronous mechanical ventilation of the neonate. *Arch. Dis. Child.*, **61**, 1190–1195
27. Greenough, A. and Milner, A. D. (1987) High frequency ventilation in the neonatal period. *Eur. J. Pediatr.*, **146**, 446–449
28. Heaf, D. P., Belik, J., Spitzer, A. R., Gewitz, M. H. and Fox, W. W. (1982) Changes in pulmonary function during the diuretic phase of respiratory distress syndrome. *J. Paediatr.*, **101**, 103–107
29. Greenough, A., Pool, J. and Gamsu, H. (1988) Weaning from high frequency positive pressure ventilation. *Proceedings of the Neonatal Society*, London, February 1988, pp. 1–2
30. Greenough, A., Elias–Jones, J. Pool, J., Morley, C. J. and Davis, J. A. (1985) The therapeutic actions of theophylline in preterm ventilated infants. *Early Hum. Dev.*, **12**, 15–22
31. Forbes, A. R. (1973) Humidification and mucus flow in the intubated trachea. *Br. J. Anaesth.*, **45**, 874–878
32. Burton, J. D. K. (1962) Effects of dry anaesthetic gases on the respiratory mucus membrane. *Lancet*, **i**, 235–238
33. Lomholt, N., Cooke, R. and Lunding, M. (1968) A method of humidification in ventilator treatment of neonates. *Br. J. Anaesth.*, **40**, 335–339
34. British Standards Institution (1970) Specifications for humidifiers for use with breathing machines (BS 4494), London, British Standards Institution
35. Tarnow–Mordi, W. O., Fletcher, M., Sutton, P. and Wilkinson, A. R. (1986) Evidence of inadequate humidification of inspired gas during artificial ventilation of newborn infants in the British Isles. *Lancet*, **ii**, 909–910
36. Greenough, A., Wood, S., Morley, C. J. and Davis, J. A. (1984) Pancuronium prevents pneumo-

thoraces in ventilated premature infants who actively expire against positive pressure inflation. *Lancet*, **i**, 1–4

37. Greenough, A., Morley, C. J. and Johnston, P. (1986) An active expiratory reflex in preterm ventilated infants. In *The Physiological Development of the Fetus and Newborn* (eds C. T. Jones and P. W. Nathaniels), Academic Press, London, pp. 259–262
38. Etches, P. C. and Scott, B. (1978) Chest physiotherapy in the newborn: effect on secretions removed. *Pediatrics*, **62**, 713–715
39. Prendiville, A., Thomson, A. and Silverman, M. (1986) Effect of tracheobronchial suction on respiratory resistance in intubated preterm babies. *Arch. Dis. Child.*, **61**, 1178–1183
40. Simbruner, G., Coradello, H., Fodor, M., Havelec, L., Lubec, G. and Pollak, A. (1981) Effect of tracheal suction on oxygenation, circulation and lung mechanics in newborn infants. *Arch. Dis. Child.*, **56**, 326–330
41. Cordero, L. and Hon, E. H. (1971) Neonatal bradycardia following nasopharyngeal stimulation. *J. Pediatr.*, **78**, 441–447
42. Storm, W. (1980) Transient bacteraemia following endotracheal suctioning in ventilated newborns. *Pediatrics*, **65**, 487–490
43. Alpan, G., Glick, B., Peleg, O., Amit, Y. and Eyal, F. (1984) Pneumothorax due to endotracheal tube suction. *Am. J. Perinatol.*, **1**, 345–348
44. Rojas, J., Green, R. S., Fannon, L. *et al.* (1982) A quantitative model for hyaline membrane disease. *Pediatr. Res.*, **16**, 35–39
45. Avery, M. E., Tooley, W. H., Keller, J. B. *et al.* (1987) Is chronic lung disease preventable? A survey of eight centers. *Pediatrics*, **79**, 26–30
46. Baker, R. J. and Nelder, J. A. (1978) *The GLIM (General Linear Interactive Modelling) System: Release 3*, Numerical Algorithms Group, Oxford
47. Campbell, R. (1970) Interpulmonary interstitial emphysema: a complication of hyaline membrane disease. *AJR*, **110**, 449–456
48. Cole, S. K. (1987) SMR 11, Scottish Health Service Common Services Agency, Edinburgh
49. Tarnow-Mordi, W. O., Reid, E., Griffiths, P. and Wilkinson, A. R. (1989) Low inspired gas temperature and respiratory complications in very low birth weight infants. *J. Paediatr.* (in press)

Chapter 7

Pulmonary air leak

Anne Greenough

Introduction

Pulmonary air leak (PAL) is a common problem in the neonatal period [1,2], frequently complicating the course of preterm infants receiving respiratory support [3,4]. Unfortunately, until this decade only small numbers of ELBW infants survived [5,6] and relatively little data on the incidence of PAL amongst such infants exist, but it appears to be between 20 and 40% if all forms of PAL are included [7–9].

The largest series of 230 infants with birth weight between 500 and 999 g from an eight-year period (1977–1984) reported an incidence of 41% [7], very similar to the 36% incidence amongst 59 infants reported from Cambridge between 1980 and 1983 [8]. More recently, 21% of ELBW infants during a twelve-month period at King's College Hospital developed PAL (A. Greenough, NICU Statistics 1985–86, King's College Hospital).

The most common form of PAL amongst ELBW infants is pulmonary interstitial emphysema (PIE), the incidence varying from 14 to 35% [7,9,10], whereas pneumothorax occurs in 11–20% [7,9]. Other forms of PAL – pneumomediastinum (PM), pneumopericardium – are relatively uncommon (less than 3%) as in other birth weight groups [7].

Madansky *et al.* reported that the incidence of all forms of PAL increased with decreasing gestational age [3]. However, although it is now well recognized that PIE is much more common in the ELBW infant, the effect of maturity on the likelihood of a pneumothorax is a much more open question. Thibeault *et al.* [11] demonstrated a significant difference in the type of PAL according to maturity, with the highest incidence of pneumothorax in term infants and PIE increasingly common with decreasing gestational age. Adler and Wyszogroski [12] also reported a similar association of increased pneumothorax with increased maturity and this was confirmed by evidence from their subsequent animal study [12]. The lungs of rabbit fetuses were inflated after death and the inflating pressures necessary to rupture the lung were found to be significantly higher in the more immature animals. This finding was explained by the lower resistance of the lung at term to rupture due to the reduction in both elastic and surface forces within the lung with increasing maturity.

Two of the most recent clinical studies have shown a very poor relationship between the incidence of pneumothorax and birth weight [7,8] (Table 7.1). In contrast, there is an obvious inverse relationship between the incidence of PIE and birth weight [7,9] (Table 7.1). This is explained by the high connective tissue content of the immature lung [13], as in other species such as the cow which has a high

Table 7.1 Relationship between birth weight and PAL (expressed as a percentage)

	Pneumothorax		*PIE*	
Birth weight (kg)	*Greenough and Roberton*[8]	*Yu* et al.[7]	*Hart* et al.[9]	*Yu* et al.[7]
< 1.0	35	24	42	32
1.0–1.5	35	17	26	22
1.5–2.0	27			

interstitial tissue content, the lung is more susceptible to widespread PIE [14]. Unfortunately this is worsened, as in RDS, by a high interstitial water content which impedes the flow of gas into the perivascular spaces – this then blocks the formation of a PM which is necessary to decompress the interstitial emphysema [15].

Mortality and morbidity

Mortality and morbidity in ELBW infants with PAL is greatly increased; the mortality is high, 47% of infants with PIE and all infants with pneumothorax dying in one series [7] and 53% in another [8]. Mortality associated with PAL decreases with increasing birth weight: 53% with birth weight < 1000 g, 33% with birth weight < 1500 g, and only 8% for infants between 1500 and 2000 g [8]. Low birth weight infants without air leak have significantly higher survival rates [7]. Survival amongst ELBW infants without PAL has improved as shown by one study comparing results in the period 1981–1984 with 1977–1980, but not for infants with PAL [7]. This stresses the need for improvements in both the treatment and, more importantly, the prevention of PAL.

The association of PAL and periventricular haemorrhage (PVH) is well known [16,17]. Among 36 ELBW infants ventilated at King's College Hospital last year, of the eight infants who developed PAL all either died or developed an IVH or both occurred, compared to only 13 of the 28 infants without PAL ($P < 0.02$).

The other important sequel of PAL is an increased incidence of chronic lung disease (CLD) [18]. Two recent studies have confirmed this important association; Escobedo and Gonzalez [19] reported 58% of ELBW infants with CLD had had at least one pneumothorax and Bhat and Zikos-Labropoulou [20] that 35% had had air leak syndrome. Amongst 16 of 107 ELBW infants with bronchopulmonary dysplasia (BPD) reported by Yu *et al.* [21] PIE was a significant perinatal association ($P < 0.0005$) CLD was commoner amongst infants with PAL, 16 of 34 ventilated survivors with PAL in one series developing CLD compared to only 29 of 86 without PAL [21]. As a consequence, among survivors with PAL the median duration of ventilation was 34 days (range 2–115 days) and median duration of treatment with oxygen was 49 days (range 6–243 days) [21].

Aetiology

There have been no studies reported investigating the aetiological associations of PAL exclusively amongst infants with birth weight < 1000 g. From studies of preterm infants, including ELBW babies, four main factors have been incriminated:

(1) Peak inspiratory pressure (PIP).
(2) Positive end expiratory pressure (PEEP).
(3) Inflation time (TI).
(4) Spontaneous respiratory activity.

The association between high PIP and PAL was first reported by Oh and Stern [22] and confirmed more recently by Greenough, Dixon and Roberton [10] (Figure 7.1). Attempts to ventilate the lower peak pressures in one study did not result in a reduction in the incidence of PAL [23], but PIP was documented only just before the air leak and this may not have been a true representation of the PIP used throughout the period of ventilation up to then. Equally important, if PIP is reduced without other compensatory maneouvres to maintain mean airway pressure (MAP), some estimation must be made of the probable increased infant's respiratory effort, as the latter is known to be associated with the development of PAL [24]. Among 36 ELBW infants ventilated at King's College Hospital in the twelve-month period 1985–86, both the mean PIP and MAP were significantly elevated ($P<0.05$ and <0.02 respectively) between birth and air leak compared to the median PIP and MAP during the first week of life of infants without air leak.

The addition of PEEP during ventilation is beneficial; it is a method of improving oxygenation in infants suffering from RDS [25] and can conserve surfactant [26]. Too much, however, or 'inadvertent PEEP' results in air trapping, with reduction in compliance and CO_2 retention [27,28]. In one study the introduction of PEEP during IPPV was associated with an increased incidence of both pneumothorax and BPD [29], but this study was neither randomized nor did it compare two simultaneous time periods.

In a retrospective study comparing ventilator settings of infants with and without air leaks, Primak [30] found that although MAP was higher amongst infants developing PAL, only differences in TI between the two groups reached statistical significance. Two physiological studies have confirmed an association between TI and PAL [31,32]. Both have shown that 'active expiration' (a respiratory pattern significantly associated with PAL [24]) during positive pressure inflation can be reduced in

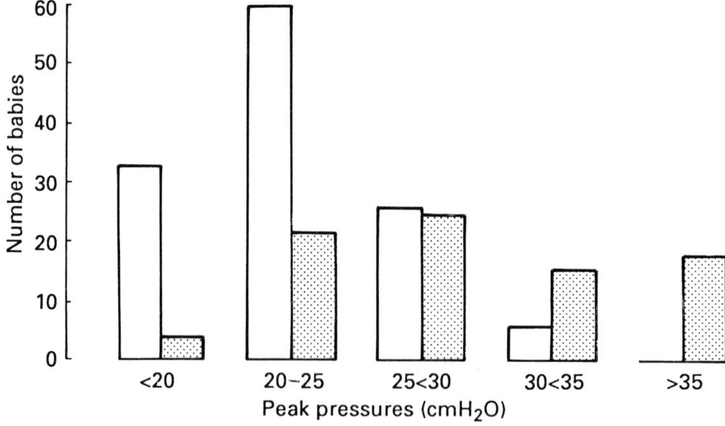

Figure 7.1 Relationship between PIP and development of PAL in infants ventilated for RDS: □ no air leak, ▦, air leak

some infants by increasing ventilator rate or reducing TI alone. More recently we have shown that the duration of the plateau of positive pressure inflation is significantly longer in infants who actively expire [33].

The association of 'fighting the ventilator' clinically observed and the occurrence of PAL has long been recognized [34]. Unfortunately, until recently the nature of such respiratory efforts could not be determined and it had been postulated that the most likely mechanism for alveolar rupture during artificial ventilation would be simultaneous inspiratory efforts with inflation as this would generate the largest transpulmonary pressure swings [35]. However, a detailed study of infants' respiratory efforts during ventilation has demonstrated that the development of PAL seems to relate to expiratory rather than inspiratory efforts during positive pressure inflation [24]. Infants who developed PAL had shown, prior to its development, a consistent respiratory interaction, i.e. they were in expiration during positive pressure inflation and the flow of gas into their lungs was either reduced or in some cases even reversed compared to that which occurred during passive positive pressure inflation. The pattern (reflex) was therefore designated the 'active expiratory reflex'. The reflex occurred in infants with the stiffest lungs and did not seem related to gestational age or birth weight [36]. It did occur in ELBW infants, although such babies with large PVHs tended to be apnoeic during ventilation. This 'expiratory reflex' was provoked if the start of positive pressure inflation occurred during a respiratory window (± 0.2 s) around end-inspiration [36]. Using a square wave pressure waveform such a combination would generate the largest transpulmonary pressure swings, and this may have been the mechanism for production of PAL. The active expiratory reflex which follows inflation of the lungs at end-inspiration may be an alternative mechanism or it may simply be a very reliable marker [37] and hence predictor of infants at high risk of developing this important condition.

Prevention

Two preventative measures have been extensively employed to try and reduce the incidence of PAL – paralysis and high frequency ventilation.

A number of potentially serious problems have been associated with the use of paralysis, e.g. hypoventilation [38], blood pressure abnormalities [39,40], fluid retention and a possible increased incidence of PVH [41]. Until recently, although a variety of beneficial effects such as reduction in IVH [42], reduction in mortality [43], and reduction in CLD [35] had been claimed for this treatment, it had not been associated with a reduction in PAL [35,42,43]. However, selective paralysis, i.e. giving pancuronium only to those infants at high risk of developing air leak, was confirmed in two independent studies [37,44] as an effective method of preventing PAL. Unfortunately, in one of the two studies a statistically significant reduction in PAL occurred only in 'more mature' infants [44] and in the second study the only infant who sustained pneumothorax during paralysis was 24 weeks gestational age (birth weight < 1000 g) [37].

High frequency ventilation (> 60/min) has been used as an alternative method of preventing pneumothoraces. High frequency oscillation and high frequency jet ventilation have not yet been used with this aim, but both methods are already associated with improvements in oxygenation amongst infants with severe air leak unresponsive to conventional ventilation [45,46]. High frequency positive pressure ventilation (HFPPV) using conventional ventilators has been associated with a reduced incidence of PAL in three studies [47–49]. In the study of Heicher, Kastings and Richards [48], rates of 60/min and a TI of 0.5 s was associated with approximately half the incidence of PAL. In a recently reported multi-centre randomized study, similar ventilator settings when compared to slower rates (30/40/min and a longer TI) were associated with a significant reduction in PAL [49]. Even amongst infants with PIE, HFPPV reduces the incidence of pneumothorax [10], although PIE actually worsens on fast rates as in the absence of a pneumothorax or PM the PIE cannot decompress.

The association of a lower incidence of PAL and fast rates may be due to a number of mechanisms. Using certain ventilators an increase in ventilator rates increases MAP [50] and thus PIP and could be lowered without impairing oxygenation and thus barotrauma would be reduced. Increasing ventilator rates in two physiological studies [31,32] has been associated with a reduction in the active expiratory reflex. In a recent study [51] it has been found that among infants breathing during ventilation, fast rates (120/min) were associated with improved oxygenation and a reduction in CO_2 and this was the result of synchronous respiration with ventilation at the increased rate. Investigation of the spontaneous respiratory rate of low birth weight infants with RDS revealed it to be inversely related to gestational age (Figure 7.2) [52]. Thus, among ELBW infants fast rates (> 100/min) mimic their spontaneous respiratory frequency and thus would be most likely to induce synchronous respiration, improving oxygenation and reducing the likelihood of PAL.

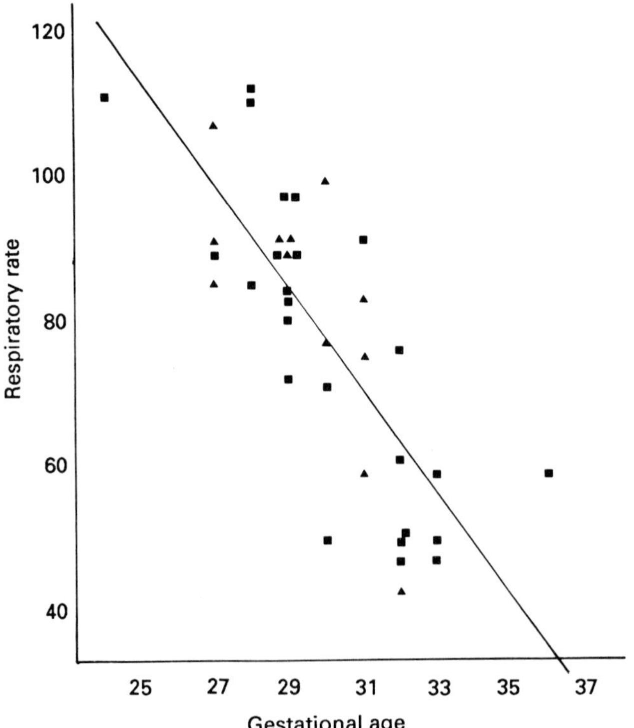

Figure 7.2 Relationship between spontaneous respiratory rate and gestational age in infants ventilated for RDS during first 24 h; ▲, male; ■, female; $r = -0.76$

Conclusion

Pulmonary air leak is a common problem in the infant with birth weight under 1000 g and is an important cause both of mortality and morbidity. Indeed the development of PAL in such infants has much more devastating effects than in any other weight group. An accurate understanding of the aetiology of this condition is hampered by a lack of studies concentrating exclusively on ELBW infants. Trials which have included such infants, however, along with those with birth weight over 1000 g, have demonstrated that barotrauma, either due to artificial ventilation or the infant's respiratory efforts, is important in the development of PAL.

Effective methods of treatment of both pneumothorax and PIE do not differ according to birth weight. Large pneumothoraces should be urgently and adequately drained using under water-sealed drains (with or without suction as necessary) positioned to lay anteriorly in the thoracic cavity [53]. Fast rate ventilation, using either conventional ventilators [10] or newer techniques [45], is beneficial in PIE, improving oxygenation. In severe unilateral PIE selective intubation has been advocated [54] but is particularly difficult in the ELBW infant; however, attention to positioning of the baby with 'good' lung uppermost provides a simple non-invasive method of improving oxygenation [55]. In bilateral severe interstitial emphysema, where oxygenation has proved difficult, treatment by lung puncture has been resorted to successfully [56].

Unfortunately, despite such therapeutic maneouvres, the severe collapse, often associated with the development of PAL in the ELBW infant, will already have resulted in serious long-term complications. Thus the development of more effective preventative methods must be the challenge for neonatologists interested in this condition. Both selective paralysis and HFPPV have had some success in this respect, but perhaps the best way forward would be the introduction of a method of ventilation designed exclusively for the infant with birth weight < 1000 g.

References

1. Ogata, E. S., Gregory, G. A., Kitterman, J. A., Phibbs, R. H. and Tooley, W. H. (1979) Pneumothorax in the respiratory distress syndrome. Incidence and effect on vital signs, blood gases and pH. *Pediatrics*, **58**, 177–182
2. Steele, T. W., Metz, J. R., Bass, J. W. and DuBas, J. J. (1971) Pneumothorax and pneumomediastinum in the newborn. *Pediatr. Radiol*, **98**, 629–632
3. Madansky, D. L., Lawson, E. E., Chernick, V. and Taeusch, H. W. (1979) Pneumothorax and other forms of pulmonary air leak in newborns. *Am. Rev. Resp. Dis.*, **120**, 729–737
4. Yu, V. Y. H., Liew, S. W. and Roberton, N. R. C. (1975) Pneumothorax in the newborn. *Arch. Dis. Child.*, **50**, 449–454
5. Yu, V. Y. H. and Hollingsworth, E. (1980) Improving prognosis for infants weighing 1000 g or less at birth. *Aust. Paediatr. J.*, **15**, 152–159
6. Yu, V. Y. H., Zhao, S. M. and Bajuk, B. (1982) Results of intensive care of 375 very low birth weight infants. *Aust. Paediatr. J.*, **18**, 188–192
7. Yu, V. Y. H., Wong, P. Y., Bajuk, B. and Szymonowicz, W. (1986) Pulmonary air leak in extremely low birth weight infants. *Arch. Dis. Child.*, **61**, 239–241
8. Greenough, A. and Roberton, N. R. C. (1985) Morbidity and survival in neonates ventilated for the respiratory distress syndrome. *Br. Med. J.*, **290**, 597–600
9. Hart, S. M., McNair, M., Gamsu, H. R. and Price, J. F. (1983) Pulmonary interstitial emphysema in very low birth weight infants. *Arch. Dis Child.*, **58**, 612–615

10. Greenough, A., Dixon A. D. and Roberton, N. R. C. (1984) Pulmonary interstitial emphysema. *Arch. Dis. Child.*, **19**, 1046–1051
11. Thibeault, D. W., Lachman, R. S., Laul, V. R. and Kwong, M. S. (1973) Pulmonary interstitial emphysema, pneumomediastinum and pneumothorax occurrence in the newborn period. *Am. J. Dis. Child.*, **126**, 611–614
12. Alder, S. M. and Wyszogroski, I. (1973) Pneumothorax as a function of gestational age: clinical and experimental studies. *J. Pediatr.*, **87**, 771–775
13. Reid, L. and Rubino, L. (1959) The connective tissue septa in the fetal human lung. *Thorax*, **14**, 3–12
14. Reid, L. (1959) The connective tissue septa in the adult human lung. *Thorax*, **14**, 138–150
15. Thibeault, D. W. (1978) Pulmonary barotrauma. In *Neonatal Pulmonary Care* (eds D. W. Thibeault and G. A. Gregory), Addison Wesley, London, pp. 307–317
16. Lipscomb, A. P., Thorburn, R. J., Reynolds, E. O. R. *et al.* (1981) Pneumothorax and cerebral haemorrhage in preterm infants. *Lancet*, **i**, 414–418
17. Hill, A., Periman, J. M. and Volpe, J. J. (1982) Relationship of pneumothorax to occurrence of intraventricular haemorrhage in the premature newborn. *Pediatrics*, **69**, 144–149
18. Stahlman, M. T., Cheatham, W. and Gray, M. E. (1979) The role of air dissection in bronchopulmonary dysplasia. *J. Pediatr.*, **95**, 878–885
19. Escobedo, M. B. and Gonzalez, A. (1986) Bronchopulmonary dysplasia in the tiny infant. *Clin. Perinatol.*, **13**, 315–326
20. Bhat, R. and Zikos-Labropoulou, E. (1986) Resuscitation and respiratory management of infants weighing less than 1000 g. *Clin. Perinatol.*, **13**, 285–297
21. Yu, V. Y. H., Orgill, A. A., Lim, S. B., Bajuk, B. and Astbury, J. (1983) Bronchopulmonary dysplasia in very low birth weight infants. *Aust. Paediatr. J.*, **19**, 233–236
22. Oh, W. and Stern, L. (1977) Diseases of the respiratory system. In *Neonatal and Perinatal Medicine: Diseases of the Fetus and Infant* (ed. R. E. Behrman), C. V. Mosby, St. Louis, p. 558
23. Tarnow-Mordi, W. O., Narang, A. and Wilkinson, A. R. (1985) Lack of association of barotrauma and airleak in hyaline membrane disease. *Arch. Dis. Child.*, **60**, 555–560
24. Greenough, A., Morley, C. J. and Davis, J. A. (1983) The interaction of the infant's spontaneous respiration with ventilation. *J. Pediatr.*, **103**, 769–773
25. Cumavasamy, N., Nussli, R., Vischer, D., Dangel, P. and Duc, G. (1973) Artificial ventilation in hyaline membrane disease. The use of positive end expiratory pressure and continuous positive airways pressure. *Pediatrics*, **51**, 629–653
26. Wyszogrodski, I., Kyeboagye, K. and Taeusch, H. W. (1975) Surfactant inactivation by hyperventilation, conservation at end-expiratory pressure. *J. Appl. Physiol.*, **38**, 461–464
27. Simburner, G. (1986) Inadvertent positive end expiratory pressure in mechanically ventilated infants. Detection and effect on lung mechanics and gas exchange. *J. Pediatr.*, **108**, 589–595
28. Pepe, P. E. and Marini, J. J. (1982) Occult positive end expiratory pressure in mechanically ventilated patients with airflow obstruction. *Am. Rev. Resp. Dis.*, **126**, 166–170
29. Berg, T. J., Pagtakhan, R. D., Reed, M. H., Langston, C. and Cherick, V. (1975) Bronchopulmonary dysplasia and lung rupture in hyaline membrane disease. Influence of continuous distending pressure. *Pediatrics*, **55**, 51–55
30. Primak, R. A. (1983) Factors associated with pulmonary air leak in premature infants receiving mechanical ventilation. *J. Pediatr.*, **102**, 764–769
31. Field, D. J., Milner, A. D. and Hopkin, I. E. (1985) Manipulation of ventilator settings to prevent active expiration against positive pressure ventilation. *Arch. Dis. Child.*, **60**, 1036–1040
32. Greenough, A., Morley, C. J. and Pool, J. (1986) Fighting the ventilator – are fast rates an effective alternative to paralysis? *Early Hum. Dev.*, **13**, 189–194
33. Greenough, A., (1988) The premature infant's response to mechanical ventilation. *Early Human Development*, **17**, 1–5
34. Stark, A. R., Bascomb, R. and Frantz, I. D. (1979) Muscle relaxation in mechanically ventilated infants. *J. Pediatr.*, **94**, 439–443
35. Pollitzer, M. J., Reynolds, E. O. R., Shaw, D. G. and Thomas, R. M. (1981) Pancuronium during mechanical ventilation speeds recovery of the lungs with hyaline membrane disease. *Lancet*, **i**, 346–348
36. Greenough, A., Morley, C. J. and Johnson, P. (1985) An active expiratory reflex in preterm ventilated infants. In *The Physiological Development of the Fetus and Newborn* (eds C. T. Jones and P. W. Nathanielsz), Academic Press, New York pp. 259–263

37. Greenough A., Wood, S., Morley, C. J. and Davis, J. A. (1984) Pancuronium prevents pneumothoraces in ventilated premature babies who actively expire against positive pressure inflation. *Lancet*, **i**, 1–4
38. Bourgeois, J., Beithler, J. C., Cottancin, G., Milan, J. J. and Bethenod, M. (1982) Dangers de la caransation au cours de la ventilation artificielle chez le nouveau-né. *Pediatrie*, **37**, 101–112
39. Driscoll, D. J., Fukushige, J., Hartley, C., Lewis, R. M. and Entman, M. L. (1975) Hemodynamic effects of pancuronium in chronically instrumented dogs. *Crit. Care Med.*, **10**, 41–45
40. Cabal, L. A., Siassi, B., Artal, R., Gonzalez, F., Hodgman, J. and Plajstek, C. (1985) Cardiovascular and catecholamine neonates. *Pediatrics*, **75**, 284–287
41. Bancalari, E., Gerhardt, T., Feller, R. *et al.* (1980) Muscle relaxation during IPPV in prematures with RDS. *Pediatr. Res.*, **14**, 590
42. Perlman, J. M., McMenamin, J. B. and Volpe, J. J. (1983) Fluctuating cerebral blood flow velocity in respiratory distress syndrome. *N. Engl. J. Med.*, **309**, 204–208
43. Henry, G. W., Stevens, D. C., Schreier, R. L., Grosfield, J. L. and Ballantine, T. V. N. (1979) Respiratory paralysis to improve oxygenation and mortality in large newborn infants with respiratory distress. *J. Pediatr. Surg.*, **94**, 481–487
44. Cooke, R. W. I. and Rennie, J. M. (1984) Pancuronium and pneumothorax. *Lancet*, **i**, 286–287
45. Frantz, I. D., Stark, A. R. and Westhammer, J. (1981) Improvement in pulmonary interstitial emphysema in high frequency ventilation. *Pediatr. Res.*, **15**, 719
46. Ng, K. P. K. and Easa, D. (1979) Management of interstitial emphysema by high frequency low pressure ventilation in the neonate. *J. Pediatr.*, **95**, 117–118
47. Bland, R. D., Kim, M. H. and Light, M. J. (1980) High frequency mechanical ventilation in severe hyaline membrane disease: an alternative therapy? *Crit. Care Med.*, **8**, 275–280
48. Heicher, D. A., Kastings, D. S. and Richards, J. R. (1981) Prospective clinical comparison of two methods for mechanical ventilation of neonates: rapid rates and short inspiratory times versus slow rate and long inspiratory time. *J. Pediatr.*, **98**, 957–961
49. Pohlandt, F., Bernsau, V., Feilen, K. D. *et al.* (1985) Reduction of barotrauma in ventilated neonates by increase in ventilation frequency. First results of a prospective collaborative and randomised trial of two different ventilator techniques. *Pediatr. Res.*, **19**, 1077 (abstract)
50. Boros, S. J., Bing, D. R. and Mammel, M. C. (1984) Using conventional infant ventilators at unconventional rates. *Pediatrics*, **74**, 487–492
51. Greenough, A., Pool, J., Greenall, F., Morley, C. and Gamsu, H. (1989) Spontaneously breathing ventilated infants have improved oxygenation at fast rates. *Acta Paediatr. Scand.*, **76**, 706–712
52. Greenough, A., Greenall, F. and Gamsu, H. (1988) Synchronous ventilation: which rate is best? *Acta Paed. Scand.*, **76**, 713–718
53. Allen, R. W., Jung, A. L. and Lester, P. D. (1981) Effectiveness of chest tube evacuation of pneumothorax in neonates. *J. Pediatr.*, **99**, 629–634
54. Brooks, J. G., Bustamante, S. A. and Knoops, B. L. (1977) Selective bronchial intubation for the treatment of severe localised pulmonary interstitial emphysema in newborn infants. *J. Pediatr.*, **91**, 648–653
55. Cohen, R. S., Smith, D. W., Stevenson, D. K., Moskowitz, P. S. and Graham, C. B. (1984) Lateral decubitus position as therapy for persistent focal pulmonary interstitial emphysema in neonates: a preliminary report. *J. Pediatr.*, **104**, 441–443
56. Milligan D. W. A., Issler, H., Massam, M. and Reynolds, E. O. R. (1984) Treatment of neonatal pulmonary interstitial emphysema by lung puncture. *Lancet*, **i**, 1010–1011

Chapter 8

Chronic lung disease

Robert Dinwiddie

Introduction

Chronic lung disease is unfortunately all too common in the baby under 1000 g. Because of their size and maturity the lungs are not usually sufficiently developed to cope with extrauterine life without difficulty. Modern methods of surfactant stimulation or replacement and acute resuscitation at birth have made great strides in helping these infants to cope with the demands which are made on their lungs in the first few hours and days of life. While a considerable number cope remarkably well a sizeable minority develop chronic lung disease and can remain persistently symptomatic for weeks, months or even years. These babies may tax our physical, financial and emotional resources to the limits and their disease presents one of the major outstanding problems in perinatal and infant care.

Incidence

The incidence of chronic lung disease is difficult to compare between centres because of the lack of a standard definition of what separates ‘recurrent acute’ lung disease from chronic lung disease. Those who have tried to find a definition have focused on bronchopulmonary dysplasia (BPD) whereas many infants under 1000 g show features of a number of lung conditions acting together. The term chronic lung disease of prematurity (CLP) seems more appropriate in these cases. Most authors are agreed that chronic lung disease is present when there is persistent dependence on oxygen and usually, but not always, a need for ventilation, in the presence of chronic chest X-ray changes at the age of four weeks.

Causes

The list of conditions which can cause these problems is shown in Table 8.1. These will be considered separately although they frequently overlap in clinical practice.

Bronchopulmonary dysplasia (BPD)

This was first outlined in its classical form by Northway, Rosan and Porter [1] in 1967. They described the typical progression of the lung changes from hyaline

Table 8.1 Causes of chronic lung disease of prematurity (CLP)

Bronchopulmonary dysplasia
Acute or chronic infection (bacterial or viral)
Retained lung secretions
Hypersecretory state
Patent ductus arteriosus
Recurrent aspiration
Wilson–Mikity syndrome
Metabolic bone disease of prematurity

Table 8.2 Factors in the aetiology of chronic lung disease in infants weighing less than 1000 g at birth

Pulmonary immaturity	Recurrent infection
Birth asphyxia	Artificial ventilation
Oxygen therapy	Poor mucociliary clearance (usually from endotracheal intubation)
High fluid intake	Patent ductus arteriosus
Surfactant deficiency (hyaline membrane disease)	Vitamin deficiency (A, D or E)
Pulmonary air leak (interstitial emphysema)	Persistent fetal circulation

membrane disease through a period of pulmonary plethora to a bubbly cystic appearance finally emerging into the classical pattern of overinflated lower lobes with patchy and often linear streaky opacities throughout the upper zones. More recently Yu [2] has pointed out that these changes are by no means clear-cut and one period often merges into the other. The following definition is useful clinically.

(1) Intermittent positive pressure ventilation (IPPV) during the first week and lasting at least three days.
(2) Chronic respiratory distress characterized by tachypnoea, retractions and râles persisting for over 28 days.
(3) Oxygen therapy for more than 28 days to maintain $P\text{ao}_2$ levels above 6.7 kPa (50 mmHg).
(4) X-ray changes showing strands of increased density alternating with areas of increasing lucency.

The incidence of BPD in infants under 1000 g at Queen Charlotte's Maternity Hospital, London in 1984–85 was 15%. This agrees with the estimates of 15–23% found by others [2–4].

The aetiology of BPD is multifactorial and the possible factors involved are shown in Table 8.2. The major precipitating factors are the presence of hyaline membrane disease requiring the administration of oxygen and artificial ventilation [5]. Many of the other factors shown act together to increase the lung injury. It should be noted that a number of these are avoidable or responsive to aggressive treatment. This may be important in prevention.

Argument has raged for many years whether barotrauma from ventilation or oxygen toxicity is the most important causative factor in BPD. Stocks and Godfrey [6] showed that ventilated infants have increased airway resistance up to at least one year of age. A number of clinical studies however have not consistently demonstrated a relationship of BPD to high ventilator pressures alone [7]. Most studies to date have only included small numbers of ELBW infants. It seems likely, however, that the positive pressure ventilation used to treat RDS in infants of this size, if not the sole cause of chronic lung disease, is a major contributory factor. High oxygen concentrations are known to be potentially toxic to the lungs at any age and this too must be an important factor in pathogenesis.

The role of intrinsic protection against oxygen toxicity in these infants by enzymes such as superoxide dysmutase is not clear and requires further study [8]. High oxygen concentrations also produce an acute inflammatory response in the lung which undoubtedly contributes to the chronic changes which are seen. The use of antioxidants such as vitamin E has not been shown to be beneficial in prevention of BPD [7]. Apart from ventilation and oxygen therapy other contributory factors to the development of BPD are also known to include patent ductus arteriosus, pulmonary oedema and chronic lower respiratory tract infection (Table 8.2). These other factors may be of particular relevance to the baby under 1000 g who often needs prolonged airway support because of immaturity of the respiratory centres or recurrent apnoea.

Treatment

Treatment of BPD and CLP is complex and requires attention to all aspects of the baby's general condition as well as the need for respiratory support. The ultimate cure for this disease is the natural growth and maturation of the normal lung which occurs with increasing maturity and overall weight gain when adequate nutrition can be provided. The treatments available for BPD and CLP are shown in Table 8.3.

Oxygen therapy is required by definition. It is useful to maintain $P\text{aO}_2$ above 8 kPa (60 mmHg, 90% saturation) and to provide adequate levels during periods of stress. Cutaneous monitoring of $\text{P}_{\text{TC}}\text{O}_2$ or saturation is helpful in assessing the quantity required. Oxygen can usefully be administered by nasal catheter once ventilation is no longer required [9,10]. Low flow oxygen may be needed for several months in those with the worst disease who may be successfully managed at home at this stage (Figure 8.1).

Fluid restriction is often required in very small infants with BPD as there is an element of interstitial pulmonary oedema present. This will be exacerbated in those with a patent ductus arteriosus when there is a left-to-right shunt present. Closure of the duct early in the illness will remove this contribution to the interstitial changes. Diuretics are also useful; many infants exhibit diuretic dependency and become more hypoxic if these agents are withdrawn. Their use, however, in conjunction with fluid

Table 8.3 Treatment of chronic lung disease of prematurity

Oxygen	Antibiotics for infections
Ventilation	Adequate vitamin supplements (A, D and E)
Fluid restriction	Diuretics
Closure of PDA	Adequate nutrition
Theophylline	Bronchodilators (ipratropium)
Steroids	

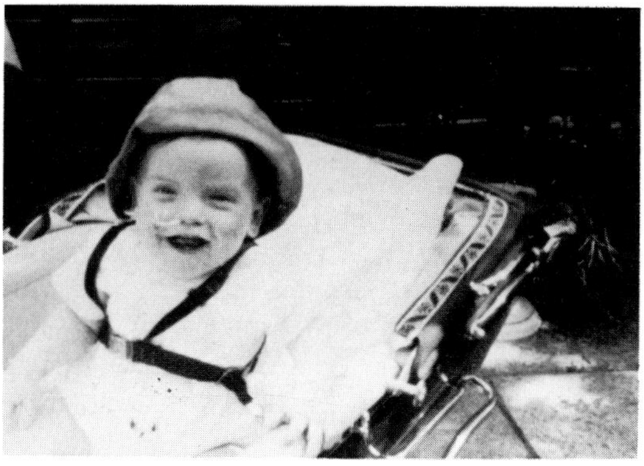

Figure 8.1 Child receiving nasal oxygen at home

restriction may limit nutritional input and contribute to electrolyte and calcium loss in the urine thus increasing the risks of metabolic bone disease of prematurity. Theophylline is usually given to those who are being weaned from ventilation. It may function in various ways including the reduction of diaphragm fatigue, stimulation of central drive, diuresis and bronchodilation [11]. Many of these infants develop acute wheeziness due to airway obstruction and bronchodilators such as ipratropium bromide or sympathomimetic agents may be beneficial [12].

Chronic infection almost inevitably supervenes in the patients who need prolonged respiratory support and appropriate antibiotic therapy is often needed with an aminoglycosid or one of the newer penicillins or cephalosporins active against *Pseudomonas aeruginosa*. The possible ototoxic effects of the aminoglycosides should be remembered in this particularly vulnerable group of infants. Acute infections also exacerbate the chronic lung disease and viruses such as respiratory syncytial virus (RSV) are especially dangerous. Care should be taken to prevent nosocomial spread during epidemic periods. Other agents such as cytomegalovirus (CMV) and chlamydia are discussed later.

Prevention of vitamin deficiency is another important part of treatment. Adequate intake of vitamin A [13], vitamin D [14] and vitamin E are essential in the efforts to minimize lung damage. These vitamins should be replaced to physiological levels especially when overall nutritional intake is often deficient. The use of vitamin E in pharmacological doses has not been shown to be effective in the prevention of BPD [15].

Steroids have been shown to be effective in BPD. Mammel *et al.* [16] showed a response in six infants with a mean birth weight of 1049 g. All were weaned from ventilation but three later died from infection. Steroid therapy may have to be given over an extended period with all the associated complications that this may produce. The role of steroids in BPD requires further evaluation and this is being undertaken at present by means of a large multicentre trial.

Wilson–Mikity syndrome

This condition which was first described by Wilson and Mikity in 1960 [17] is typically seen in VLBW infants. They usually have mild respiratory distress initially and do not require ventilation. Subsequently they develop chronic respiratory distress beginning towards the end of the first or second week of life. X-ray shows a bubbly appearance with streaky shadows alternating with more obviously cystic areas within the lung. Some infants show multiple rib fractures as well. The aetiology is unclear but it probably represents the effects of a number of stress factors on the immature lung.

Treatment is supportive with oxygen therapy and occasionally ventilation, especially during intercurrent respiratory infections. Those with the worst disease may develop cor pulmonale but this is unusual. Most infants show a gradual resolution of their symptoms over a period of several months. The long-term outlook for those who survive this period is excellent.

Retained lung secretions

All infants who have required intubation for ventilation during the first few days of life will have disturbance of the mucociliary lining of the respiratory tract. High oxygen concentrations are also known to cause epithelial damage [8]. These changes result in the retention and poor clearance of lung secretions, especially during infections. If present for more than a short period there is an associated hypersecretion of mucus which can contribute to the pulmonary difficulties. This may produce a hazy *white-out* appearance on the chest X-ray. One variant of this condition seen in babies under 1200 g is described as chronic pulmonary insufficiency of prematurity [18]. Treatment includes the avoidance of unnecessarily prolonged endotracheal intubation, reduction of inspired oxygen when tolerated, antibiotics for infection and regular chest physiotherapy to aid the clearance of the lung secretions.

Infection

Infection plays a major role in the chronic lung disease of prematurity especially in infants under 1000 g. They are particularly prone to this for a number of reasons including disturbance of mucociliary function, introduction of pathogenic hospital organisms, endotracheal intubation, interstitial pulmonary oedema, relative immaturity of the immune system and lack of transfer of maternal antibodies. Some infants, especially very small ones, have acquired chronic pulmonary infection with CMV via blood transfusion [19]. Human immune deficiency virus (HIV) has also been introduced by blood transfusion, before screening was routine, and it led to the subsequent development of opportunistic lung infection.

The agents responsible may be bacterial or viral. They most commonly include hospital pathogens such as staphylococci, streptococci, *E. coli*, *Klebsiella* spp. and *Pseudomonas* spp. Fungi such as *Candida albicans* are increasing in frequency. RSV is a major problem in these children. Other viruses such as CMV may also be present in the respiratory tract at birth [20] and can lead to chronic lung disease manifested by interstitial pneumonitis initially [2] or later by recurrent wheezing in infancy. *Chlamydia trachomatis* is another agent which can cause chronic lung disease in very preterm infants.

Patients with chronic lung disease therefore frequently require antimicrobial therapy with antibiotics and increasingly with antifungal and antiviral agents. Many of these have potential toxic side effects and the measurement of blood concentrations, especially when aminoglycosides are used, is essential.

Very preterm infants should be protected against pertussis as this can be fatal to this group especially in the first few months to life. Immunization should begin three months after birth whatever the gestation.

Aspiration

The ELBW infant has poorly developed swallowing and sucking reflexes; there is also a poor cough. These conditions predispose to the aspiration of upper respiratory secretions and milk feeds, which may have been regurgitated up to the pharynx, into the lower respiratory tract. The presence of a relatively lax gastro-oesophageal sphincter and large diaphragmatic movements increases the risk of aspiration. Particular caution should be observed in feeding infants who have recently been extubated since they may be unable to secure glottic closure at this stage.

Prevention of this aspect of chronic lung disease consists of a graded transfer from intravenous or nasojejunal feeding to nasogastric feeds. Keeping the baby propped up at an angle of 30 degrees and the use of thickened feeds or the relatively early introduction of solids into the diet are also helpful. These infants are often limited in the volume they are able to tolerate, so high energy thickened feeds may be very useful in the early stages.

Metabolic bone disease of prematurity

This condition is common in ELBW infants under 1000 g [14]. The effects on breathing are shown by softening of the bony structure of the rib cage. One of the diagnostic features of this condition is the presence of multiple rib fractures on the chest X-ray. The rib cage becomes soft and this results in indrawing and subcostal recession causing a Harrison's sulcus. Where there is chronic lung disease these changes may be accentuated secondary to the high negative intrathoracic pressures which are required to ventilate relatively non-compliant lungs [6]. Diaphragm function is also compromised by the floppy chest wall.

There is considerable debate regarding prevention and treatment of metabolic bone disease. Measurement of serial alkaline phosphatase may be one practical method of screening those at risk [21]. Adequate intake of calcium, phosphate and vitamin D is important, but this is often difficult to provide in those whose tolerance of feeds is restricted by underlying pulmonary oedema or cor pulmonale.

Long-term prognosis

The long-term outlook for very small infants with chronic lung disease is not yet known. Short-term studies have shown a higher incidence of sudden death in infants under 1000 g in whom the incidence of BPD was 45% [22]. There is an increased incidence of lower respiratory tract infection in the first two years of life and a large proportion are under weight and height for age although head circumference is normal [23]. It is likely that in the longer term there will be marked variation in the outcome for lung function. Those with relatively mild disease may expect to have normal lungs particularly as extensive growth of new alveoli occurs during the first few years. Those with the worst disease may well have permanent disturbance of lung function although not all will be limited in their physical activity or exercise tolerance.

Bronchial hyper-reactivity is not uncommon [24] and may require appropriate treatment with bronchodilators.

The very smallest infants with the worst disease place the greatest emotional burden on their parents and also on the nursing and medical staff devoted to their care. The psychological support required for all of those involved, both during an extended hospital period fraught with many crises and in the early days at home, is a major part of the management of these patients.

Hopefully the overall morbidity from chronic lung disease in infants under 1000 g will reduce as better techniques of ventilation and greater understanding of the pathogenesis occurs with time.

References

1. Northway, W. H., Rosan, R. C. and Porter, D. Y. (1967) Pulmonary disease following respiratory therapy for hyaline membrane disease. Bronchopulmonary dysplasia. *N. Engl. J. Med.* **276**, 357–368
2. Yu, V. Y. H., (1986) Chronic lung disorders. In *Respiratory Disorders of the Newborn*, (ed. V. Y. H. Yu), Churchill Livingstone, Edinburgh, pp. 109–122
3. Wung, J., Koons, A. H., Driscoll, J. M. and James, L. S. (1979) Changing incidence of bronchopulmonary dysplasia. *J. Pediatr.*, **95**, 845–847
4. Hodson, W. A., Truog, W. E., Maycock, D. E., Lyrene, R. and Woodrum, D. E. (1979) Bronchopulmonary dysplasia: the need for epidemiological studies. *J. Pediatr.*, **95**, 848–851
5. Coalson, J. J. (1986) Animal models for bronchopulmonary dysplasia research, particulary primate studies. In *Bronchopulmonary Dysplasia and Related Chronic Respiratory Disorders* (eds P. M. Farrell and L. M. Taussig), Ross Laboratories, Columbus, Ohio, p. 7
6. Stocks, J. and Godfrey, S. (1976) The role of artificial ventilation, oxygen and CPAP in the pathogenesis of lung damage in neonates: assessment by serial measurement of lung function. *Pediatrics*, **57**, 352–356
7. Bancalari, E. (1985) Bronchopulmonary dysplasia. In *Neonatal and Pediatric Respiratory Medicine* (eds A. D. Milner and R. J. Martin), Butterworths, London, pp. 54–80
8. O'Brodovich, H. M. and Mellins, R. B. (1985) Bronchopulmonary dysplasia. Unresolved acute neonatal lung injury. *Am. Rev. Resp. Dis.*, **132**, 694–709
9. Dinwiddie, R. (1981) Long term oxygen therapy via nasal catheter. *J. Mat. Child Health*, **6**, 426
10. Campbell, A. N., Zarfin, Y., Groenveld, M. and Bryan, M. H. (1983) Low flow oxygen therapy in infants. *Arch. Dis. Child.*, **58**, 795–798
11. Rooklin, A. R., Moomjian, A. S., Shutack, J. G., Schwartz, J. G. and Fox, W. W. (1979) Theophylline therapy in bronchopulmonary dysplasia. *J. Pediatr.*, **95**, 882–885
12. Kao, L. C., Warburton, D., Platzker, A. C. G. and Keens, T. C. (1984) Effect of isoproterenol inhalation on airway resistance in chronic bronchopulmonary dysplasia. *Pediatrics*, **73**, 509–514
13. Zachman, R. D. (1986) Vitamin A. In *Bronchopulmonary Dysplasia and Related Chronic Respiratory Disorders* (eds P. M. Farrell and L. M. Taussig), Ross Laboratories, Columbus, Ohio, pp. 86–96
14. Editorial (1987) Metabolic bone disease of prematurity. *Lancet*, **i**, 200
15. Bell, E. F. (1986) Prevention of bronchopulmonary dysplasia: vitamin E and other antioxidants. In *Bronchopulmonary Dysplasia and Related Chronic Respiratory Disorders* (eds P. M. Farrell and L. M. Taussig), Ross Laboratories, Columbus, Ohio, pp. 77–85
16. Mammel, M. C., Green, T. P., Johnston, D. E. and Thompson, T. R. (1983) Controlled trial of dexamethasone therapy in infants with bronchopulmonary dysplasia. *Lancet*, **i**, 1356–1358
17. Wilson, M. E. and Mikity, Y. G. (1960) A new form of respiratory disease seen in premature infants. *Am. J. Dis. Child.*, **99**, 489–499
18. Krauss, A. N., Klain, D. B. and Auld, P. A. M. (1975) Chronic pulmonary insufficiency of prematurity (CPIP). *Pediatrics*, **77**, 27–36
19. Yeager, A. S., Grumet, F. C., Halfleigh, E. B., Arvin, A. M., Bradley, J. S. and Prober, C. G. (1981) Prevention of transfusion acquired cytomegalovirus infections in newborn infants. *J. Pediatr.*, **98**, 281–287

20. Peckham, C. S., Chin, K. S., Coleman, J. C., Henderson, K., Hurley, R. and Preece, P. M. (1983) Cytomegalovirus in pregnancy: preliminary findings from a prospective study. *Lancet*, **i**, 1352–1355
21. Kovar, I., Mayne, P. and Barltrop, D. (1982) Plasma alkaline phosphatase activity: a screening test for rickets in preterm infants. *Lancet*, **i**, 308–310
22. Saigal, S., Rosenbaum, P., Stoskopf, B. and Sinclair, J. C. (1984) Outcome in infants 501–1000 g birth weight delivered to residents of the McMaster Health Region. *J. Pediatr.*, **105**, 969–976
23. Yu, V. Y. H., Orgill, A. A., Lim, S. B., Bajuk, B. and Astbury, J. (1983) Growth and development of very low birthweight infants recovering from bronchopulmonary dysplasia. *Arch. Dis. Child.*, **58**, 791–794
24. Smyth, J. A., Tabachni, E., Duncan, W. J., Reilly, B. and Levison, H. (1981) Pulmonary function and bronchial hyper-reactivity in long term survivors of bronchopulmonary dysplasia. *Pediatrics*, **68**, 336–340

Chapter 9

The hazards of an immature skin

Nicholas Rutter

The skin is an important barrier between man and his environment. It keeps out noxious agents and keeps in the main body constituent, water. If there is extensive skin loss, as a result of trauma or disease, death commonly results. In most preterm infants problems due to immaturity of the skin do not occur. Illness and outcome are largely determined by delivery, resuscitation and the development of cerebral, respiratory and bowel complications. Babies born before 30 weeks gestation however, especially those below 28 weeks gestation (who will usually weigh less than 1000 g), suffer from profound immaturity of all the organ systems of the body including the skin. Immaturity of the skin as a barrier leads to major clinical problems of fluid and heat loss, accidental absorption of toxic agents and superficial trauma.

Structure of the skin

The outer layer of the skin, the epidermis, provides its barrier properties. Epidermal cells are produced in the basal layer, migrate upwards, flatten, become filled with a fibrous protein (keratin) and die. The dead keratinized cell plates are tightly interlocked and overlapping, forming the stratum corneum. It is this layer which resists the escape of water or the entry of toxic agents. The development of keratinization of the fetal epidermis starts at about 18 weeks when the periderm starts to disappear [1,2]. By about 26 weeks the development of a keratinized stratum corneum involves the whole body surface but the epidermis is only two or three cells thick and a keratinized stratum is barely visible. In the last trimester the epidermis increases in thickness, keratinization becomes more marked and the stratum corneum well defined, so that by term the epidermis resembles that of an adult [3] (Figure 9.1). However, these maturational changes which occur in the last trimester are greatly accelerated if the infant is born prematurely. No matter how immature the infant is at delivery, by the time he reaches two weeks of age the epidermis resembles that of a term infant (Figure 9.2). Thus the epidermis of an infant of 25 weeks gestation at two weeks of age is similar to that of a term infant, rather than an infant of 27 weeks gestation.

Birth therefore triggers a rapid acceleration of epidermal maturation, similar to the changes which are seen in adult skin which has been damaged by stripping or by superficial burns. The very immature infant is a water dwelling animal forced prematurely to live on dry land. Presumably the stimulus to the hastened epidermal maturation is exposure to air but the mechanism by which it occurs is unknown. It

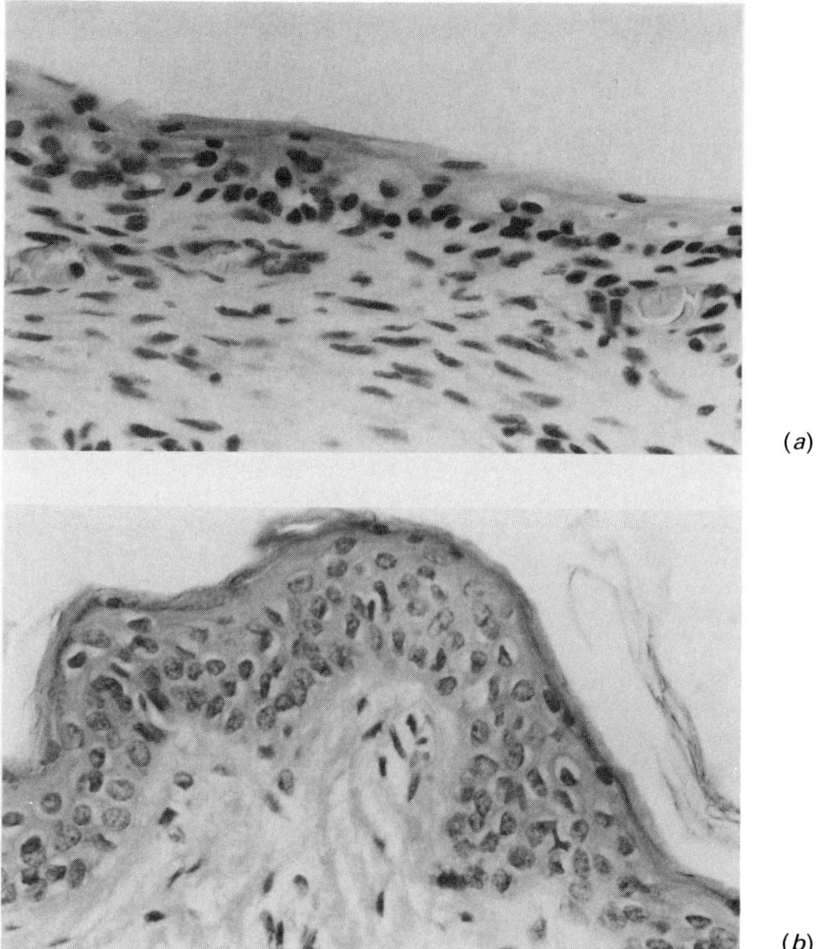

Figure 9.1 The effect of gestation on maturation of the epidermis. (*a*) Section of abdominal skin of an infant born at 26 weeks gestation who died shortly after delivery. Note the thin epidermis, 2–3 cells thick, with little formation of a keratinzied stratum corneum. (*b*) The abdominal skin of an infant delivered at 40 weeks gestation who died in labour. There is a well developed epidermis. Magnification × 90. (Reproduced with with permission [57])

means, however, that clinical problems associated with an immature skin are only relevant in the early neonatal period.

Barrier properties of immature skin

Transepidermal water loss (TEWL)

Water is lost from the skin by two routes – secretion of sweat via the sweat ducts and passive diffusion of water through the epidermis (transepidermal water loss). Babies

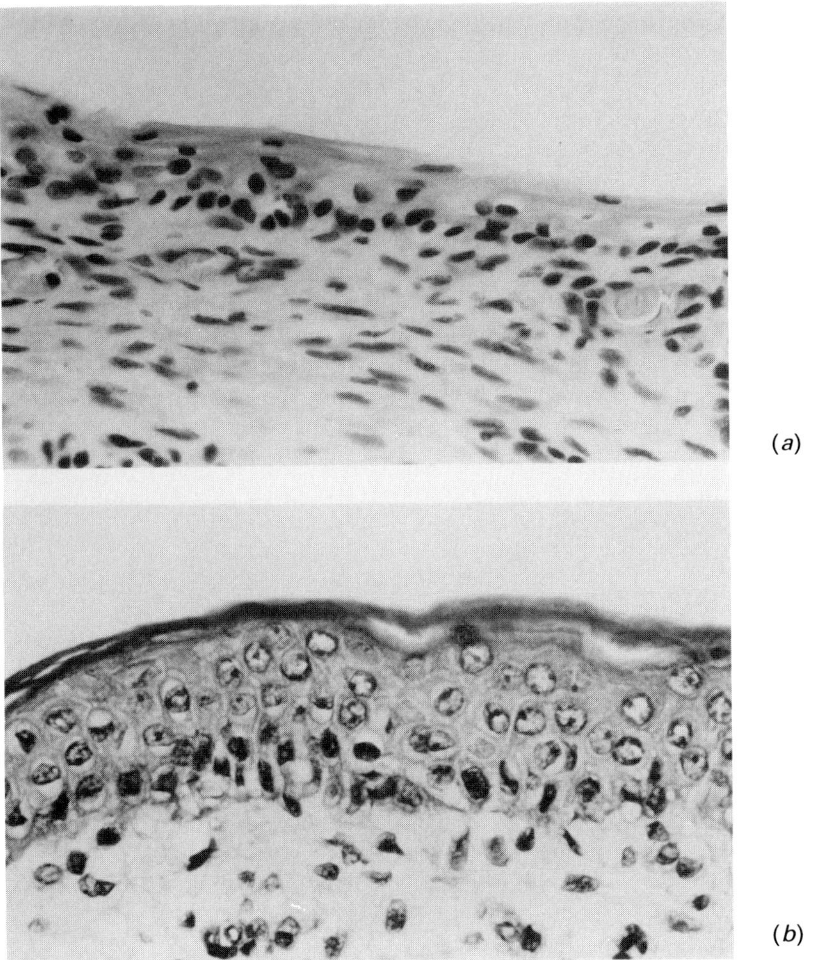

Figure 9.2 The effect of extrauterine existence on maturation of the epidermis. (*a*) From an infant born at 26 weeks gestation who died shortly after delivery (Figure 9.1). (*b*) The abdominal skin of an infant born at 26 weeks gestation who died at 16 days. The epidermal development is comparable to that of a term infant. Magnification ×90. (Reproduced with permission [57])

born before 36 weeks gestation are unable to sweat in the early neonatal period [4–6] so that all skin water loss is through the epidermis.

TEWL and the effect of gestational age

Gestational age has a very marked effect on TEWL [7,8] as would be expected from the epidermal histology. Losses rise exponentially before 30 weeks, and can reach values of 100 $g/m^2/h$ in infants of 24 weeks gestation on the first day or so of life. By 32 weeks gestation losses are lower, and by term have fallen to about 6 $g/m^2/h$ (Figure 9.3).

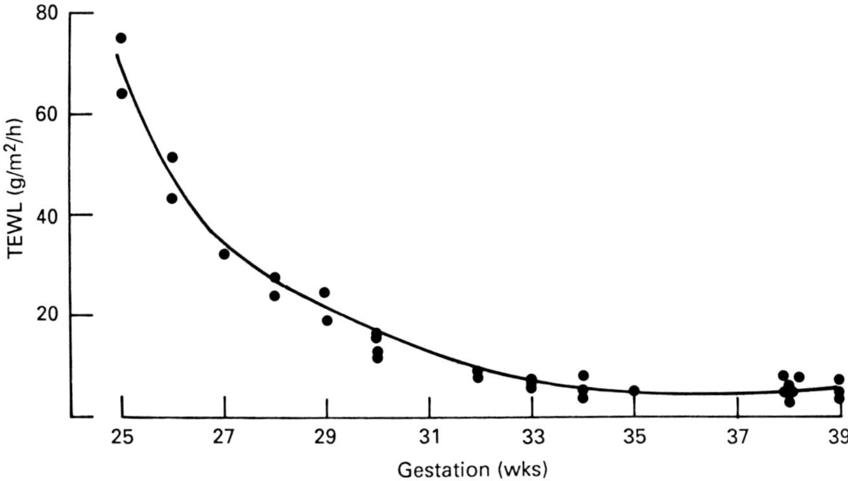

Figure 9.3 The effect of gestation on transepidermal water loss (TEWL). TEWL was measured at three representative skin sites on the first day of life (ambient relative humidity 50%). Redrawn from the data of Hammarlund and Sedin [8]

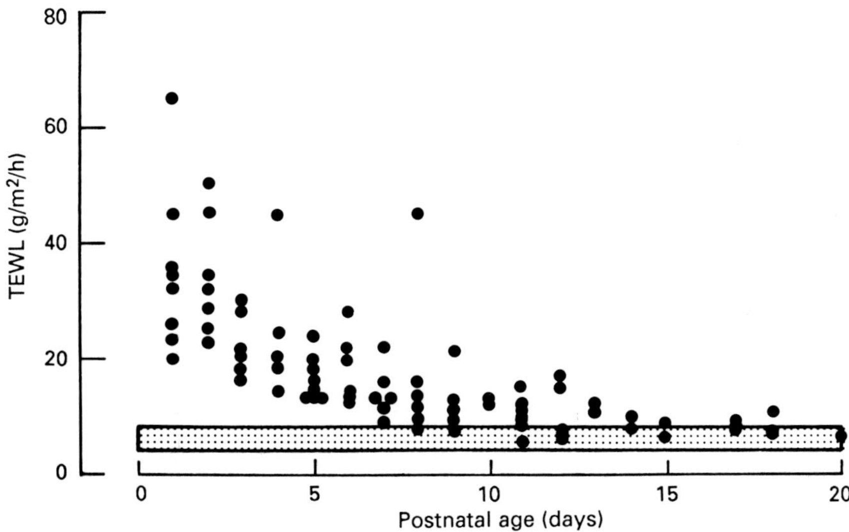

Figure 9.4 The effect of extrauterine existence on transepidermal water loss (TEWL). Serial measurements were made from the abdominal skin of 17 infants born between 25 and 29 weeks gestation. The shaded part represents values of TEWL found in full term infants. Redrawn from the data of Harpin and Rutter [11]

TEWL and the effect of postnatal age

There is an accelerated fall in TEWL after birth in babies born before 30 weeks gestation so that by about two weeks of age losses are only a little higher than those of a term infant [7,9–11]. This parallels the acceleration in epidermal maturation (Figure 9.4).

TEWL and the effect of environmental factors

TEWL is a physical process and not under physiological control. It is determined not only by the effectiveness of the epidermal barrier, but also by environmental factors.

TEMPERATURE

The temperature of the skin and air is positively related to TEWL [12], although the effect is not great over the narrow range of skin and air temperatures found in a neonatal unit.

AIR SPEED

This is positively related to TEWL. When air speed is low, natural convection exists and there is a boundary layer of still air close to the skin. This becomes relatively saturated and reduces TEWL. When air speed is high, the boundary layer is lost and TEWL is higher [13–15]. These conditions of forced convection are found when infants below 30 weeks gestation are nursed naked in incubators or under radiant warmers, and therefore exposed to draughty air.

HUMIDITY

Ambient humidity is a powerful determinant of TEWL; at low relative humidity TEWL is high, at 100% relative humidity TEWL is abolished. The relationship is linear and the effect more marked in the most immature infants [8,16] (Figure 9.5).

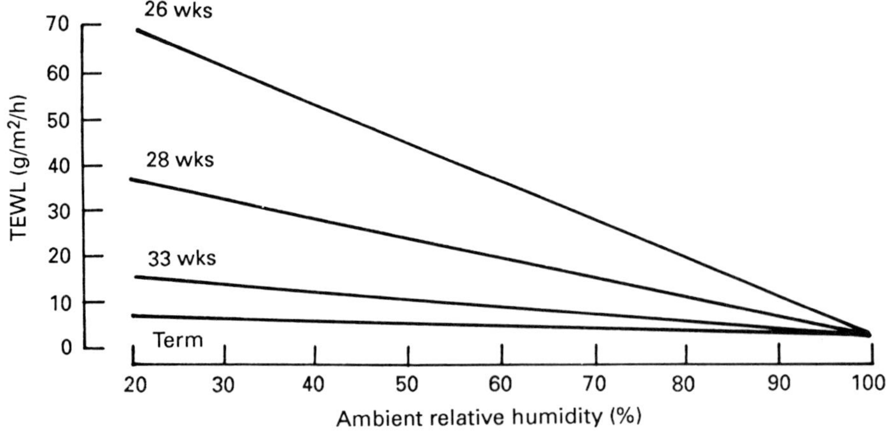

Figure 9.5 The effect of ambient relative humidity on transepidermal water loss (TEWL). Redrawn and modified from the data of Hammarlund and Sedin [8]

RADIATION

Exposure of the skin to radiant energy increases TEWL. This is important in very immature infants nursed under radiant warmers or phototherapy. Radiant warmers increase TEWL by a factor of 0.5–2.0 [17,18,19], phototherapy by 0.4–2.0 [18,20]. The two together have an additive effect [21]. Although part of the increase in TEWL can be explained by the higher skin temperatures, higher air speeds and lower ambient humidity which occur when infants are nursed under radiant warmers, there is an unexplained direct effect of radiant energy [22].

Although it is clear that very immature infants have a high TEWL when measurements are made from local areas of skin, there is disappointingly little information available about the overall water loss from the whole body – the insensible water loss. It is this parameter which would be so useful to know in planning the fluid intake of such an infant. Insensible water loss has been measured directly and indirectly (as insensible weight loss) by many investigators, but most studies have included very few infants under 1000 g birth weight or below 28 weeks gestation. Furthermore, studies based on measurement of insensible weight loss have probably overestimated water loss because the balances have been affected by temperature changes [23,24]. Table 9.1 summarizes the results of these investigations which include predominantly those infants of less than 1000 g.

Insensible water loss in the term infant is approximately 8–11 g/m^2/h. This is equivalent to about 11–15 ml/kg/day. Depending on environmental conditions, insensible water loss in very immature infants can range from 50 to 150 ml/kg/day. The highest value might be found in an infant of 24 weeks gestation nursed naked under a radiant warmer and phototherapy lamp in the immediate neonatal period.

Babies with a high TEWL pose problems in the management of fluid balance. Since heat is lost from the evaporation of water they are also difficult to keep warm [22].

Management of fluid balance

The very immature infant of less than 1000 g has a higher water content than a term infant (Figure 9.6). The result is that administration of excessive or too little fluid has a more harmful effect than in more mature infants. Over-administration of fluid is the more serious. Clinically it may result in a rapid weight gain (or a failure of the usual weight loss) and appearance of oedema, although the latter is a common finding in very immature infants. Worsening of respiratory illness may occur – respiratory distress syndrome requires more ventilation and higher inspired oxygen concentra-

Table 9.1 Measurements of insensible weight loss in preterm infants below 1000 g birth weight (note that two studies include heavier infants)

Reference	*Weight of infants* (g)	*Method of nursing*	*Insensible water loss (mean ± SEM)* (ml/kg/24 h)
Fanaroff *et al.*[25]	700–1250	Incubator	84.0 ± 16.8
Wu and Hodgman[18]	below 1000	Incubator	64.8 ± 4.8
Bell *et al.*[19]	790–1310	Incubator	38.4 ± 7.2
		Radiant warmer	58.6 ± 4.8
Baumgart *et al.*[26]	660–1000	Radiant warmer	127.2 ± 18.5

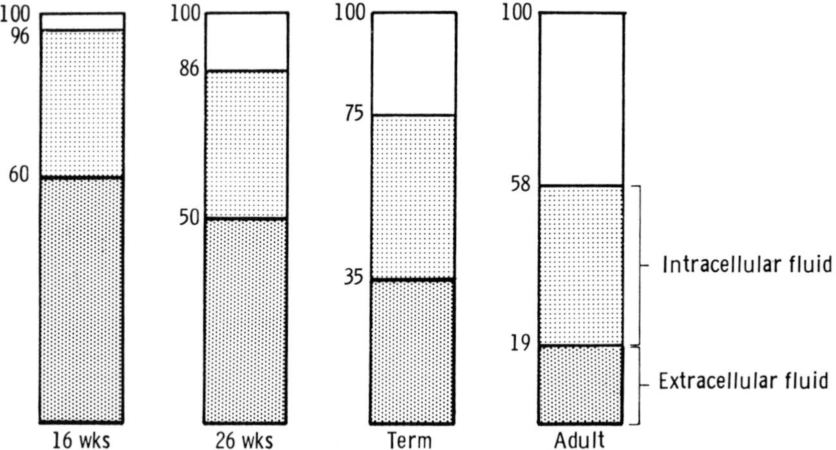

Figure 9.6 Body water content (intracellular and extracellular) as a percentage of total body weight

tions, and bronchopulmonary dysplasia is similarly made worse in its early stages. A left-to-right shunt through a patent ductus arteriosus is significantly more likely [28], and there is a possible increase in the incidence of necrotizing enterocolitis. Too little fluid results in a high weight loss, clinical dehydration, oliguria and pre-renal failure. Hypernatraemia is common and often marked [29]. Drugs, notably gentamicin, are less easily excreted.

Since the insensible water loss of an immature infant depends on so many factors, it cannot be predicted with any accuracy. Fluid balance management is greatly simplified if steps are taken to reduce the high TEWL, whether the infant is nursed in an incubator or under a radiant warmer. Assessment of fluid balance clinically and by investigation allows the infant's fluid needs to be calculated. Weight is the single most useful method of assessment and should be measured as accurately as possible. Daily or even twice daily weighing may be necessary, especially if no measures are taken to reduce TEWL. Since even the most immature infant has some ability to conserve or excrete water, measurement of the degree of concentration of the blood and urine will be useful. Guidelines are given in Table 9.2.

If TEWL is effectively reduced the fluid requirements of an immature infant will, on average, be similar to those of other preterm and term infants (60 ml/kg/day on day 1,

Table 9.2 Assessment of fluid needs in immature infants

Body weight	
Average % weight loss in first week: <26 weeks – 20% (Gill *et al.*[30])	
26–28 weeks – 15%	
Less than 10% weight loss (or no weight loss, or weight gain) suggests too much fluid	
Greater than 20% weight loss suggests too little fluid	
Blood	
Sodium: normal range, 130–145 mmol/l	lower levels suggest too much fluid
Osmolality: normal range, 260–290 mOsmol/kg	higher levels suggest too little fluid
Urine	
Osmolality: aim to maintain between 150 and 300 mOsmol/kg	
Specific gravity: aim to maintain between 1.005 and 1.010	

increasing to 150 ml/kg/day by the end of the first week). If TEWL is not reduced fluid requirements will be much higher, up to 200 ml/kg/day. It is preferable to err on the side of too little fluid rather than too much, especially in the early stages of respiratory distress syndrome when fluid restriction is advocated [31].

Temperature control

Each millilitre of water which evaporates from the skin removes 560 calories of heat. The infant below 1000 g is already at a major disadvantage because of his high surface area to weight ratio, so that heat loss by all channels is high relative to heat production. A high TEWL as well will render the very immature infant susceptible to hypothermia. In the delivery room, for example, body temperature can drop by 1 °C every five minutes in spite of the provision of supplementary heat.

The very immature infant can either be nursed in an incubator or under a radiant warmer. Since the infant is likely to be ill and require intensive care, nursing care is easier if the infant is naked. The major advantage of the radiant warmer in this situation is that the infant can be effectively kept warm whilst doctors and nurses have ready access for intubation, placing of intra-arterial and intravenous catheters, etc. Fluid balance, though, is more difficult. Immature infants can be kept warm in an incubator if carefully nursed, but practical procedures are difficult to carry out and cause cold stress.

Incubators

The very immature infant nursed naked in an incubator can only be kept warm if steps are taken to reduce the high TEWL. A high ambient temperature close to 37 °C will be necessary. Although TEWL can be reduced using a waterproof covering such as a plastic thermal bubble blanket [32] or topical soft paraffin [33,34], in practice the only effective method is to increase the ambient humidity [8,16]. It is otherwise impossible to avoid hypothermia [35]. It would require an ambient temperature in excess of 40 °C to maintain a normal body temperature in a very small and immature infant without the use of humidity. For safety reasons such a temperature is not permitted in the UK.

Some, although not all, current incubators can be very effectively humidified. A relative humidity of 85–90% can be achieved at the highest air temperature setting, a level at which TEWL is greatly reduced (Figure 9.5). The effect of providing a humid environment on temperature control is dramatic [35] (Figure 9.7). When the incubator portholes are opened for access to the infant, relative humidity falls to 50–60%, still higher though than the levels of 25–40% which are found in dry incubators. Although plastic coverings will reduce water loss from the skin by as much as 75% [32], as well as reducing heat loss by convection and radiation, they impair observation of the infant and frequently have to be removed for access. This results in episodes of very high TEWL.

The main worry about incubator humidification is a possible increased risk of bacterial infection, particularly as a result of water-borne organisms such as *Pseudomonas aeruginosa*. This can be reduced if the humidifier is drained daily, run dry for a brief spell, then filled with fresh sterile water. Use of humidification should be confined to those infants who need it (infants less than 30 weeks gestation for the first week of life) and not be extended to all preterm infants nursed in incubators. Another possible hazard of the use of high humidity is overhydration, with an increased incidence of patent ductus arteriosus.

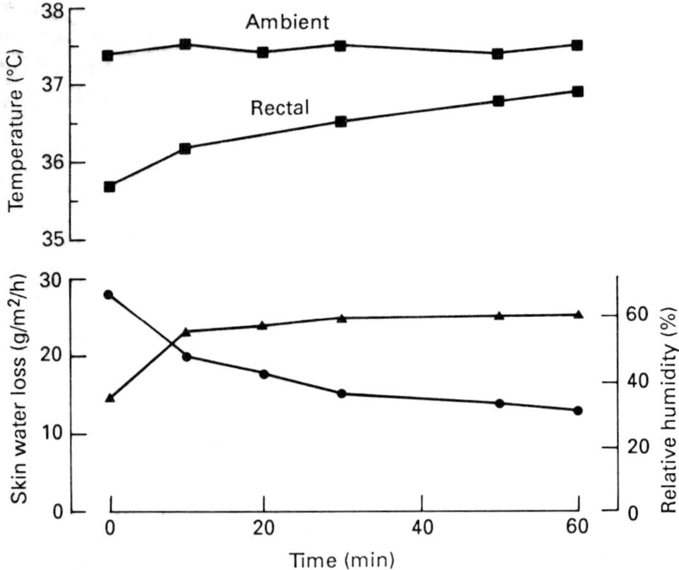

Figure 9.7 The effect of increasing ambient relative humidity within an incubator. The infant, 26 weeks gestation and birth weight 960 g, had a persistently low rectal temperature of 35.8°C at 10 h of age, despite a high incubator air temperature. When humidification is added, relative humidity (▲–▲) increases from 36% to 61%, skin water loss (●–●) falls and rectal temperature rises to normal within an hour. Reproduced with permission [35]

Radiant warmers

These devices allow very immature infants to have enormous heat losses from evaporation of water and convection without the development of hypothermia. This is achieved by providing a large amount of radiant heat to compensate for the losses. The advantages of visibility and access have been mentioned, but there is a risk of overheating unless obsessional nursing care is practised, and fluid balance is much more difficult than for infants nursed in incubators. It is both possible and desirable to reduce the high TEWL of very immature infants nursed under radiant warmers by use of plastic waterproof coverings [36–38]. Thin polyethylene film is transparent to long wave radiation but impermeable to water and is therefore a suitable material. It can be draped directly over the infant's body but this carries the risk of maceration of the moist skin and increased bacterial colonization. It is best suspended a few centimetres above the infant like a framed tent.

Absorption of drugs and chemicals

The immature epidermal barrier greatly increases the risk of absorption of topically applied agents in the early neonatal period. Significant absorption can result in systemic toxicity. This was first noted when aniline marker dyes produced met-haemoglobinaemia [39–42], but subsequent effects have been confined to the use of topical antiseptics. Hexachlorophene myelinopathy [43–46], iodine-induced goitre [47], alcohol-related skin necrosis [48,49] and neomycin ototoxicity have been described [50]. Any antiseptic agent should be used sparingly and with care. Although the commonly used chlorhexidine is not known to have any toxic effects, it is certainly systemically absorbed [51]. Any water soluble drug or chemical is rapidly absorbed through the skin of immature infants.

A major concern is that since the most immature infants are expected to have a high mortality and morbidity rate, disasters which result from percutaneous absorption of toxic agents will pass unrecognized.

Resistance to trauma

Neonatal monitoring of heart rate, respiration, temperature, transcutaneous partial pressure for oxygen (tc$P\text{O}_2$) and carbon dioxide (tc$P\text{CO}_2$) is carried out using surface probes which are stuck to the skin with adhesive. When the adhesive tape is removed the most superficial cell layer is removed with it [52]. This is not important to a term infant with an epidermal barrier several layers thick, but it is adding insult to injury in an infant whose epidermis has only two or three cell layers. TEWL and drug absorption increase and there is a possibility of entry of bacteria through the broken barrier [11]. Probes are large relative to the infant's surface area and up to 15% of the skin can be subjected to trauma each day. Although skin damage caused by monitoring probes is usually transient and can be expected to heal completely, occasional scarring can result. An ECG electrode can leave an area of roughened, irregular skin, and a heated tc$P\text{O}_2$ electrode can leave a small round shiny scar at the site of a third degree burn [53,54].

Prevention of epidermal trauma is difficult because the most immature infants are the most ill and need the most monitoring. The number of surface probes should be kept to a minimum and their area should be as small as possible. It is not necessary, for example, for an ECG electrode to be attached to the chest with a disc the size of the baby's face. New substances need to be explored which will not strip the epidermis when removed – materials used to protect the skin around ileostomies are promising in this respect. For example, the epidermis can be protected from adhesive by prior application of a spray-on copolymer dressing without interfering with the normal function of a transcutaneous gas electrode [55]. ECG electrodes made out of kuraya gum can easily be removed from the chest for easy access and then replaced; they do not damage the epidermis or cause pain when they are removed but give good quality ECG traces [56].

References

1. Holbrook, K. A. (1979) Human epidermal embryogenesis. *Int. J. Dermatol.*, **18**, 329–356
2. Holbrook, K. A. (1982) A histological comparison of infant and adult skin. In *Neonatal Skin* (ed. H. I. Maiback), Marcel Dekker, New York, pp. 3–31
3. Evans, N. J. and Rutter, N. (1986) Development of the epidermis in the newborn. *Biol. Neonate*, **49**, 74–80
4. Harpin, V. A. and Rutter, N. (1982) Sweating in preterm babies. *J. Pediatr.*, **100**, 614–619
5. Hey, E. N. and Katz, G. (1969) Evaporative water loss in the newborn baby. *J. Physiol.*, **200**, 605–619
6. Foster, K. E., Hey, E. N. and Katz, G. (1969) The response of the sweat glands of the newborn baby to thermal stimuli and to intradermal acetyl choline. *J. Physiol.*, **203**, 13–29
7. Rutter, N. and Hull, D. (1979) Water loss from the skin of term and preterm babies. *Arch. Dis. Child.*, **54**, 858–868
8. Hammarlund, K. and Sedin, G. (1979) Transepidermal water loss in newborn infants. III. Relation to gestational age. *Acta Paediatr. Scand.*, **68**, 795–801
9. Hammarlund, K., Sedin, G. and Stromberg, B. (1982) Transepidermal water loss in newborn infants.

VII. Relation to postnatal age in very preterm and full term appropriate for gestational age infants. *Acta Paediatr. Scand.*, **71**, 360–374
10. Hammarlund, K., Sedin, G. and Stromberg, B. (1983) Transepidermal water loss in the newborn. VIII. Relation to gestational age and postnatal age in appropriate and small for gestational age infants. *Acta Paediatr. Scand.*, **72**, 721–728
11. Harpin, V. A. and Rutter, N. (1983) Barrier properties of the newborn infant's skin. *J. Pediatr.*, **102**, 419–425
12. Grice, K., Sathar, H., Sharratt, M. and Baker, H. (1971) Skin temperature and transepidermal water loss. *J. Invest. Derm.*, **57**, 108–110
13. Clark, R. P., Cross, K. W., Goff, M. R., Mullen, B. J., Stothers, J. K. and Warner, R. M. (1978) Neonatal natural and forced convection. *J. Physiol.*, **284**, 22–23
14. Stothers, J. K. (1980) The effect of forced convection on neonatal heat loss. *J. Physiol.*, **305**, 778
15. Thompson, M. H., Stothers, J. K. and McLellan, N. J. (1984) Weight and water loss in the neonate in natural and forced convection. *Arch. Dis. Child.*, **59**, 951–956
16. Sedin, G., Hammarlund, K., Nilsson, G. E., Stromberg, B. and Oberg, P. A. (1985) Measurements of transepidermal water loss in newborn infants. *Clin. Perinatol.*, **12**, 79–99
17. Williams, P. R. and Oh, W. (1974) Effects of radiant warmer on insensible water loss in newborn infants. *Am. J. Dis. Child.*, **128**, 511–514
18. Wu, P. Y. K. and Hodgman, J. E. (1974) Insensible water loss in preterm infants: changes with postnatal development and non-ionizing radiant energy. *Pediatrics*, **54**, 704–712
19. Bell, E. F., Weinstein, M. R. and Oh, W. (1980) Heat balance in premature infants: comparative effects of convectively heated incubator and radiant warmer with and without plastic heat shield. *J. Pediatr.*, **96**, 460–465
20. Oh, W. and Karecki, H. (1972) Phototherapy and insensible water loss in the newborn infant. *Am. J. Dis. Child.*, **124**, 230–232
21. Bell, E. F., Neidich, G. A., Carshore, W. J. and Oh, W. (1979) Combined effect of radiant warmer and phototherapy on insensible water loss in low birthweight infants. *J. Pediatr.*, **94**, 810–813
22. Wheldon, A. C. and Rutter, N. (1982) The heat balance of small babies nursed in incubators and under radiant warmers. *Early Hum. Dev.*, **6**, 131–143
23. Darnall, R. A. (1981) Insensible weight loss measurements in newborn infants: possible over-estimation with the Potter baby scale. *J. Pediatr.*, **99**, 794–797
24. Doyle, L. W. and Sinclair, J. C. (1981) Thermal effect on a Potter baby scale. *Pediatr. Res.*, **15**, 658
25. Fanaroff, A. A., Wald, M., Gruber, HS. and Klaus, M. H. (1972) Insensible water loss in low birth weight infants. *Pediatrics*, **50**, 236–245
26. Baumgart, S., Engle, W. D., Fox, W. W. and Polin, R. A. (1981) Radiant warmer power and body size as determinants of insensible water loss in the critically ill neonate. *Pediatr. Res.*, **15**, 1495–1499
27. Baumgart, S. (1984) Reduction of oxygen consumption, insensible water loss, and radiant heat demand with use of a plastic blanket for low birthweight infants under radiant warmers. *Pediatrics*, **75**, 89–99
28. Bell, E. F., Warburton, D. and Stonestreet, B. S. (1980) Effect of fluid administration on the development of symptomatic patent ductus arteriosus and congestive heart failure in premature infants. *N. Engl. J. Med.*, **302**, 598–604
29. Jones, R. W. A., Rochefort, M. J. and Baum, J. D. (1976) Increased insensible water loss in newborn infants nursed under radiant heaters. *Br. Med. J.*, **ii**, 1347–1350
30. Gill, A., Yu, V. Y. H., Bajuk, B. and Astbury, J. (1986) Postnatal growth in infants born before 30 weeks gestation. *Arch. Dis. Child.*, **61**, 549–553
31. Costarino, A. and Baumgart, S. (1986) Modern fluid and electrolyte management of the critically ill premature infant. *Pediatr. Clin. North Am.*, **33**, 153–178
32. Marks, K. H., Friedman, Z. and Maisels, M. J. (1977) A simple device for reducing insensible water loss in low birth weight infants. *Pediatrics*, **60**, 223–226
33. Rutter, N. and Hull, D. (1981) Reduction of skin water loss in the newborn. I. Effect of applying topical agents. *Arch. Dis. Child.*, **56**, 669–672
34. Brice, J. E. H., Rutter, N. and Hull, D. (1981) Reduction of skin water loss in the newborn. II. Clinical trial of two methods in very low birthweight babies. *Arch. Dis. Child.*, **56**, 673–675
35. Harpin, V. A. and Rutter, N. (1985) Humidification of incubators. *Arch. Dis. Child.*, **60**, 219–224

36. Baumgart, S., Engle, W. D., Fox, W. W. and Polin, R. A. (1981) Effect of heat shielding on convection and evaporation and radiant heat transfer in premature infants. *J. Pediatr.*, **99**, 948–956
37. Baumgart, S., Fox, W. W. and Polin, R. A. (1982) Physiologic implications of two different heat shields for infants under radiant warmers. *J. Pediatr.*, **100**, 787–790
38. Baumgart, S. (1984) Reduction of oxygen consumption, insensible water loss, and radiant heat demand with use of a plastic blanket for low birthweight infants under radiant warmers. *Pediatrics*, **75**, 89–99
39. Rayner, W. (1886) Cyanosis in newly born children caused by aniline marking ink. *Br. Med. J.*, **i**, 294–295
40. Scott, E. P., Prince, G. E. and Rotando, C. C. (1946) Dye poisoning in infancy. *J. Pediatr.*, **28**, 713–718
41. Kagan, B. M., Mirman, B., Calvin, J. and Lundeen, E. (1949) Cyanosis in premature infants due to aniline dye intoxication. *J. Pediatr.*, **34**, 574–578
42. Fisch, R. O., Berglund, E. G., Bridge, A. G., Finley, P. R., Quie, P. G. and Raille, R. (1963) Methemoglobinaemia in a hospital nursery. *JAMA*, **185**, 760–763
43. Curley, A., Hawks, R. G., Kimbrough, R. D., Nathesson, G. and Finberg, L. (1971) Dermal absorption of hexachlorophene in infants. *Lancet*, **ii**, 296–297
44. Kopelman, A. E. (1973) Cutaneous absorption of hexachlorophene in low birth weight infants. *J. Pediatr.*, **82**, 972–975
45. Powell, H., Swarner, O., Gluck, L. and Lampert, P. (1973) Hexachlorophene myelinopathy in premature infants. *J. Pediatr.*, **82**, 976–981
46. Shuman, R. M., Leech, R. W. and Alvord, E. C. (1974) Neurotoxicity of hexachlorophene in the human. *Pediatrics*, **54**, 689–695
47. Chabrolle, J. P. and Rossier, A. (1978) Goitre and hypothyroidism in the newborn after cutaneous absorption of iodine. *Arch. Dis. Child.*, **53**, 495–498
48. Schick, J. B. and Milstein, J. M. (1981) Burn hazard of isopropyl alcohol in the neonate. *Pediatrics*, **68**, 587–588
49. Harpin, V. A. and Rutter, N. (1982) Percutaneous alcohol absorption and skin necrosis in a preterm infant. *Arch. Dis. Child.*, **57**, 477–479
50. Morrell, P., Hey, E., Mackee, I. W., Rutter, N. and Lewis, M. (1985) Deafness in a preterm baby associated with topical antibiotic spray containing neomycin. *Lancet*, **i**, 1167–1168
51. Aggett, P. J., Cooper, L. V., Ellis, S. H. and McAinsh, J. (1981) Percutaneous absorption of chlorhexidene in neonatal cord care. *Arch. Dis. Child.*, **56**, 878–880
52. Tregear, R. T. (1966) *Physical Functions of the Skin*, Academic Press, New York, pp. 21–37
53. Boyle, R. J. and Oh, W. (1980) Erythema following transcutaneous oxygen monitoring. *Pediatrics*, **65**, 333–334
54. Golden, S. M. (1981) Skin craters – a complication of transcutaneous oxygen monitoring. *Pediatrics*, **67**, 514–516
55. Evans, N. J. and Rutter, N. (1986) Reduction of skin damage from transcutaneous oxygen electrodes using a spray-on dressing. *Arch. Dis. Child.* **61**, 881–884
56. Cartlidge, P. H. T. and Rutter, N. (1987) Kuraya gum ECG electrodes for the preterm infant. *Arch. Dis. Child.*, **62**, 1281–1282
57. Rutter, N. (1987) Percutaneous drug absorption in the newborn: hazards and uses. *Clin. Perinatol.*, **14**, 911–930

Chapter 10

Monitoring

Peter Rolfe

Introduction

Nearly two decades ago, in the early pioneering days of neonatal monitoring, equipment manufacturers were unwittingly supplying adult monitoring systems for use with the ill newborn. Then followed a period of increasing awareness of the needs for apparatus designed specifically for the newborn, although reviews of the subject about one decade ago still lamented the inappropriate design of electrodes, cables and monitors even for something as basic as neonatal heart rate monitoring [1–3]. It was the greater importance of apnoea monitoring and arterial oxygen measurement and control in the ill preterm baby as compared to the adult which finally succeeded in focusing the attention of biomedical engineers and commercial organizations onto the subject of neonatal monitoring.

In spite of these earlier messages concerning the importance of matching monitoring systems to specific patient groups, the needs of the ELBW baby have not yet been adequately addressed. This is partly because although manufacturers have now largely adjusted to the 2500 g baby, most of them incorrectly assume that the 800 g baby cannot be very different, and in any case they mostly feel that 'the market cannot be big enough to justify special attention'!

Monitoring involves collecting a signal from the subject by means of a *transducer* or *sensor*, and displaying and recording the signal on a suitable *monitor*. The monitors themselves may often be used equally well with an 800 g baby as with a 2500 g baby, although sometimes smaller and noisier signals in the former demand better processing facilities than those which may be adequate for the latter. The sensors, on the other hand, must be quite different for the very small baby to take into account both size and the extreme fragility of the skin onto which many of the sensors will be attached. The design of optimally small sensors, and the development of safe, effective and convenient methods for their attachment, remain important but largely unsolved problems.

This review is unable to provide clear guidelines and recommendations for monitoring the very small baby; it can merely offer some suggestions and emphasize the areas in which improvements are still needed. It also provides an indication of research activities which are underway and which may eventually solve some of the outstanding problems.

Cardiorespiratory monitoring

Continuous monitoring of heart rate and breathing are, of course, still the minimum requirements for all babies in this category. The addition of continuous arterial pressure monitoring is considered essential by some, whilst others are content with intermittent measurements. The combination of heart rate and breathing monitoring has also attracted some attention as the basis of pattern analysis in so-called cardiorespirography. Numerous combinations of sensors have been developed for such monitoring, and in assessing their use for preterm babies certain conclusions may be drawn concerning their use with the very smallest babies.

ECG monitoring

Although modern electrocardiographic (ECG) monitoring techniques may be considered to be sophisticated from the electronics viewpoint, the evolution of ECG electrodes for very small babies has been a long and slow process. The earlier large and rigid electrodes have been replaced by smaller, flexible electrodes, but chemical adhesive attachment is at present an unhappy compromise. Aggressive adhesives are more likely to keep the electrode in place, but some skin damage seems inevitable, while the milder adhesives lead to annoying false alarms due to electrode detachment. However, the skin-compatible characteristics of the natural gum kuraya have been utilized for the fixation of neonatal ECG electrodes (Arbo, Henley's Medical) (see Figure 10.1). The moistened gum adheres quite well to even the smallest babies, and

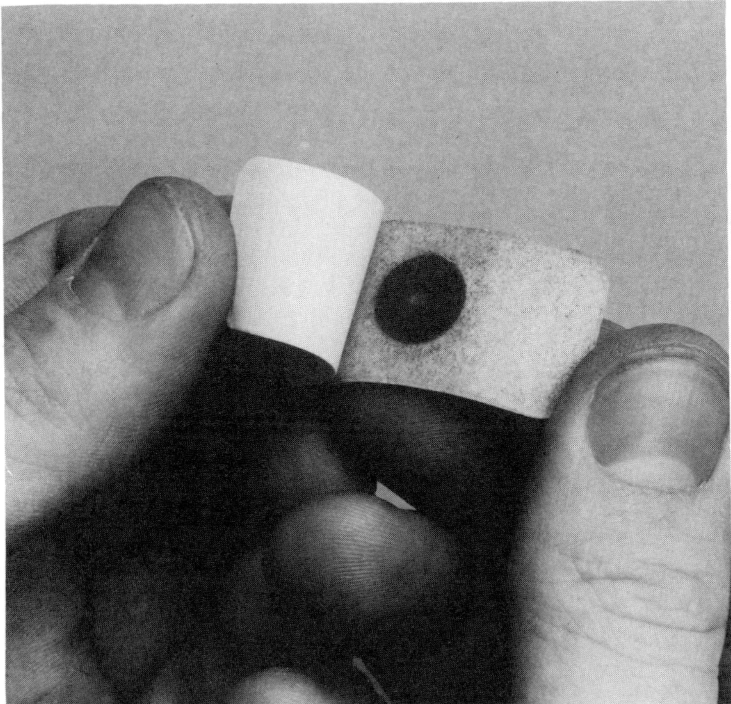

Figure 10.1 Recently introduced neonatal ECG electrode employing the natural gum kuraya for safe attachment to delicate skin

the incorporated thin silver film does not require the normal electrode-conductive gel or cream. Remoistening of the gum is needed more frequently when the baby is nursed under a radiant warmer, but the incidence of skin trauma is very low.

Most cables and leads for connecting electrodes to monitors are still not ideal. The basic arrangement of having a single relatively heavy and robust cable connected to the monitor, with a small connector block at its end for attachment of the three lighter, individual electrode leads, is a sound principle. The cable can generally withstand the harsh treatment to which it is subject in a busy neonatal unit, but electrode leads still require improvement. Very fine, light, and flexible electrode leads have some advantages for the baby under 1000 g, but they do frequently become tangled and can then make rapid access to the baby awkward and inconvenient.

Of course, once the problems of electrodes, leads and cables have been completely solved, the selection of an associated ECG and heart rate monitor has no special requirements for the ELBW baby. Nevertheless, noise and artefact produced by non-ideal electrodes and cables are less likely to be troublesome with the high quality ECG amplifiers found in monitors such as those available from, for example, Hellige and Hewlett Packard.

Future research on ECG electrodes, leads, cables and associated amplifiers and displays is undoubtedly still needed in order to produce more reliable heart rate monitoring for the very small baby. Ideally, of course, the electrode attachment and contact problem should be eliminated entirely, and there were attempts, some ten years ago, to use a thin metallized plastic plate on which to place the naked baby and thereby eliminate individual fixed electrode connections. This approach was clearly unencumbering for the baby, but signal reliability was poor. This could perhaps now be improved using modern electronic and computing techniques. An alternative approach for the elimination of electrode contact problems is to take advantage of nasogastric tubes whenever they are in place. Polymer feeding tubes can be constructed easily to incorporate small conductive 'pick-up' regions, using wire or ring elements, and very reliable oesophageal ECG monitoring can be achieved.

There is no doubt that the initial resuscitation and stabilization of the very small baby immediately following delivery could be greatly facilitated by the use of an efficient means for ECG and thus heart rate monitoring. Many approaches for the attachment of ECG electrodes have been tried for this application, including conventional adhesives, clips, clamps and even needles. The use of suction ($\sim$ 80 mmHg) applied in an annular groove around a soft plastic moulding containing a silver/silver chloride electrode has been found to be quite successful. Three of these electrodes may be placed on the resuscitation table and the baby laid directly on them, and wet skin actually improves the security of the suction attachment. The optimum design of a suction ECG electrode for this purpose has, however, not yet been produced.

Apnoea monitoring

The monitoring of breathing, primarily for apnoea detection, has improved only marginally over the past decade, and the very small baby has always presented particular problems. Once again these have largely arisen from the difficulties of constructing appropriately small, sensitive, reliable, unencumbering sensors and connecting cables. The improved ECG electrodes mentioned above (e.g. Arbo) may also be used for monitoring transthoracic electrical impedance to give a moderately reliable breathing signal. In spite of this electrode improvement further significant improvements are needed in the impedance monitors themselves to deal with movement artefacts before this method is adequate for the very small baby. A more recent technique employing abdominal surface electrodes records the diaphragm electromyogram (EMG); processing of this produces a signal which has been reported to correlate with tidal volume [4].

Dimensional changes of the chest and abdomen associated with breathing can be recorded with strain gauges, magnetometers, inflatable jackets and inductive straps [2,5–7]. However, none of these methods is ideal for the very small baby because of the necessary straps, bands or coils which must be placed around the chest or abdomen. Changes in curvature of the chest or abdominal wall during breathing can be detected by a small plastic 'pressure capsule' such as that developed by Wright and Callan [8]. This technique has acceptable performance as an apnoea detector and can be improved in terms of reliability by using two capsules, one to detect thoracic cage movement and the other abdominal movements.

The conventional lung function approach of recording intra-oesophageal pressure changes can be useful in some very small babies. Ideally, of course, an appropriate latex rubber balloon attached to a flexible plastic catheter should be used to make accurate measurements of intra-oesophageal, and thereby intrathoracic, pressure changes. However, a liquid-filled, open-ended catheter or feeding tube is almost as good for quantitative pressure monitoring, and is perfectly adequate for apnoea monitoring in the very small baby. Furthermore, the feeding tube can be further modified to carry small wire contacts to enable either EMG detection or electrical impedance monitoring of breathing via the oesophagus, and this is actually more convenient and more reliable than using surface electrodes on the chest or abdomen.

Apnoea monitoring without electrodes or other sensors attached directly to the baby first became feasible with the introduction of Lewin's air-filled multi-compartment mattress [9]. This device is still used although it lacks the sensitivity needed for very small babies. Mattress-type apnoea monitors using the same approach of detecting the weight redistribution produced by breathing have now been improved by using very sensitive, thin, pressure sensitive pads. These monitors (e.g. Draeger Medical, Eastwood and Son) perform well with the very small babies, although it is important to position the pad so that cardiac movement during apnoea does not prevent the alarm being activated.

Obstructive apnoea will not be detected by any of the methods mentioned above since all are indirect and do not sense respired gas flow. Small thermistors or thermocouples can be used to detect nasal gas flow, but this approach is not always entirely reliable and cannot easily be used as a clinical routine. Undoubtedly this is an area for further research, and consideration should perhaps be given to improved CO_2 sensors or to the use of microphones for detection of gas flow.

Arterial pressure measurement

In many centres it is still common to insert umbilical artery catheters for blood gas and pH measurement, and arterial pressure measurement via the catheter is then useful in its own right, as well as providing an important guide to catheter patency. In the very small babies it is of course necessary to use small catheters (e.g. 4 FG), and the problem of catheter lumen blockage due to thrombus formation can be significant. The phasic arterial pressure waveform can be monitored reliably through small bore catheters by means of modern low volume displacement pressure tranducers, which may be connected either direct to the luer fitting of the catheter, or at some

60 cm distance attached to saline-filled manometer tubing. Ideally the phasic pressure waveform should be displayed on a monitor screen so that smoothing and damping of the waveform due to progressive lumen blockage can be easily detected. The luer fitting transducers have been commercially available for many years [1], but only comparatively recently have single-use disposable transducers been introduced (e.g. Gould). The use of conventional blood pressure transducers (e.g. Hewlett Packard) has been greatly simplified by the introduction of disposable pressure domes, obviating the need for the cumbersome and time-consuming sterilization of the transducer which has been necessary in the past. Catheter patency can undoubtedly be improved by continuous infusion through the catheter by means of 'intra-flow' devices or similar.

In spite of these precautionary measures arterial catheters must still be regarded as potential hazards because of thrombus formation, so improved catheter materials are needed. It is now well established that plasticized polyvinyl chloride (PVC) catheters have far worse haemocompatibility characteristics than the more recently introduced material polyurethane. In spite of this PVC catheters continue to be used in many centres.

Non-invasive arterial pressure measurement is clearly desirable. Many systems are now available based on the use of limb encircling cuffs and the so-called oscillometric principle. With this technique mean arterial pressure is first measured from a measurement of the cuff pressure at which cardiac-related pulsations in the cuff reach maximum amplitude. Subsequently systolic and diastolic pressures may be obtained. These arterial pressure monitors are now widely used for semi-continuous monitoring. However, the cuff needs to be matched to the size of the baby's limb, otherwise systematic errors will be introduced. Furthermore, repeated automatic inflation of the cuff is not to be recommended in very small fragile babies with poor peripheral perfusion. Recently work has commenced on a non-invasive technique for continuous arterial pressure measurement, but further research is necessary before this technique is available for routine use [10].

Blood gas and pH measurement

The umbilical artery catheter is still widely used to allow arterial sampling for intermittent $P\text{O}_2$, $P\text{CO}_2$ and pH measurement. Laboratory blood gas analysers which have been introduced over the last five years now allow very small volumes of blood to be used, and of course this is important for the small baby. The problems associated with thrombus formation in arterial catheters have already been mentioned above, and at present these put a limitation on the time over which blood gas and pH assessment may be achieved on the basis of arterial sampling. Polyurethane catheters undoubtedly improve this problem, but substantial further research is needed to produce new polymers or surface coatings to achieve long-term haemocompatibility. This is particularly important when it is necessary to resort to the use of radial artery puncture or catheterization.

Indwelling $P\text{O}_2$ sensors have promised much over the past two decades but the reality has been disappointing. The first devices to be used in the human newborn (Figure 10.2) gave very exciting indications of abrupt changes and short-term trends in arterial $P\text{O}_2$ (Figure 10.3), in spite of the fact that these devices were based on PVC catheters and membranes which are now known to be inferior. Since those early days more is demanded of the performance of arterial $P\text{O}_2$ sensors in terms of reliability, stability and safety, and it seems clear that there is no suitable device commercially

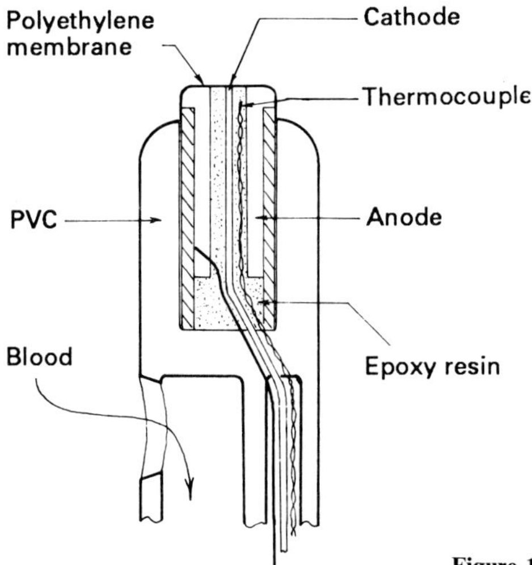

Figure 10.2 Oxygen cell with integral thermocouple (see [36])

available for use in the ELBW baby. Once again the key to success will be the utilization of modern polymers to construct 3.5–4.0 FG catheter tip $P\text{O}_2$ sensors, together with the incorporation of haemocompatible gas-permeable membranes for the active part of the sensor. Fibreoptic catheter oximeters are available for continuous arterial oxygen saturation monitoring (e.g. Oximetrix). These are available in 4 FG catheters, and the use of polyurethane together with an end-sampling eye produces quite good haemocompatible features.

The use of oxygen saturation for the control of arterial oxygen levels in the small

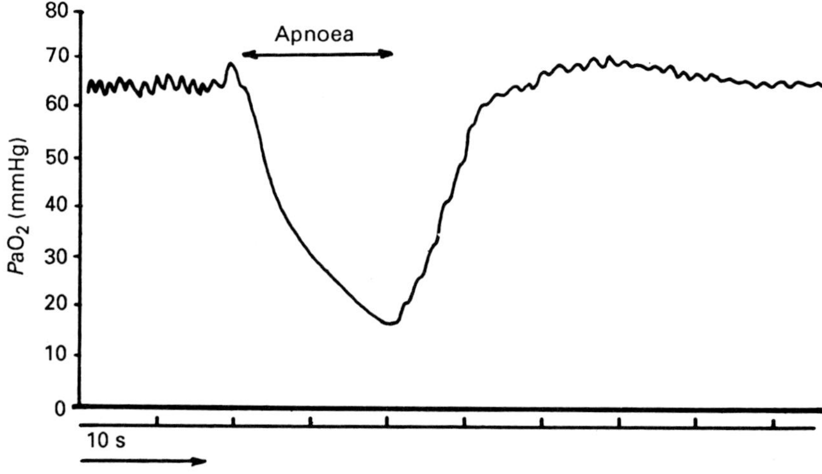

Figure 10.3 Recording from a rapid-response umbilical artery $P\text{O}_2$ sensor

preterm baby is not entirely satisfactory. The 'S' shape oxyhaemoglobin binding curve means that at relatively high levels of oxygenation very small changes in saturation accompany very large changes in oxygen partial pressure. The prevention of hyperoxaemia in terms of oxygen partial pressure is therefore very demanding of precision and accuracy in oxygen saturation measurement. This situation is worsened by the significant 'left-shifting' of the binding curve by fetal haemoglobin. Thus if one's clinical approach is to achieve control of arterial $P\text{O}_2$ by O_2 saturation monitoring it is essential, firstly, to determine the precise position of the oxyhaemoglobin binding curve and, secondly, to ensure that the precision and accuracy of the oximeter is adequate.

The direct arterial monitoring of $P\text{CO}_2$ and pH in the small newborn baby is not yet feasible as a clinical routine. Catheter tip sensors have been described in the literature [11], but as yet these have not been refined sufficiently to overcome the major problems of stability and freedom from thrombogenesis. It is possible that optical sensors based on spectrophotometric and fluorimetric techniques will eventually produce invasive sensors for $P\text{O}_2$, $P\text{CO}_2$ and pH.

Non-invasive estimation of arterial $P\text{O}_2$ and $P\text{CO}_2$ using so-called transcutaneous techniques can be used to complement intermittent arterial blood sampling. The relationships between skin surface and arterial values of $P\text{O}_2$ and $P\text{CO}_2$ are, of course, influenced by epidermal thickness and gas permeability as well as many other factors. In the very small preterm baby this leads to skin surface $P\text{O}_2$ values which may be approximately 10% above arterial $P\text{O}_2$ in the range 8–12 kPa (60–90 mmHg). Early theoretical work by Thunstrom, Stafford and Severinghaus [12] and Lubbers [13], together with more recent clinical results, has emphasized the fact that the skin surface/arterial $P\text{O}_2$ relationship is non-linear, the skin surface $P\text{O}_2$ being significantly lower than arterial $P\text{O}_2$ when it is above about 13 kPa (100 mmHg).

The electrical heating of skin surface gas sensors is critically important and can be problematical. On the one hand adequate heating of the skin is necessary to induce the maximal vasodilatation which is essential for the $P\text{O}_2$ measurement to be independent of moderate fluctuations in cutaneous perfusion. On the other hand the preterm baby's skin can be very sensitive to the required heating, and this necessitates the sensor being moved to a new site every 1–2 h depending upon the size of the baby. A skin surface temperature of 42°C is probably optimal in very small babies, but it is often not appreciated that the sensor temperature which is set on the associated monitor may be as much as 2°C higher than the skin surface temperature achieved beneath the sensor. This temperature gradient between the sensor and the skin surface also varies according to the precise design of the sensor and will therefore differ from manufacturer to manufacturer. For these reasons it is essential for centres to evaluate the overall performance which is being achieved with the sensors, instrumentation and protocols being employed.

Skin surface $P\text{CO}_2$ monitoring is by no means as widely used as skin surface $P\text{O}_2$ monitoring. Generally the sensor temperature is less critical for $P\text{CO}_2$ monitoring, although maximal vasodilatation must still be achieved. Once again it is essential for individual centres to establish their own protocols for this method to produce useful information.

When both skin surface $P\text{O}_2$ and $P\text{CO}_2$ are to be monitored there is a certain practical advantage in employing a single sensor which combines means for both $P\text{O}_2$ and $P\text{CO}_2$ measurement (e.g. Radiometer). This of course reduces the number of devices which must be attached to the relatively small exposed surface area of the baby, and furthermore it is obviously much less demanding in terms of sensor calibration, membrane changing, and application site rotation.

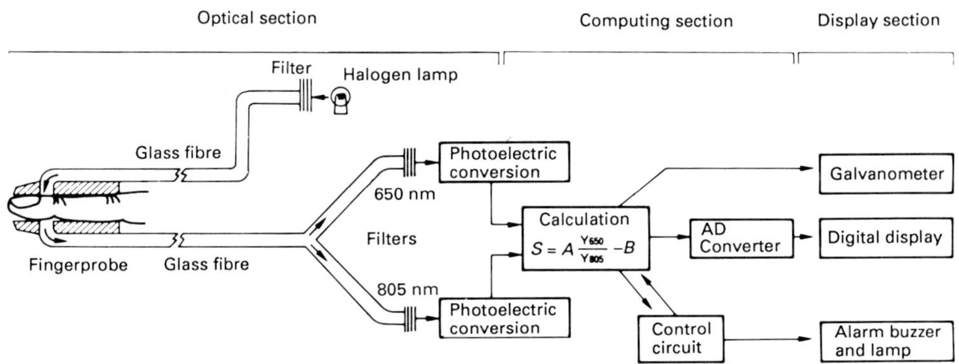

Figure 10.4 Diagrammatic scheme for measurement of arterial oxygen saturation by pulse oximetry (From [14] with permission)

There is now considerable interest in the use of non-invasive techniques for arterial oxygen saturation measurement by means of so-called pulse oximetry. This method, originally developed for use in adults [14], utilizes the pulsatile blood volume change in a digit or palm to calculate, spectrophotometrically, oxygen saturation. The method has become popular because it is very much easier to use than conventional transcutaneous gas monitoring (Figure 10.4). The sensors do not need to be heated and the optical sensors are much more stable than the electrochemical sensors for $P\text{O}_2$ and $P\text{CO}_2$ measurement. However, pulse oximetry should be used with caution in preterm babies due to the limitations imposed by the shape of the oxyhaemoglobin binding curve at high levels of oxygenation referred to above. The precision and accuracy of the various commercially available pulse oximeters has not yet been established in detail, and it is therefore not clear at what level of oxygen saturation nominal safety thresholds should be set. Once again there is an urgent need for users to assess the performance and limitations of the means which they employ before basing clinical management on the data derived.

Cerebral monitoring

There have been significant research activities over the past decade focusing on the problems of cerebral haemorrhage and hypoxic ischaemic brain injury. Some interesting new methodologies have emerged, although most of these remain research tools and do not play a major part in routine clinical monitoring. This situation is likely to continue until it becomes firmly established that there is some real benefit to clinical management through the monitoring of one or more of the relevant variables. Beyond the obvious importance of detecting such abnormalities as haemorrhage or hydrocephalus using appropriate scanning methods (see Chapter 19), there continues to be interest in the investigation and assessment of cerebral circulation. In this respect the study of intracranial pressure and cerebral blood flow are relevant.

Intracranial pressure (ICP) monitoring

Knowledge of mean arterial pressure and intracranial pressure allows the cerebral perfusion pressure to be calculated, and this can be important in deciding whether or not some intervention is required to ensure adequate cerebral perfusion. Invasive and non-invasive techniques have been used in small preterm babies with varying degrees of success. Levene and Evans [15] have evolved an invasive technique for the newborn which had originally been developed for adult monitoring by Lundberg [16]. The method involves passing a 16 G intravenous cannula through the lateral margin of the anterior fontanelle into the subarachnoid space. Pressure is then measured via the cannula, either with a miniature luer fitting pressure tranducer or by a conventional blood pressure transducer connected to the cannula by a saline-filled manometer tube. Several groups of infants have been monitored with this invasive technique, and in a small group of babies who had failed to develop regular breathing immediately after birth and who had convulsions and were being mechanically ventilated, maximum pressures ranged from 10–48 mmHg (13.6–65.3 cmH_2O) [15]. Using this method, babies with ICP raised above 10 mmHg (13.6 cmH_2O) were treated with mannitol or dexamethasone [17].

Although when used with great care the invasive technique is an acceptable method for deriving important clinical data, an appropriate non-invasive technique must be preferred in terms of both safety and convenience. Many attempts have been made since the late 1960s to develop satisfactory sensors which might be attached to the anterior fontanelle to derive a reliable estimate of ICP. The very earliest sensors [18] were relatively large, and were held manually in place over the anterior fontanelle to make single measurements. The principle utilized by these and subsequent non-invasive sensors is that of applanation. With this method the bulging fontanelle is flattened by the sensor, and in this situation the externally applied pressure exactly balances the ICP. Continuous non-invasive ICP monitoring became more of a reality when the Ladd miniature sensor became available [19]. This sensor was originally developed for invasive monitoring in adults, but may be fixed to the anterior fontanelle in very small babies. However the method of fixation is not straightforward and can introduce errors [20] and furthermore the system is high cost. A small pneumatic sensor was developed [21] and this had the advantage of being low cost, although quantitative performance has not been good [22]. The refinement of a sensor originally developed for non-invasive intravenous pressure in adults has now been found to give good correlations with direct invasive measurements as no errors are associated with attachment, and it is very low cost [23] (Figure 10.5*a* and *b*). This sensor is small and light, is attached with collodion to the anterior fontanelle, and allows continuous monitoring of pressure for several days if necessary.

Cerebral blood flow

A knowledge of arterial pressure and of intracranial pressure is useful in making assessments of cerebral perfusion. However there has long been a desire for a method with which cerebral blood flow could be monitored continuously in small newborn babies. It is still the case that no method exists which will allow such continuous monitoring, although for research purposes it is possible to use one or more of a range of methods to obtain some information [24]. Of the available methods, Doppler ultrasound and cranial electrical impedance are the two which are most likely to allow clinical monitoring to any extent.

It is relatively straightforward to use Doppler ultrasound systems to obtain a qualitative indication of short-term pulsatile changes of arterial or venous blood velocity. Small ultrasound sensors can be positioned to direct a beam of ultrasound at the carotid arteries, the jugular veins, the anterior cerebral arteries, the sagittal sinus, and the middle cerebral artery. In order to derive a quantitative measure of

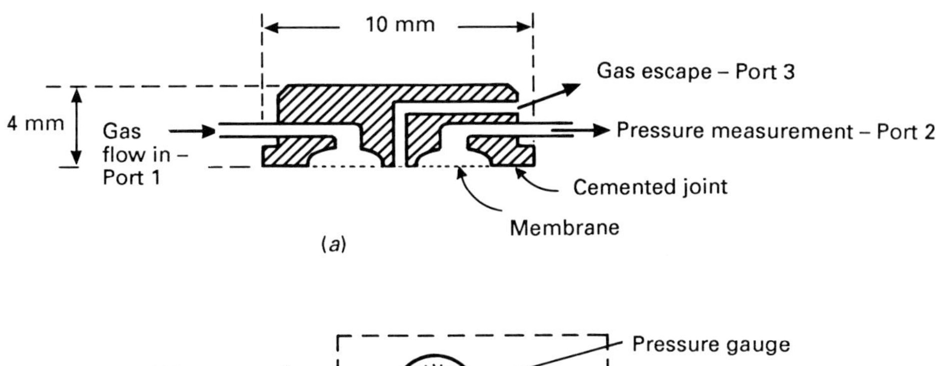

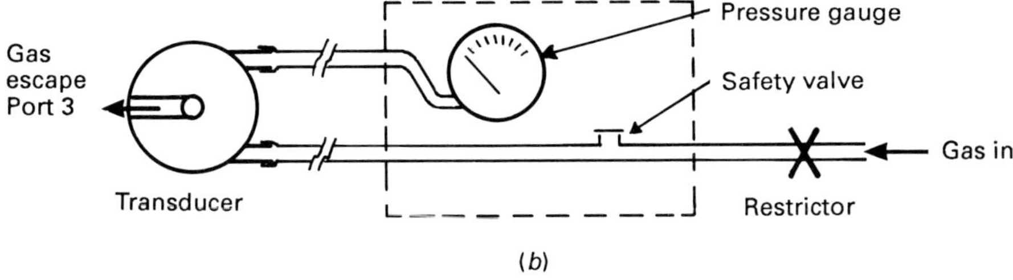

Figure 10.5 (*a*) and (*b*) Diagrammatic representation of sensor for measurement of intracranial pressure

volumetric blood flow (i.e. ml/100 g/min) it is essential to know the angle between the ultrasound beam and the direction of blood flow, the internal diameter of the blood vessel, including pulsatile changes throughout the cardiac cycle, and the distribution of blood flow across the vessel diameter – the velocity profile. Some of these problems can be overcome when the Doppler ultrasound system is combined with a real-time ultrasound scanner to produce the so-called Duplex system. In the very small preterm baby it is important to be sure that the resolution of the Doppler ultrasound system is adequate for the very small blood vessels of interest. The ultrasound scanner allows beam-vessel angle to be determined, as well as enabling individual vessels to be visualized and the depth selectivity of so-called range-gated systems to be adjusted optimally. Nevertheless, in the very small baby lateral and depth resolution of the ultrasound system may be inadequate to separate flow in adjacent vessels. Research and development in this field continues, and improvements to resolution and to the methods of processing the Doppler signals are being made. In the absence of quantitative measures there have been attempts to derive indices from the blood velocity waveforms, e.g. pulsatility index, but these must be used with caution [25].

The electrical impedance of the head, measured with four small EEG-type electrodes, is determined by the relative proportions of the main components, i.e. scalp, skull, CSF, brain tissue, blood. Accumulation of blood in the lateral ventricles will produce a change in the electrical impedance, and this may be detected by an impedance monitor, or may be displayed as a crude image using electrical impedance imaging techniques [25,26]. With each cardiac cycle there is a small reduction in the electrical impedance of the head due to the pulsatile blood volume increase. By means of computer processing techniques this signal can be monitored for several days continuously [27]. Thus pulsatile impedance signal has been found to exhibit a useful correlation with other non-invasive estimates of cerebral blood flow, and at present this method is the one which most closely approaches the requirement of a routine

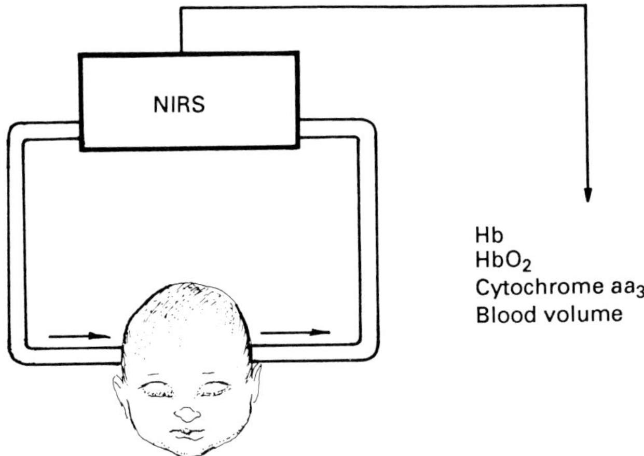

Figure 10.6 Measurement of cerebral metabolism by near infrared spectroscopy (NIRS)

clinical monitor although it must be emphasized that it cannot provide quantitative measures of cerebral blood flow.

Cerebral metabolism

There has been considerable interest in the investigation of cerebral metabolism in connection with brain haemorrhage and hypoxic ischaemic brain injury. Magnetic resonance spectroscopy (MRS) can provide important information on the relevant phosphorus-linked compounds involved in intracellular metabolic processes [28]. However, MRS does not allow clinical monitoring and there is therefore more hope in the prospect of using the emerging technique of near infrared spectroscopy [29]. This method involves passing near infrared energy at four wavelengths through the head and measuring the absorption by oxy- and deoxyhaemoglobin and by the key respiratory enzyme cytochrome aa_3. Processing of the signals allows estimation of cerebral oxygen saturation, changes of cerebral blood volume, and changes in the redox state of cytochrome aa_3 (Figure 10.6). Optical fibres are attached to the baby's head in order to make the measurements, and improvements to the method of attachment are needed before long-term continuous monitoring can be achieved. Since cytochrome aa_3 is responsible for the utilization of 95% of cellular oxygen in the brain, continuous monitoring could possibly provide a more pertinent guide to oxygen therapy and the general management of very small babies at risk of haemorrhage and hypoxic ischaemic injury [30–35].

Multiple sensors

There is clearly an advantage when monitoring the baby under 1000 g to consider the use of sensors in which a single device may contain the means for measuring more than one variable. This approach means that less space is required on the baby for attachment of sensors, and also less time is needed by nursing and clinical staff for sensor attachment and subsequent management. There have already been some attempts to produce multiple sensors, but most of these have not yet been produced as commercially available devices.

The multiple sensor [36] consists of a biluminal catheter with a PO_2 sensor and a thermocouple at its tip, blood pressure being measured through one catheter lumen and heart rate derived from the phasic blood pressure waveform.

Combined PO_2 and PCO_2 sensors have been produced for both invasive and non-invasive use. Parker, Delpy and Reynolds [37] described a catheter sensor which contained a PO_2 electrode and a pH electrode for indirect PCO_2 measurement. Combined O_2/CO_2 transcutaneous sensors are now available commercially.

It has long been recognized in adult monitoring that the placement of devices within the oesophagus can form the basis of reliable monitoring. As mentioned above, neonatal feeding tubes can be modified to contain ECG electrodes and these may also be used simultaneously for electrical impedance monitoring of breathing activity. The feeding tube may also contain a thermocouple or thermistor for core temperature monitoring. The lumen of the feeding tube can be used to monitor oesophageal pressure changes associated with breathing. In the adult it has also proved possible to include ultrasound crystals to measure aortic blood flow.

Transillumination of the neonatal head with near infrared energy has the potential to provide circulatory, blood gas and metabolic information. The attachment of optical fibre bundles, one either side of the head, could be combined with a pair of ECG electrodes and a temperature sensor, thus providing a great deal of the information needed for routine monitoring.

Conclusions

The most important difference between monitoring techniques for babies less than and greater than 1000 g relates to the sensors required for detecting the variables of interest. Improvements have occurred in recent years such as the design of ECG electrodes and their attachment, but significant improvements are still required. The limited surface area available for the attachment of external sensors is a strong motivation for the development of multiple sensors which, in a single device, have means for detecting several variables. The very real problem of attaching any sensor to the skin surface is also an incentive to develop improved biocompatible materials for multiple sensor devices for use in the umbilical artery, the oesophagus and attached to the head. Successful research and development along these lines must then, of course, be followed by effective commercialization in order that the approach may be widely adopted. This must be the focus of attention during the coming decade as the task of monitoring ELBW babies becomes more common.

References

1. Rolfe, P. (1975) Monitoring in newborn intensive care. *Biomed. Eng.*, **10**, 339–404, 413
2. Rolfe, P. (1976) Monitoring equipment for the neonate. *Br. J. Hosp. Med.*, **1**, 189–205
3. Rolfe, P. (1977) Instruments for the care of ill newborn babies. *Electronics and Power*, **23**, 32–39
4. O'Brien, M. J. *et al.* (1983) Monitoring respiratory activity in infants – a non-intrusive diaphragm EMG technique. In *Non-Invasive Physiological Measurements*, Vol. 2 (ed. P. Rolfe), Academic Press, London pp. 131–177

5. Rolfe, P. (1986) Neonatal critical care monitoring. *J. Med Eng. Technol.*, **10**, 115–120
6. Milner, A. D. (1970) The respiratory jacket. *Lancet*, **i**, 80
7. Milledge, J. S. and Stott, M. (1977) Inductive plethysmography – a new respiratory transducer. *J. Physiol.*, **267**, 4P–5P
8. Wright, B. M. and Callan, K. (1979) A new respiratory recording and monitoring system. In *ISAM*, Academic Press, London, pp. 329–335
9. Lewin, J. E. (1969) An apnoea alarm mattress. *Lancet*, **ii**, 667
10. Rolfe, P., Kanjilal, P. P., Murphy, C. and Burton, P. J. (1987) Continuous non-invasive beat-by-beat blood pressure (BP) measurement in the newborn. In *Proceedings of the 3rd International Symposium on Continuous Transcutaneous Monitoring, Zurich*, (eds G. Rooth, A. Huch and R. Huch), Plenum Press, New York, pp. 128–132
11. Peterson, J. I., Fitzgerald, R. V. and Buckhold, D. K. (1984) Fibreoptic probe for *in vivo* measurement of oxygen partial pressure. *Anal. Chem.*, **56**, 62–67
12. Thunstrom, A. M., Stafford, M. J. and Severinghaus, J. W. (1979) A two temperature, two Po_2 method of estimating the determinants of tcPo_2. In *Continuous Transcutaneous Blood Gas Monitoring* (eds A. Huch, R. Huch and J. F. Lucey), Alan R. Liss Inc., New York, pp. 167–182
13. Lubbers, D. W. (1979) Cutaneous and transcutaneous Po_2 and Pco_2 and their measuring conditions. In *Continuous Transcutaneous Blood Gas Monitoring* (eds A. Huch, R. Huch and J. F. Lucey), Alan R. Liss Inc., New York, pp. 13–31
14. Yoshiya, I., Shimada, Y. and Tanaka, K. (1980) Spectrophotometric monitoring of arterial oxygen saturation in the fingertip. *Med. Biol. Eng. Comput.*, **18**, 27–32
15. Levene, M. I. and Evans, D. H. (1983) Continuous measurement of subarachnoid pressure in the severely asphyxiated newborn. *Arch. Dis. Child.*, **58**, 1013–1015
16. Lundberg, N. (1960) Continuous recording and control of ventricular fluid pressure in neurosurgical practice. *Acta Psychiatr. Neurol. Scand.*, **36** (Suppl. 149), 1–193
17. Levene, M. I. and Evans, D. H. (1986) Direct measurement of intracranial pressure in the newborn. In *Neonatal Physiological Measurements* (ed. P. Rolfe), Butterworths, London, pp. 174–179
18. Robinson, R. O., Rolfe, P. and Sutton, P. (1977) Non-invasive method for measuring intracranial pressure in normal newborn infants. *Dev. Med. Child Neurol.*, **19**, 305–308
19. Vidyasagar, D. and Raju, T. N. K. (1977) A simple non-invasive technique of measuring intracranial pressure in the newborn. *Pediatrics*, **59**, 957–961
20. Horbar, J. D., Yeager, S., Philip, A. G. S. and Lucey, J. F. (1980) Effect of application force on non-invasive measurements of intracranial pressure. *Pediatrics*, **66**, 455–457
21. Whitelaw, A. G. L. and Wright, B. M. (1982) A pneumatic applanimeter for intracranial pressure measurements. *J. Physiol.*, **336**, 3–4
22. Kaiser, A. M., Whitelaw, A. G. L. and Besag, F. M. C. (1986) An evaluation of fontanelle pressure measurements. In *Neonatal Physiological Measurements* (ed. P. Rolfe), Butterworths, London, pp. 167–173
23. Rochefort, M. J., Rolfe, P. and Wilkinson, A. R. (1986) Non-invasive continuous estimation of intracranial pressure in the newborn by a new pneumatic applanation fontanometer. *Arch. Dis. Child.*, **62**, 152–155.
24. Rolfe, P., Persson, B. and Zetterstrom, R. (1983) An appraisal of techniques for studying cerebral circulation in the newborn. *Acta Paediatr. Scand.*, (Suppl.) **311**, 5–13
25. Tarassenko, L. and Rolfe, P. (1984) Electrical impedance tomography: a new method to image the head continuously in the newborn. *Proceedings of the 6th Nordic Meeting on Medical and Biological Engineering*, (ed. Ake Oberg), IFMBE, Linkoping, pp.84–88
26. Tarassenko, L. and Rolfe, P. (1984) Imaging distributions of electrical resistivity; an alternative approach. *Electronics Lett.*, **20**, 574–575
27. Murphy, D., Tarassenko, L., Barry, J. and Rolfe, P. (1986) Digital processing of the impedance plethysmogram. In *Progress Reports on Electronics in Medicine and Biology* (ed. K. Copeland), The Institution of Electronic and Radio Engineers, London pp. 217–224
28. Hope, P. L., Costello, A. M. de L., Cady, E. B. *et al.* (1986) Cerebral metabolism in newborn infants studied by phosphorus nuclear magnetic resonance spectroscopy. In *Neonatal Physiological Measurements* (ed. P. Rolfe), Butterworths, London, pp. 382–389

29. Rea, P. A., Crowe, J., Wickramasinghe, Y. and Rolfe, P. (1985) Non-invasive optical methods for the study of cerebral metabolism in the human newborn: a technique for the future? *J. Med. Eng. Technol.*, **9**, 160–166
30. Crowe, J., Rea, P. A., Wickramasinghe, Y. and Rolfe, P. (1986) Towards non-invasive monitoring of cerebral metabolism. In *Neonatal Physiological Measurements* (ed. P. Rolfe), Butterworths, London, pp. 150–156
31. Wickramasinghe, Y., Crowe, J. and Rolfe, P. (1985) Optical method adaptable for cerebral monitoring in the newborn. *Med. Biol. Eng. Comput.*, **23**, 468–469
32. Wickramasinghe, Y., Crowe, J. and Rolfe, P. (1986) Laser source and detector with signal processor for a near infra-red medical application. In *Progress Reports on Electronics in Medicine and Biology*, (ed. K. Copeland), The Institution of Electronic and Radio Engineers, pp. 209–215
33. Wickramasinghe, Y, Crowe, J. and Rolfe, P. (1986) Near infra-red technique for monitoring metabolism and blood oxygen saturation. *Proceedings of the Eighth Annual Conference of the IEEE Engineering in Medicine and Biology Society* (Dallas, Fort Worth), (eds C. J. Robinson and G. V. Krondaske), IEEE, Piscataway, New Jersey. pp. 1172–1174
34. Wyatt, J. S., Cope, M., Delpy, D. T., Wray, S. and Reynolds, E. O. R. (1986) Quantification of cerebral oxygenation and haemodynamics in sick newborn infants by near infra-red spectroscopy. *Lancet*, **ii**, 1063
35. Brazy, J. E., Lewis D. V., Mitnick, M. H. and Jobsis, F. E. (1985) Noninvasive monitoring of cerebral oxygenation in preterm infants: preliminary observations. *Pediatrics*, **75**, 217
36. Rolfe, P. (1976) Arterial oxygen measurement in the newborn with intravascular transducers. In *IEE Medical Electronics Monographs*, Nos. 18–22, Vol. 4, (eds D. W. Hill and B. Watson), Peter Peregrine Ltd, Stevenage
37. Parker, D., Delpy, D. and Reynolds, E. O. R. (1979) Single electrochemical sensor for transcutaneous measurement of Po_2 and Pco_2. In *National Foundation – Birth Defects: Original Article Series*, Vol. XV (4), (eds A. Huch, R. Huch and J. F. Lucey), A. R. Liss, New York pp. 109–116

Chapter 11

Jaundice

Neena Modi

Jaundice is common in the LBW baby in whom, unlike the mature neonate, it may persist for up to four weeks. Approximately 60% of babies of less than 2000 g birth weight develop a serum bilirubin in excess of 170 µmol/l [1] with peak levels on the fourth and fifth days of life. Current management, with early therapeutic intervention at lower bilirubin levels, makes it difficult to assess the natural history of jaundice in infants weighing less than 1000 g.

Physiology

The development of jaundice is influenced by most of the factors also found in more mature infants [2] though there are differences. Physiological jaundice in the term infant results primarily from a combination of increased bilirubin load and immaturity of the hepatic functions of uptake, conjugation and excretion [3]. In preterm infants increased bilirubin production, due to ineffective erythropoiesis and accelerated turnover of non-erythropoietic haem such as the cytochromes, does not appear to be as important [3]. However bruising does occur more readily; preterm red blood cells have a life span of approximately 40 days [4] in contrast to 70 days in the term infant [5] and 120 days in the adult; a hypocaloric intake is common in the first few days of life and the slow intestinal transit time increases the effect of the enterohepatic circulation. Of hepatic functions the major deficiency in the preterm infant is immaturity of UDP-glucuronyl transferase activity [3]. Though rhesus isoimmunization may pose a significant problem, the red blood cells of very immature infants have a reduced ABH antigenicity [4] and these infants are unlikely to develop haemolysis in the presence of ABO incompatibility.

Toxicity

The yellow staining of the cerebral nuclei, originally termed kernicterus by Schmorl [6], is believed to be the pathological correlate of bilirubin encephalopathy, a phrase coined by Zetterstrom and Ernster [7] to describe the clinical syndrome of bilirubin toxicity. Clinical manifestations of bilirubin neurotoxicity, both acute and long-term, and pathological findings present a relatively clear picture in the mature infant, but a simple extrapolation to the extremely immature baby has not proved possible. In this group the risk that hyperbilirubinaemia poses is a matter of current controversy [8–10].

Acute manifestations

In the term infant, acute bilirubin toxicity is manifest as initial lethargy and hypotonia, followed by irritability, hypertonia, temperature instability, convulsions and opisthotonos, and it may progress to death [11]. Clinical assessment of ELBW babies is frequently impossible because of paralysis for ventilation. Even in infants who are not paralysed, clinical assessment is unlikely to be sufficiently sensitive; even major disturbances such as convulsive activity occur far more frequently than are recognized clinically. In sick infants the possible influences upon behavioural changes are numerous and could not reliably be attributed to changes in bilirubin concentration.

Late sequelae

The classical syndrome of post-icteric encephalopathy – the tetrad of high tone deafness, impairment of upward gaze, athetoid cerebral palsy and dental dysplasia [12] – is rarely seen in ELBW survivors, nor does a conclusive picture emerge from attempts to evaluate the risk of brain damage due to hyperbilirubinaemia from follow-up studies. Though the spectrum of bilirubin-related brain damage probably does include subtle manifestations [13], the absence of a distinctive syndrome makes it difficult to attribute a given abnormality of the brain to bilirubin toxicity rather than to some other adverse influence. Duara *et al.* [14], in a follow-up study to detect sensorineural hearing loss in infants discharged from a tertiary care centre, found that birth weight of less than 1500 g, perinatal asphyxia and respiratory illness emerged as significant risk factors, but a serum bilirubin exceeding 225 μmol/l did not. Conversely Bergman *et al.* [15] found in a study of bilateral hearing loss in less than 1500 g survivors that maximum serum bilirubin emerged as a significant predictor on multivariate testing. They make the additional point that as 61% of the infants with hearing loss had no additional disability, the influence of hypoxia, ischaemia or haemorrhage was unlikely to have been contributory.

Pape *et al.* [16], in a follow-up study of 43 infants of birth weight less than 1000 g of whom only one had a serum bilirubin in excess of 255 μmol/l, found no association between peak serum bilirubin and poor neurological outcome. Other authors, studying a wider range of low birth weight infants, also found no significant association between serum bilirubin and developmental outcome [17–20]. Hyman *et al.* [21] and Koch *et al.* [22] found such an association only with total serum bilirubin levels in excess of 340 μmol/l. Naeye [23] and Scheidt *et al.* [24] described an association at levels of total serum bilirubin from 120 μmol/l and 170 μmol/l. The latter authors, however, failed to present convincing evidence in those less than 1500 g and, in addition, stated that 'birth weight and gestational age appear to be more powerful determinants of poor test performance than maximum serum bilirubin'.

The clinical studies of the past must be interpreted with caution. No allowance was made or, given the knowledge of the day, could have been made, for obvious confounders such as the adverse effect on neurological outcome of hypoxia, ischaemia and haemorrhage. Though associations between hyperbilirubinaemia of varying degree and poor outcome may exist, association should not be allowed to imply causation. It has been shown, for example, that infants with intraventricular haemorrhage have higher serum bilirubin levels [25]. Developmental studies have further drawbacks – the long follow-up period results inevitably in high drop out rates and as small changes in outcome are being studied in the face of many variables, only an extremely large study would have the statistical power to detect significance.

Pathological findings

Following the recognition of a serum bilirubin of 340 μmol/l as the level requiring intervention in the full-term baby with haemolytic disease, reports appeared suggesting increased susceptibility to bilirubin toxicity in preterm infants [26–28]. The impetus to intervene earlier was provided by accounts of *post mortem* kernicterus in immature babies without haemolysis, with peak total serum bilirubin levels of less than 340 μmol/l [29–31]. Ritter *et al.* [32] described such an infant with a peak serum bilirubin of 45 μmol/l and Gartner *et al.* [33], going one better, two such babies with no jaundice. These *post mortem* diagnoses vary in the extent to which various histological changes such as neuronal degeneration, demyelination and gliosis were demonstrated in addition to macroscopic staining and the extent to which these features reflect clinical morbidity is therefore unclear [34,35]. Macroscopic staining may simply represent bilirubin uptake by previously damaged neural tissue, a point which was recognized in the early accounts of kernicterus [36]. Yellow staining has now been produced experimentally in rats without associated EEG evidence of encephalopathy [37]. Turkel *et al.* [38], comparing 32 matched pairs of infants with and without yellow staining of the basal ganglia, found no significant difference in 'risk factors', clinical course and bilirubin levels between the two groups and concluded that yellow staining could not be equated with clinical toxicity. Additionally the absence of staining may not preclude clinical disease: Perl *et al.* [39] have demonstrated acute clinical toxicity suggestive of classical bilirubin encephalopathy in newborn rabbits without staining. The conclusion in the ELBW infants must be that the incidence of bilirubin toxicity cannot be assessed from *post mortem* findings.

Risk factors

'Risk factors' such as acidosis, asphyxia, hypercarbia and hypothermia were purported to increase the likelihood of bilirubin encephalopathy [29–31,33] in the preterm infant. It is notable that these studies all related to ill babies and took no account of other possible influences leading to an adverse outcome. Attempts to define infants at greater risk on the basis of the presence of 'risk factors' have proved unsuccessful [32,40–42] but decisions regarding intervention points in clinical practice often incorporate the presence or absence of such factors and the level of free or unbound bilirubin. The rationale for this lies in current concepts regarding the mechanism of bilirubin toxicity.

Free bilirubin

Bilirubin depresses cellular respiration, uncouples oxidative phosphorylation at mitochondrial level [7,43] and inhibits numerous enzyme systems. Two theories exist to explain the initial toxic step, believed to be the passage of bilirubin into neural tissue. The *free bilirubin theory* is based on the hypothesis that the albumin/bilirubin complex in plasma is non-diffusible and that therefore only free bilirubin is toxic with albumin exerting its protective effect so long as its molar concentration is more than that of bilirubin. The increased vulnerability of very immature infants may in part be due to albumin levels that are lower and a low bilirubin binding capacity [44,45]. Sulphonamides, which are known to increase the toxicity of bilirubin [46], displace bilirubin from albumin and the higher risk of toxicity in haemolytic compared to non-haemolytic jaundice is attributed to competitive binding by haematin. Free fatty acids, also bound by albumin, are increased during hypoxia, hypothermia, hypoglycaemia and sepsis. Serious illness in preterm babies is associated with a reduced bilirubin binding capacity and affinity and an increased risk of *post mortem* kernicterus [47]. Attempts have therefore been made to correlate free bilirubin levels or assessment of bilirubin binding capacity and bilirubin affinity with clinical outcome with a view to using such measurements in deciding intervention points. This has proved a disappointing exercise, not least because of the number of binding tests in use, of which Cashore [48] has provided a useful review.

Zamet *et al.* [49] found an association between free bilirubin and kernicterus diagnosed clinically and at post-mortem examination, and furthermore an increased susceptibility in preterm infants to raised free bilirubin concentrations. Odell *et al.* [20], studying infants of less than 1500 g birth weight at the age of five years, found a significant correlation between neurological abnormalities and the saturation of serum proteins. Nakamura *et al.* [50] have shown abnormalities in the auditory brainstem-evoked responses in term neonates to be related to the level of unbound bilirubin. However Ritter *et al.*, [32], also using a *post mortem* diagnosis of kernicterus in a study of infants less than 1500 g, found no difference in free bilirubin between those affected and those not affected. In so far as a practical application is concerned, the concept of a stable concentration of free bilirubin that may be reliably measured would appear simplistic: albumin binding is reversible with bound and free bilirubin molecules continuously undergoing exchange. Certain other observations are also inconsistent with the free bilirubin theory alone; analbuminaemic humans do not develop kernicterus [51] and the concentration of bilirubin in the brains of Gunn rats does not correlate with serum free bilirubin.

Blood-brain barrier

The second theory proposes that all that is necessary are the appropriate physical conditions at cell membrane level permitting the passage of albumin bound bilirubin – the *opening of the blood-brain barrier hypothesis*. Barrier 'opening' occurs in several disease states such as meningitis, hyperosmolality and hypoxia and may be produced experimentally [52]. Though there is evidence to support the widely held belief that the blood-brain barrier matures with postnatal age [53], classical kernicterus has developed in older infants and children with glucose-6-phosphate deficiency and Crigler-Najjar syndrome. Albumin bound bilirubin may be shown to enter the brain during experimental opening [54]. However, whether any ensuing brain dysfunction is due to bilirubin itself or whether it is due to the underlying pathological precipitant, with bilirubin merely serving as a coloured marker of opening, is undecided. Wennberg and Hance [37], have shown that bilirubin staining in a rat model, without EEG changes of encephalopathy, occurred when the blood-brain barrier was open but that blood-brain barrier opening in association with an increased free bilirubin concentration maximized the risk of encephalopathy.

A question that has not been examined is that of variations in cell susceptibility to a given bilirubin load under varying clinical conditions.

Objective assessment of neurological function

Little exists in the way of objective assessment of neurological function in the newborn. Abnormalities in the acoustic properties of the cry of hyperbilirubinaemic infants have been found [55] and recently there has been interest in the role of brain-evoked responses. Abnormalities in auditory-evoked responses attributable to hyperbilirubinaemia have been documented in otherwise well infants [50,56,57]. Of interest is that each of these authors stresses both the variability of susceptibility and the transient nature of the abnormality. The latter observation suggests an initial reversible phase of bilirubin toxicity. Ahlfors *et al.* [58], studying rhesus primate newborns, while stressing variable susceptibility, also described a progressive pattern to auditory brainstem response changes and presented limited data obtained from nuclear magnetic resonance spectroscopy, supporting a global toxic effect of hyperbilirubinaemia.

Given then the wide variations in susceptibility, the occurrence of an initial reversible phase of toxicity and the numerous additional insults infants may be exposed to, it would appear that evidence of acute cerebral dysfunction holds the best promise for the objective assessment of bilirubin toxicity against which criteria for treatment may be evaluated.

Management

Unfortunately, despite these reservations regarding assessment of toxicity and chiefly because of the unsubstantiated spectre of minimal brain damage [12], clinical practice has evolved into intervention at lower and lower levels of total serum bilirubin, culminating in the advocacy of prophylactic phototherapy for high-risk groups [2,59] and has also seen the proliferation of charts and nomograms which use a selection of criteria to decide intervention points. The rationality of current clinical practice must therefore be questioned.

The extent of current confusion regarding management is revealed by Robertson *et al.* [60] who show that no agreement exists between five methods used to decide when to perform exchange transfusion. Commonly used charts are those introduced by Gartner [2] and Maisels [61] and formulae considered incorporate total bilirubin, bilirubin binding capacity, total albumin and birth weight. Of these methods, only one, the Gartner chart, has been subjected to any evaluation [62]. A fall in the *post mortem* prevalence of kernicterus over two periods, 1966–1967 and 1971–1976, was described. The authors attributed this to the introduction, at the start of the second period, of a more aggressive policy of management. Prophylactic phototherapy was used for infants of less than 1500 g birth weight and exchange transfusion performed in infants weighing less than 1250 g at a total serum bilirubin of 220 μmol/l if the clinical course was uncomplicated and 170 μmol/l if one of several risk factors was present. Unfortunately such a study provides far from conclusive answers. Kernicterus in this series was defined loosely as yellow discolouration of cerebral nuclei with or without microscopic changes and therefore subject to the criticisms discussed above. Neonatal intensive care has become considerably more sophisticated over the periods in question and a historical study cannot allow for changes in outcome secondary to improvements in care rather than lower serum bilirubin levels.

Conclusions

1. In the ELBW infant, the incidence of bilirubin encephalopathy cannot be assessed from post-mortem findings.
2. Follow-up studies have not provided, and are unlikely to provide, an objective correlation between jaundice and developmental outcome because of the difficulty of mounting a study with sufficient statistical power.
3. There is little objective basis to current management criteria.
4. Both free bilirubin and factors opening the blood-brain barrier influence the development of encephalopathy. The question of variations in brain cell susceptibility, both regional and under differing clinical conditions, has not to date been addressed.
5. The best promise for the future lies with the development of methods of assessing acute cerebral dysfunction.

There is, therefore, no objective justification for the current aggressive management of jaundice at low levels of bilirubin. Attention would be better paid to more intensive monitoring and stabilization of perfusion, temperature, blood gas, hydration and acid-base variables. Given, however, that such management has entered medical lore, controlled trials of early versus late intervention are now ethically unacceptable.

Best guess advice to the clinician caring for infants of less than 1000 g is to start phototherapy at a total serum bilirubin level of 100 μmol/l, ensuring it is maximally effective phototherapy (see below). Guidelines for exchange transfusion are even more difficult, but in the presence of effective phototherapy and the absence of active haemolysis, it is unlikely to be of benefit at a total serum bilirubin of less than 250 μmol/l.

Obstructive jaundice

The level of conjugated bilirubin does not normally exceed 40 μmol/l in the ELBW infant but, when seen, occurs most often in infants who have received total parenteral nutrition for over three weeks. The precise reason is unclear but several theories have been advanced. Hughes *et al.* [63] suggested that cholestasis is secondary to the suppression of trophic gut hormones due to the absence of enteral nutrition. Absent enteral nutrition is also associated with mucosal atrophy [64] which, in the extremely immature infant, may further increase intestinal permeability to hepatotoxins [65]. The neonate has been described as being in a state of ‘physiological cholestasis’ [66] with a reduced rate of bile synthesis and excretion and this may lower the threshold for further cholestasis. Liver biopsies show both hepatocellular injury and bile duct proliferation as seen in biliary atresia [67]. Long-term sequelae such as fibrosis or cirrhosis appear rare and when described have occurred following periods of total parenteral nutrition exceeding six months or in association with abdominal sepsis [68,69]. The early introduction of enteral feeds even in small volume may prevent this complication and a possibility for the future is the administration of trophic gastrointestinal hormones when prolonged total parenteral nutrition is necessary. Cholelithiasis has also been described as a possible complication of parenteral nutrition [70]. Other causes of a conjugated hyperbilirubinaemia are well described and investigation should follow the lines suggested for mature neonates [71]. Phototherapy should not be used in the presence of obstructive jaundice as the accumulation and degradation of pigmented photoproducts will result in the bronze baby syndrome [72].

Treatment

Phototherapy

The use of light to clear unconjugated bilirubin was first described by Cremer *et al.* in 1958 [73,74]. It is now the method of choice for the initial treatment of jaundice in the newborn, though there remain several areas of uncertainty as to its mode of action and optimal application.

When light is used therapeutically, the prescription should specify wavelength, irradiance and duration of exposure and documentation of these parameters should form part of standard nursery procedure. The visible spectrum extends from 380 to 770 nm with the blue-green spectrum – the area of interest as regards phototherapy – from 425 to 550 nm. Irradiance is a measure of radiant flux impinging on a unit area or power density. It should not be confused with illuminance which is the radiant flux visible waveband as perceived by a standard human eye. Irradiance is measured by a spectroradiometer and expressed in mW/cm^2; illuminance, the objective measure of the sensation of brightness, is measured by a light meter and expressed in footcandles or lux. Though only an approximation, as the actual irradiance impinging on the baby will vary with time due to changing ambient illumination and changes in the position of the baby, the product of duration of exposure and irradiance will give a measure of the total radiant energy to which an infant has been exposed.

Mode of action

Native bilirubin, 4Z,15Z bilirubin IXa [75] is composed of four pyrrole rings. Phototherapy was initially assumed to act via the photo-oxidation of bilirubin to water-soluble breakdown products such as mono and dipyrroles. It appears that though photo-oxidation does occur during phototherapy [76] it is not the most important mode of action. The most rapid photochemical reaction is the formation of unstable, reversible configurational isomers of bilirubin that are polar and therefore able to be excreted directly in bile where they appear as a native unconjugated bilirubin. A non-reversible isomer termed lumirubin is also formed, though at a slower rate [77].

When using phototherapy it is important to avoid exposing an infant to wavelengths of light of no therapeutic benefit in clearing bilirubin, but which might have significant effects of their own. An obvious example is the filtering out of ultraviolet and infrared light. The optimal wavelengths for phototherapy in the human newborn baby are currently a matter for debate. Although the absorption spectrum for bilirubin *in vitro* centres around 460 nm, at which wavelength bilirubin absorbs maximally, the action spectrum defining the wavelengths most effective in producing the desired therapeutic effect is dependent *in vivo* on many factors such as competitive absorption by other compounds, skin penetration and the rate of clearance of the various photoproducts. The action spectrum for bilirubin clearance *in vivo* is still not known. Additionally, species differences exist and data pertaining to the Gunn rat model cannot be directly extrapolated to the human neonate. Blue wavelengths (425–475 nm) are undoubtedly effective in clearing bilirubin; what is not known is whether other, possibly safer, wavelengths are also effective. When phototherapy is commenced the formation of configurational isomers of bilirubin, the major photoproduct in the human neonate [78,79], proceeds rapidly reaching photoequilibrium and a stable concentration, but excretion proceeds slowly with a serum half life of 15 h [78]. The formation of lumirubin, the non-reversible structural isomer of bilirubin, is slower but excretion is more rapid (serum half life < 2 h [78]) and takes place both in bile and urine. It has therefore been proposed [80,81] that the ideal light source for phototherapy should promote lumirubin formation and green light has been suggested as effective in this respect [80–82].

Optimal use

There are several ways in which to increase the effectiveness of phototherapy: the emission spectra of lamps used must include therapeutic wavelengths in effective dose – a suitable irradiance is a minimum of 1 mW/cm^2 in the 425–475 nm waveband – and as a saturation effect is believed to exist, 3 mW/cm^2 (60 μW/cm^2/nm) should not be exceeded [83,84]. The rate-limiting factor would appear to be the excretion of photoproducts into bile and possibly urine. Irradiance may be increased by ensuring the baby is not covered in unnecessary clothing, by nursing near a window and by decreasing the distance between light source and baby. Failure to achieve an adequate irradiance, especially when nursing LBW infants in radiant heat cradles, has been shown to be responsible for therapeutic failures [85]. Changes in line voltage may decrease light emission and the output from both fluorescent tubes and halogen lamps decays with time and should be checked regularly.

Phototherapy is more effective the higher the bilirubin concentration [86]. In babies with an initial serum bilirubin concentration of greater than 250 μmol/l, an approximate decline of 30–40% should be achieved after 24 h of appropriate phototherapy. In this regard prophylactic phototherapy has been shown to be of no benefit [87]. Intermittent phototherapy has been advocated as both efficient and involving less exposure to light [86,88] but as the spectral band most efficient in producing DNA breaks is that from 420 to 500 nm, precisely the band that bilirubin best absorbs [89], increasing the number of light cycles during which breaks occur and dark cycles during which repair occurs might in theory increase the risk of wrongly repairing a break [90]. However, neither permanent cellular damage nor carcinogenesis has been attributable to phototherapy.

Hazards

Though numerous theoretical and experimental hazards exist [91,92] no serious toxicity attributable to phototherapy has been seen in all the years of its use. Babies have, however, been exposed to a large variety of light intensities and wavelengths, all loosely termed phototherapy, without further specification. It is not surprising that babies exposed to conventional phototherapy have manifest no serious side effects – it is possible to receive more radiant energy from exposure to sunlight than from many a conventional unit. Any rational consideration of the question of toxicity must take into account the precise characteristics of the light used. With the increasing use of high intensity, narrow spectra the problem of toxicity may have to be reconsidered.

It is important to point out here that the constant high intensity ambient lighting that many tiny neonates are exposed to for prolonged periods poses a significant health hazard in its own right regardless of additional phototherapy. Effects on biological rhythms, infant behaviour and the development of retinopathy of prematurity have all been described [93,94]. In practice, the following precautions should be observed during phototherapy:

(a) careful temperature monitoring especially when using a halogen burner;
(b) shielding of eyes;
(c) compensation for the increased fluid lost – from 30–60 ml/kg/day and occasionally more – principally as insensible water but occasionally in the ELBW infant as increased stool water loss as well.

Exchange transfusion

Exchange transfusion remains the definitive treatment for unconjugated hyperbilirubinaemia. It is, however, a hazardous procedure, perhaps all the more so as certain sequelae may not be immediately evident. A standard two-volume exchange transfusion (two volume = twice circulating blood volume, i.e. 85 ml/kg doubled = 170 ml/kg) will exchange over 90% of the infant's blood and should reduce the serum bilirubin by approximately 50%. The exchange may be performed as a *push-pull* procedure via the umbilical vein or artery or as a continuous withdrawal via a central vessel with concurrent continuous infusion via a vein. The latter is the preferred technique as it is likely to result in less haemodynamic fluctuation. If the umbilical vein is used, the catheter tip must be positioned in the inferior vena cava and should not be used if wedged in a hepatic branch vessel. During push-pull exchange each cycle of input and output should take a minimum of 5 min, withdrawing and infusing slowly. Each aliquot should not exceed 5 ml/kg [95]. Too rapid a rate of exchange results in a progressive fall in blood pressure. The ELBW baby (and ideally all babies) undergoing an exchange transfusion should have continuous monitoring of ECG, BP, CVP, blood gases and temperature. Blood glucose, packed cell volume (PCV) and serum bilirubin, calcium, sodium and potassium should be checked pre, mid and post exchange. The blood used should fulfil the following requirements: CPD stored; less than 48 h old; cytomegalovirus negative; partially packed with a PCV of 40–50. For rhesus incompatibility use low titre O negative blood cross-matched against maternal serum or rhesus negative blood of the same ABO group as the baby cross-matched against baby's serum. Though a theoretical risk of graft versus host disease exists and has infrequently been described [96], in practice it does not appear necessary to irradiate donor blood.

Following exchange transfusion the infant's platelet count is likely to be low, but platelets should not be transfused unless there is evidence of disseminated intravascular coagulation or active bleeding, manifest as oozing, from venepuncture sites. The 24–48 hours following exchange transfusion requires careful monitoring especially in rhesus isoimmunized or hydropic infants. These babies are initially hypoalbuminaemic to varying degrees and after exchange, with the consequent improvement in intravascular oncotic pressure, oedema fluid is progressively drawn into the circulation. The intravascular volume may expand sufficiently to result in acute left ventricular failure and catastrophic pulmonary haemorrhage. A careful watch should therefore be kept on the CVP post exchange and any rise above 10 cmH_2O (7.4 mmHg) treated by venesection and intravenous frusemide. Pulmonary haemorrhage, in particular, is invariably due to left ventricular failure and should be treated by venesection and not with further transfusion of blood.

Other methods

Adjunctive methods of managing hyperbilirubinaemia include earlier feeding to promote the passage of meconium and earlier provision of fluid and calories [97] to prevent dehydration and acidosis. Methods which have not gained acceptance are:

(a) phenobarbitone to induce glucuronyl transferase activity [3,98,99];
(b) infusions of albumin to augment bilirubin binding capacity;
(c) riboflavin, a singlet oxygen generator, used concomitantly with phototherapy to increase the photo-oxidative route of bilirubin clearance [100];
(d) vitamin E used in haemolytic jaundice to reduce red cell breakdown by increasing membrane stability [101];
(e) absorbent materials such as cholestyramine [102] and agar [103] to trap unconjugated bilirubin in the upper intestine thus reducing the effect of the enterohepatic circulation.

Though these methods have suffered an eclipse other avenues continue to be investigated, e.g. the administration of tin protoporphyrin IX lowers bilirubin levels in newborn rats by inhibiting the haem oxygenase system and thereby slowing the conversion of haem to bilirubin [104,105].

References

1. Brown, K. A., Kim, M. H., Wu, P. *et al.* (1985) Efficacy of phototherapy in prevention and management of neonatal hyperbilirubinaemia. *Pediatrics*, **75** (Suppl.), 393–400
2. Gartner, L. (1983) Jaundice and liver disease. In *Behrmann's Neonatal-Perinatal Medicine: Diseases of the Fetus and Infant* (eds A. A. Fanaroff and R. J. Martin), C. V. Mosby, St. Louis, pp. 753–784
3. Gartner, L. M., Lee, L. S., Vaisman, S. L. *et al.* (1977) Development of bilirubin transport and metabolism in the newborn rhesus monkey: Part I. The functional basis of physiological jaundice in the newborn. Part II. Effect of prenatal and neonatal administration of phenobarbital. *J. Pediatr.*, **90**, 513–531
4. Mollison, P. L. (1983) In *Blood Transfusion in Clinical Medicine*, 7th edn., Blackwell Scientific Publications, Oxford, p. 105
5. Pearson, H. A. (1967) Lifespan of the fetal red blood cell. *J. Pediatr.*, **70**, 166–171
6. Schmorl, G. (1903) Zur kentniss des icterus neonatorum. *Verh Deutsche Pathol.*, **6**, 109
7. Zetterstrom, R. and Ernster, L. (1956) Bilirubin, an uncoupler of oxidative phosphorylation in isolated mitochondria. *Nature*, **178**, 1335
8. Levine, R. L. (1979) Bilirubin: worked out years ago? *Pediatrics*, **64**, 380–385
9. Lucey, J. F. (1982) Bilirubin and brain damage – a real mess. *Pediatrics*, **69**, 381–382
10. McDonagh, A. F. (1985) 'Like a shrivelled blood orange' – bilirubin, jaundice and phototherapy. *Pediatrics*, **75**, 443–455
11. Van Praagh, R. (1961) Diagnosis of kernicterus in the neonatal period. *Pediatrics*, **28**, 870–876
12. Perlstein, M. A. (1960) The late clinical syndrome of posticteric encephalopathy. *Pediatr. Clin. North Am.*, **7**, 665–687
13. Hansen, T., Sagvolden, T. and Bratlid, D. (1986) Transient hyperbilirubinaemia causes long term changes in the open field behaviour of young rats. *Pediatr. Res.*, **20**, 462A (abstract)
14. Duara, S., Suter, C. M., Bessard, K. *et al.* (1986) Neonatal screening with auditory brainstem responses: results of follow up audiometry and risk factor evaluation. *J. Pediatr.*, **108**, 276–281

15. Bergman, I., Hirsch, I. P., Fria, T. S. *et al.* (1985) Cause of hearing loss in the high risk premature infant. *J. Pediatr.*, **106**, 95–101
16. Pape, K. E., Buncic, R. J., Ashby, S. *et al.* (1978) The status at two years of low birth weight infants born in 1974 with birth weights less than 1000 g. *J. Pediatr.*, **92**, 253–260
17. Shiller, J. G. and Silverman, W. A. (1961) 'Uncomplicated' hyperbilirubinaemia of prematurity: the lack of association with neurological deficit at three years of age. *Am. J. Dis. Child.*, **101**, 587–592
18. Crichton, J. U., Dunn, H. J., McBurney, A. K. *et al.* (1972) Long term effects of neonatal jaundice on brain function in children of low birth weight. *Pediatrics*, **49**, 656–670
19. Wishingrad, L., Cornblath, M., Takakuwa, T. *et al.* (1965) Studies of non-haemolytic hyperbilirubinaemia in premature infants. I. Prospective randomised selection for exchange transfusion with observations on the levels of serum bilirubin with and without exchange transfusion and neurologic evaluation one year after birth. *Pediatrics*, **36**, 162–172
20. Odell, G. B., Storey, G. N. and Rosenberg, L. A. (1970) Studies in kernicterus III.The saturation of serum proteins with bilirubin during neonatal life and its relationship to brain damage at five years. *J. Pediatr.*, **76**, 12–21
21. Hyman, C. B., Keaster, J., Hanson, V. *et al.* (1969) CNS abnormalities after neonatal hyperbilirubinaemia: a prospective study of 405 patients. *Am. J. Dis. Child.*, **117**, 395–405
22. Koch, C. A., Jones, D. V., Dine, M. S. *et al.* (1959) Hyperbilirubinaemia in preterm infants: a follow up study. *J. Pediatr.*, **55**, 23–29
23. Naeye, R. L. (1978) Amniotic fluid infections, neonatal hyperbilirubinaemia and psychomotor impairment. *Pediatrics*, **62**, 497–503
24. Scheidt, P. C., Mellits, E. D., Hardy, J. B. *et al.* (1977) Toxicity of bilirubin in neonates. Infant development during the first year in relation to maximum neonatal serum bilirubin concentration. *J. Pediatr.*, **91**, 292–297
25. Lucey, J. F., Pasnick, M. and Horbar, J. F. (1982) Hyperbilirubinaemia and intracranial haemorrhage in low birth weight infants. *Pediatr. Res.*, **16**, 336A
26. Aidin, R., Corner, B. and Tovey, G. (1950) Kernicterus and prematurity. *Lancet*, **i**, 1153–1154
27. Zuelzer, W. W. and Mudgett, R. T. (1950) Kernicterus: aetiologic study based on an analysis of 55 cases. *Pediatrics*, **6**, 452–474
28. Harris, R. C., Lucey, J. F. and MacLean, J. R. (1958) Kernicterus in premature infants associated with low concentrations of bilirubin in plasma. *Pediatrics*, **21**, 875–883
29. Stern, L. and Denton, R. L. (1965) Kernicterus in small premature infants. *Pediatrics*, **35**, 483–485
30. Ackerman, B. D., Dyer, G. Y. and Leydorf, M. M. (1970) Hyperbilirubinaemia and kernicterus in small premature infants. *Pediatrics*, **45**, 918–925
31. Keenan, W. J., Perlstein, P. H., Light, I. J. *et al.* (1972) Kernicterus in small sick premature infants receiving phototherapy. *Pediatrics*, **49**, 652–655
32. Ritter, D. A., Kenny, J. D., Norton, H. J. *et al.* (1982) A prospective study of free bilirubin and other risk factors in the development of kernicterus in premature infants. *Pediatrics*, **69**, 260–266
33. Gartner, L. M., Snyder, R. N., Chabon, R. S. *et al.* (1970) Kernicterus: high incidence in premature infants with low serum bilirubin concentrations. *Pediatrics*, **45**, 906–917
34. Ahdab-Barmada, M. (1983) Neonatal kernicterus: neuropathologic diagnosis. In *Hyperbilirubinaemia in the Newborn* (Report of the 85th Ross Conference on Paediatric Research), (eds R. L. Levine and M. J. Maisels), Ross Laboratories, Columbus, Ohio, pp. 2–10
35. Turkel, S. B. (1963) Clinical and pathological correlations with kernicterus and yellow pulmonary membranes. In *Hyperbilirubinaemia in the Newborn* (Report of the 85th Ross Conference on Paediatric Research), (eds R. L. Levine and M. J. Maisels), Ross Laboratories, Columbus, Ohio, pp. 11–18
36. Gerrard, J. (1952) Kernicterus. *Brain*, **75**, 526–570
37. Wennberg, R. P. and Hance, A. J. (1986) Experimental bilirubin encephalopathy: importance of total bilirubin, protein binding and blood-brain barrier. *Pediatr. Res.*, **20**, 789–792
38. Turkel, S. B., Miller, C. A., Guttenberg, M. E. *et al.* (1982) A clinical pathologic reappraisal of kernicterus. *Pediatrics*, **69**, 267–272
39. Perl, H., Nijjar, A., Ebara, H. *et al.* (1982) Bilirubin toxicity without CNS staining. *Pediatr. Res.*, **16**, 303A

40. Turkel, S. B., Guttenberg, M. E., Moynes, D. R. *et al.* (1980) Lack of identifiable risk factors for kernicterus. *Pediatrics*, **66**, 502–506
41. Kim, M. H., Yoon, J. J., Sher, J. *et al.* (1980) Lack of predictive indices in kernicterus: a comparison of clinical and pathologic factors in infants with or without kernicterus. *Pediatrics*, **66**, 852–858
42. Cashore, W. J. and Oh, W. (1982) Unbound bilirubin and kernicterus in low birth weight infants. *Pediatrics*, **69**, 481–485
43. Wennberg, R. P., Pal, N. and Bessman, S. P. (1986) Effects of blood-brain barrier disruption and bilirubin on cerebral metabolism. *Pediatr. Res.*, **20**, 469A
44. Kapitulnik, J., Horner–Mibashan, R., Blondheim, S. H. *et al.* (1975) Increase in bilirubin binding affinity of serum with age of infant. *J. Pediatr.*, **86**, 442–445
45. Ebbesen, F. and Nyboe, J. (1983) Postnatal changes in the ability of plasma albumin to bind bilirubin. *Acta Paediatr. Scand.*, **72**, 665–670
46. Silverman, W. A., Anderson, D. H., Blanc, W. A. *et al.* (1956) A difference in mortality rate and incidence of kernicterus in premature infants allotted to two prophylactic antibacterial regimens. *Pediatrics*, **18**, 616–624
47. Cashore, W. J. (1980) Free bilirubin concentrations and bilirubin binding affinity in term and preterm infants. *J. Pediatr.*, **96**, 521–527
48. Cashore, W. J. (1983) Bilirubin binding tests. In *Hyperbilirubinaemia in the Newborn* (Report of the 85th Ross Conference on Paediatric Research), (eds R. L. Levine and M. J. Maisels), Ross Laboratories, Columbus, Ohio, pp. 101–115
49. Zamet, P., Nakamura, H., Perez–Robles *et al.* (1975) The use of critical levels of birth weight and 'free bilirubin' as an approach for the prevention of kernicterus. *Biol. Neonate*, **26**, 274–282
50. Nakamura, H., Takada, S., Shimabuku, R. *et al.* Auditory nerve and brainstem responses in newborn infants with hyperbilirubinaemia. *Pediatrics*, **75**, 703–708
51. Carmode, E. J., Lyster, D. M. and Israels, S. (1975) Analbuminaemia in a neonate. *J. Pediatr.*, **86**, 862–867
52. Rapoport, S. I. (1983) Reversible osmotic opening of the blood brain barrier for experimental and therapeutic purposes. In *Hyperbilirubinaemia in the Newborn* (Report of the 85th Ross Conference on Paediatric Research), (eds R. L. Levine and M. J. Maisels), Ross Laboratories, Columbus, Ohio, pp. 116–124
53. Lee, C., Stonestreet, B. S., Outerbridge, E. *et al.* (1986) Postnatal maturation of the blood brain barrier for unbound bilirubin in piglets. *Pediatr. Res.*, **20**, 353A
54. Levine, R. L. Fredricks, W. R. and Rapoport, S. I. (1982) Entry of bilirubin into the brain due to opening of the blood brain barrier. *Pediatrics*, **69**, 255–259
55. Golub, H. L. and Corwin, M. J. (1982) Infant cry: a clue to diagnosis. *Pediatrics*, **69**, 197–201
56. Stein, L., Ozdamar, O., Kraus, N. *et al.* (1983) Follow up of infants screened by auditory brainstem response in the neonatal intensive care unit. *J. Pediatr.*, **103**, 447–453
57. Perlman, M., Fainmesser, P., Sohmer, H. *et al.* (1983). Auditory nerve brainstem evoked responses in hyperbilirubinaemic infants. *Pediatrics*, **72**, 658–664
58. Ahlfors, C. E., Bennett, S. H., Shoemaker, C. T. *et al.* (1986) Changes in auditory brainstem response associated with intravenous infusion of unconjugated bilirubin into infant rhesus monkeys. *Pediatr. Res.*, **20**, 511–515
59. Lucey, J. (1972) Neonatal jaundice and phototherapy. *Pediatr. Clin. North Am.*, **19**, 827–839
60. Robertson, A. F., Karp, W. B., Davis, H. C. *et al.* (1983) Predicting the need for exchange transfusion in newborn infants. *Clin. Pediatr.*, **22**, 533–536
61. Maisels, M. J. (1972) Bilirubin. *Pediatr. Clin. North Am.*, **19**, 447–501
62. Pearlman, M. A., Gartner, L. M., Lee, K. *et al.* (1978) Absence of kernicterus in low birth weight infants from 1971 through 1976: comparison with findings in 1966 and 1967. *Pediatrics*, **62**, 460–464
63. Hughes, C. A., Talbot, I. C., Ducker, D. A. *et al.* (1983) Total parenteral nutrition in infancy: effect on the liver and suggested pathogenesis. *Gut*, **24**, 241–248
64. Hughes, C. A. and Dowling, R. H. (1980) Speed of onset of adaptive mucosal hypoplasia and hypofunction in the intestine of parenterally fed rats. *Clin. Sci.*, **59**, 317–327
65. Tanner, M. S., Stocks, R. J. and McNeish, A. S. (1984) Adaptation to extrauterine life – a

commentary. In *Neonatal Gastroenterology, Contemporary Issues* (eds M. S. Tanner and R. J. Stocks), Intercept Publications, Newcastle upon Tyne, pp. 209–210

66. Balistreri, W. F., Heubi, J. E. and Suchy, F. J. (1983) Immaturity of the enterohepatic circulation in early life: factors predisposing to 'physiologic' maldigestion and cholestasis. *J. Pediatr. Gastroenterol. Nutr.*, **2**, 346–354
67. Dahms, B. B. and Halpin, T. C. (1981) Serial liver biopsies in parenteral nutrition-associated cholestasis of early infancy. *Gastroenterology*, **81**, 136–144
68. Peden, V. H., Witzleben, C. L. and Skelton, M. A. (1971) Total parenteral nutrition. *J. Pediatr.*, **78**, 180–181
69. Cohen, C. C. and Olsen, M. M. (1981) Pediatric total parenteral nutrition. *Arch. Pathol. Lab. Med.*, **105**, 152–156
70. Whitington, P. F. and Black, D. D. (1980) Cholelithiasis in premature infants treated with parenteral nutrition and furosemide. *J. Pediatr.*, **97**, 647–649
71. Johnston, D. I. (1984) Neonatal cholestasic jaundice. In *Neonatal Gastroenterology, Contemporary Issues* (eds M. S. Tanner and R. J. Stocks), Intercept Publications, Newcastle upon Tyne, pp. 139–153
72. Onishi, S., Itoh, S., Isobe, S. *et al.* (1982) Mechanism of development of bronze baby syndrome in neonates treated with phototherapy. *Pediatrics*, **69**, 273–276
73. Cremer, R. J., Perryman, P. W. and Richards, D. H. (1958) Influence of light on the hyperbilirubinaemia of infants. *Lancet*, **i**, 1094–1097
74. Dobbs, R. H. and Cremer, R. J. (1975) Phototherapy. *Arch. Dis. Child.*, **50**, 833–836
75. Ennever, J. F. (1986) Phototherapy in a new light. *Pediatr. Clin. North Am.*, **33**, 603–620
76. Lightner, D. A., Linnane, W. P. and Ahlfors, C. E. (1984) Bilirubin photooxidation products in the urine of jaundiced neonates receiving phototherapy. *Pediatr. Res.*, **18**, 696–700
77. McDonagh, A. F., Palma, L. A. and Lightner, D. A. (1982) Phototherapy for neonatal jaundice: stereospecific and regioselective photoisomerization of bilirubin bound to human serum albumin and NMR characterisation of intramolecular cyclized photoproducts. *J. Am. Chem. Soc.*, **104**, 6867–6869
78. Ennever, J. F., Knox, K., Denne, S. C. *et al.* (1985) Phototherapy for neonatal jaundice: *in vivo* clearance of bilirubin photoproducts. *Pediatr. Res.*, **19**, 205–208
79. Costarino, A. T., Ennever, J. F., Baumgart, S. *et al.* (1985) Bilirubin photoisomerization in premature neonates under low and high dose phototherapy. *Pediatrics*, **75**, 519–522
80. Pratesi, R., Agati, G., Fusi, F. *et al.* (1985) Laser investigation of bilirubin – photobilirubin photoconversion. *Pediatr. Res.*, **19**, 166–171
81. Ennever, J. F., Knox, I. and Speck, W. T. (1986) Differences in bilirubin isomer composition in infants treated with green and white light phototherapy. *J. Pediatr.*, **109**, 119–122
82. Vecchi, C., Donzelli, G. P., Sbrana, G. *et al.* (1986) Phototherapy for neonatal jaundice: clinical equivalence of fluorescent green and 'special' blue lamps. *J. Pediatr.*, **108**, 452–456
83. Tan, K. L. (1982) The pattern of bilirubin response to phototherapy for neonatal hyperbilirubinaemia. *Pediatr. Res.*, **16**, 670–674
84. Modi, N. and Keay, A. J. (1983) Phototherapy for neonatal hyperbilirubinaemia: the importance of dose. *Arch. Dis. Child.*, **58**, 406–409
85. Bonta, B. W. and Warshaw, J. B. (1976) Importance of radiant flux in the treatment of hyperbilirubinaemia: failure of overhead phototherapy units in intensive care units. *Pediatrics*, **57**, 502–506
86. Jahrig, K., Jahrig, D. and Meisel, P. (1982) Dependence of the efficiency of phototherapy on plasma bilirubin concentration. *Acta Paediatr. Scand.*, **71**, 293–299
87. Curtis-Cohen, M., Stahl, G. E., Costarino, A. T. *et al.* (1985) Randomized trial of prophylactic phototherapy in the infant of very low birth weight. *J. Pediatr.*, **107**, 121–124
88. Lau, S. P. and Fung, K. P. (1984) Serum bilirubin kinetics in intermittent phototherapy of physiological jaundice. *Arch. Dis. Child.*, **59**, 892–894
89. Sideris, E. G., Papageorgiou, G. C., Charalampous, S. C. *et al.* (1981) A spectrum response study on single strand DNA breaks, sister chromatid exchanges and lethality induced by phototherapy lights. *Pediatr. Res.*, **15**, 1019–1023
90. Speck, W. T., Santella, R. M. and Rosenkranz, H. S. (1977) Intermittent phototherapy: effect on intracellular DNA. *Pediatr. Res.*, **11**, 542A

91. Cohen, A. N. and Ostrow, J. D. (1980) New concepts in phototherapy: photoisomerization of bilirubin IXa and potential toxic effects of light. *Pediatrics*, **65**, 740–750
92. Sisson, T. R. C. and Vogl, T. P. (1982) Phototherapy of hyperbilirubinaemia. In *The Science of Photomedicine* (eds J. D. Regan and J. A. Parrish), Plenum Press, New York and London, pp. 477–509
93. Sisson, T. R. C. (1981) Molecular basis of hyperbilirubinaemia and phototherapy. *J. Invest. Dermatol.*, **77**, 158–161
94. Glass, P., Avery, G. B., Kolinjavadi, N. *et al.* (1985) Effect of bright light in the hospital nursery on the incidence of retinopathy of prematurity. *N. Engl. J. Med.*, **313**, 401–404
95. Aranda, J. V. and Sweet, A. Y. (1977) Alterations in blood pressure during exchange transfusion. *Arch. Dis. Child.*, **52**, 545–548
96. Cochran, W. D. (1978) Increasing safety of exchange transfusions. *Pediatr. Res.*, **12**, 462
97. Wu, P. Y., Hodgman, J. E., Kirkpatrick, B. V. *et al.* (1985) Metabolic aspects of phototherapy. *Pediatrics*, **75** (Suppl), 427–433
98. Wallin, A. and Boreus, L. O. (1984) Phenobarbital prophylaxis for hyperbilirubinaemia in preterm infants. A controlled study of bilirubin disappearance and infant behaviour. *Acta Paediatr. Scand.*, **73**, 488–497
99. Segni, G., Polidori, G. and Romagnoli, C. (1977) Bucolome in prevention of hyperbilirubinaemia in preterm infants. *Arch. Dis. Child.*, **52**, 549–550
100. Pascale, J. A., Mims, L., Greenberg, M. H. *et al.* (1976) Riboflavin and bilirubin response during phototherapy. *Pediatr. Res.*, **10**, 854
101. Gross, S. J. (1979) Vitamin E and neonatal bilirubinaemia. *Pediatrics*, **64**, 321–323
102. Tan, K. L., Jacob, E. and Karim, S. M. (1984) Cholestyramine and phototherapy for neonatal jaundice. *J. Pediatr.*, **104**, 284–286
103. Odell, G. B., Gutcher, G. R., Whitington, P. F. *et al.* (1983) Enteral administration of agar as an effective adjunct to phototherapy of neonatal hyperbilirubinaemia. *Pediatr. Res.*, **17**, 810–814
104. Samonte, D., Peng, C., Veng, F. *et al.* (1986) Effect of tin-protoporphyrin on neonatal Gunn rat bilirubin. *Pediatr. Res.*, **20**, 417A
105. Whitington, P. F., Moscioni, D. A. and Gartner, L. M. (1986) Tin protoporphyrin and bilirubin excretion in rat bile. *Pediatr. Res.*, **20**, 364A

Chapter 12

Feeding

Anthony F. Williams

Although a great deal has been written about the feeding of preterm infants, little relates specifically to the feeding of those weighing under 1000 g at birth. Why should this subgroup warrant separate attention, and in what respects might their requirements differ from those of more mature preterm infants?

Our current understanding of preterm infant feeding draws upon evidence from three major sources. First, the fetus has been viewed as a model upon which optimal nutrition and growth of the preterm baby may be based [1]. Second, studies of small numbers of selected infants have led to an understanding of basic physiological aspects of feeding, helping to clarify the relationship between nutrient intake and utilization [2,3]. Third, clinical trials comparing outcome in unselected infants randomly allocated to alternative feeding regimens [4,5] have been of the greatest importance in determining appropriate management.

However, none of these sources alone is wholly satisfactory as an indicator of the preterm infant's requirements. For example, questions exist about the applicability of the fetus as a growth model, and generalization from physiological studies carried out under controlled conditions on selected infants may also be misleading. No clinical trial of sufficient statistical power has yet studied infants who were all under 1000 g. Many factors may account for this: morbidity is frequent, numbers in individual centres are small and the outcome can be difficult to measure with precision. Additionally, it is increasingly realized that feeding plays many roles other than nutrient supply in postnatal adaptation and much remains to be learned about its immunological and endocrine aspects. It is conceivable that these may have a more important clinical role in more immature and vulnerable infants, though clinical outcome has not been examined in these terms.

Consequently, any proposition for the feeding of infants under 1000 g must at present be based on inference rather than the results of any formal test. This chapter therefore principally seeks to identify the general problems of feeding very small infants in order to suggest ways in which feeding regimens for more mature preterm infants may rationally be modified. In the absence of absolute demonstration of the superiority of any particular method, the 'correct' approach must depend on the viewpoint adopted in individual nurseries, but a detailed account of the practice adopted in one nursery may be found in a recently published review [6].

What can be learnt from the fetus?

The assumption implicit in the *reference fetus* [1] approach to the definition of nutrient requirements is that fetal growth represents an optimum for the preterm infant in both quantitative and qualitative terms. By combining data about birth weight and body composition at a given gestational age a pattern of fetal biochemical accretion may be composed and used as a guideline to the extrauterine requirements of growing preterm babies.

This assumption raises several questions. Firstly, which growth charts should be used? Charts in common use in the UK do not give data for infants born before 28 weeks of gestation, but three recently published studies [7–9] fill this gap. One set of data [9] is very different from the other two, probably because a hospital population was studied rather than one defined in geographical terms. The inclusion of growth-retarded infants, increasingly delivered electively by caesarean section [7], clearly affects birth weight distribution making it important to use data drawn from spontaneous deliveries only.

Further questions about the *quality* of growth are inseparable from those about *quantity*. For example, the fetus will double in weight between 24 and 28 weeks of gestation [7,8]; should an infant born at 24 weeks show a similar change if optimally nourished? Clearly this cannot be the case since major changes in water and electrolyte balance after birth imply that an 800 g baby must have a greater proportion of body weight attributable to protein and fat than a fetus of equal weight. Much remains to be learned about the relationship between weight change and nutrient utilization in the immediate postnatal period. For example, the fetus does not deposit fat in significant quantities until a body mass of 800 g has been exceeded [10] but there are no data as yet upon the body composition of growing preterm infants of equivalent size.

The implication of these arguments is that rigid reproduction of the pattern of intrauterine weight gain in infants at this maturity may be an elusive aim. Indeed, such evidence as we have from the study of more mature preterm infants suggests that the attainment of intrauterine rates of weight gain is achieved by excessive deposition of fat rather than lean tissue [11].

Ultimately the definition of an optimal early growth pattern and early nutrition must depend upon the correlation of observed trends with long-term physical and psychomotor development [4,5].

Physiology of the ELBW infant

Feeding and the development of the gastrointestinal tract

Many aspects of the physiology of the ELBW infant may constrain nutrient supply (see Chapter 18) or affect requirements (see Chapters 9 and 14) but some consideration of the structural and functional development of the gut at birth is clearly central to a discussion of enteral feeding.

Most small bowel structures of importance to the absorptive process are present by the end of the fourth month of gestation, and by 20 weeks the gut can be considered anatomically differentiated [12]. Functionally it remains immature in many important respects.

Small bowel transit

It is known that transit of fetal intestinal contents does not occur until week 30 [13]. Similarly, longitudinal studies of peristaltic activity in the newborn have suggested that small intestinal motor activity is disorganized and luminal transit inefficient or absent between weeks 27 and 30. Rhythmical peristaltic activity may not appear until sucking and swallowing are seen at around 34 weeks of gestation [14].

Absorptive mechanisms

Since disaccharidases may be identified on the brush border as early as 12 weeks of gestation, it is surprising that lactase (β-galactosidase) is not present in significant quantities until the considerably later gestational age of 30–34 weeks [12]. Lactase activity nevertheless increases rapidly after birth even in very immature infants, probably as a result of enteral feeding [15]. The potential of the immature gut for such adaptive change is a subject of central importance to the feeding of very small infants. The recent demonstration (albeit in relatively mature preterm infants) that even minimal quantities of human milk may induce endocrine changes characteristic of adaptation [16] corroborates the belief that early luminal nutrient supply is important even if total requirements cannot be met by the enteral route. Animal studies imply that colostrum may be more effective than artificial formulae in inducing such changes [17] but it is not yet known whether such qualitative aspects of feeding have relevance to the extremely immature human infant.

Mucosal macromolecular permeability

The macromolecular permeability of the gastrointestinal mucosa appears greater in more immature infants [18] and it has been shown that the plasma concentration of β-lactoglobulin (the principal whey protein of cow's milk) is higher in artificially fed infants under 33 weeks gestation than in more mature preterm infants [19]. Furthermore, basophils from artificially fed VLBW infants released histamine when challenged with β-lactoglobulin *in vitro* suggesting that sensitization may occur as a consequence [20]. It should nevertheless be stressed that the relationship of these observations to the pathogenesis of allergic disease is only speculative at present and much remains to be learnt about the immunology of feeding. Since β-lactoglobulin is frequently present in human milk as a contaminant [21], mechanisms other than simple antigen avoidance may be operative and little is known about the relevance of the antigen dose in induction of tolerance or sensitization.

Feeding and the metabolic milieu of the small infant

There are insignificant fat deposits in the immature infant; at 24 weeks gestation fat accounts for only 1% of body weight at birth, while at 28 weeks the corresponding figure is 3.5% and at term 12% or more [10]. The clear implication of this observation is that energy stores are very limited. Calculations indicate that non-protein energy stores (including glycogen) in the ELBW infant will amount to only 110 Cal/kg (462 kJ/kg), and the caloric reserve (taken to include non-protein energy and one-third of body protein) cannot exceed 200 Cal/kg (840 kJ/kg). If assumptions about energy expenditure are made it can be shown that the unfed infant could not be expected to survive more than four days [22]. The immediate provision of basal requirements will therefore be essential to the maintenance of biochemical homeostasis after birth: maintenance energy requirements under optimal environmental conditions in the first week will approximate 40–50 Cal/kg/day (168–210 kJ/kg/day) but the requirements of an individual infant could be increased by such factors as excessive transepidermal water loss with concomitant rise in evaporative heat loss. The obligatory nitrogen requirement (that necessary to replace unavoidable losses) is approximately 150 mg/kg/day (equivalent to 1.0 g/kg/day of amino acid or protein) [23], though the tolerable nitrogen load will vary according to the availability of energy to support net protein synthesis. Protein turnover rates are greater in less mature infants [24], presumably because protein accounts for a greater proportion of body mass. Although low non-protein energy reserves and high rates of nitrogen flux lead to an increased tendency to protein catabolism, the capacity to synthesize urea from nitrogen liberated during gluconeogenesis from catabolized protein may be limited by reduced argininosuccinase activity which, before 30 weeks of gestation, is only half that present at term [25].

Implications for clinical practice

The preceding sections have suggested that, although the ELBW newborn infant is poorly equipped for survival without immediate feeding, substantial problems exist in the immediate adoption of the enteral route as the sole source of nutrient supply. This dilemma implies that the aim of enteral feeding in the very immature infant is dependent upon the postnatal stage attained.

Early enteral feeding

The principal aims of feeding after birth are the maintenance of biochemical homeostasis and the establishment of gastrointestinal function in preparation for full enteral feeding. Parenteral and enteral feeding should be viewed as complementary, and not mutually exclusive, strategies. It is of interest that 80% of infants in this weight group were *exclusively* parenterally fed according to a recent survey [26]. Since parenteral feeding is discussed elsewhere (Chapter 13) we shall principally discuss the approach to early enteral feeding at this point. The main questions relate to the type of feed and the route of administration most suitable.

An inductive case may be made to support the use of human milk, preferably the mother's own, in the initiation of feeding. Whilst its nutritional value may be uncertain, requirements at this stage can be met by the parenteral route. Human milk may have important advantages when used as a component in such a complementary strategy, reducing antigen exposure and providing growth factors and anti-inflammatory mediators. Whilst it is accepted that any such advantages which might accrue to an individual infant are currently unquantified, there are certainly no reasons to suppose *a priori* that an artificial formula would be superior in conferring these non-nutritional functions.

Arguments about the role of enteral feeding in inducing adaptation similarly influence the choice between the intragastric and transpyloric routes of administration. Intragastric infusion of less than 0.5 ml/kg/h of human milk may achieve this aim [16]. Weight gain in transpylorically fed infants is lower than in those intragastrically fed [27], but it is unclear whether this reflects reduced fat absorption or alteration of the endocrine milieu. Limited studies suggest the latter to be unaffected [28].

It has also been suggested that, where intravenous feeding is prolonged, minimal enteral feeding may play an important role in reducing the incidence of cholestasis [29] in small infants.

Later enteral feeding

If the infant is able to tolerate an enteral intake of 150 ml/kg/day, intravenous nutrient supply presents an unnecessary hazard. The management of feeding at this juncture will clearly be influenced by the availability of the mother's own milk. If this is not available, requirements are unlikely to be met by human milk collected from donors in mature lactation. Several clinical studies performed on VLBW infants support this viewpoint [4,5,30] and there is no reason to suppose that the nutritional requirements of the infant weighing less than 1000 g at birth will differ substantially. Whilst no randomized studies have examined the growth of infants fed mother's own milk, a study utilizing banked human milk from mothers delivered prematurely suggested that it is likely to be nutritionally adequate [30]. Furthermore, studies employing nutritional balance techniques have shown mother's own milk to be capable of supporting acceptable physical growth and macronutrient accretion [2,3].

Protein and energy supplements

Energy or protein supplements have been used as an alternative to the introduction of preterm formula. In this context carbohydrate polymers may prove useful permitting achievement of high caloric density without the cost of high osmolality or presentation of an excessive lactose load. Although pancreatic amylase is not produced in significant quantities at this gestation a brush border glucoamylase [12] is known to be present. Randomized crossover feeding studies of infants under 1500 g (mean birth weight 969 ± 123 g) indicated a growth advantage to accrue from supplementation of human milk or artificial formula with carbohydrate polymer [31].

Protein supplementation of human milk with bovine or human milk proteins has also been practised and a commercial preparation of the former is available. There has been no formal clinical evaluation of this procedure in the feeding of very immature infants and those in infants under 1500 g are few [32,33]. Milk produced by the mothers of preterm infants is highly variable in its protein:energy content. Measurements of the protein content of milk samples collected from an unselected population of mothers delivering infants weighing under 1800 g at birth indicated the range in protein content two weeks after birth to be from 12 to over 20 g/l [34]. In practice this means that the addition of a standard quantity of protein to all milk is not logical: in some cases the effect might be simply to stress further a metabolically vulnerable infant, particularly if the energy content of the milk is low.

Conclusions

Any clinical recommendations about the enteral feeding of the infant under 1000 g are necessarily based on inference from observations about the fetus, the physiology of very immature infants and extrapolation from clinical trials of alternative regimes in more mature infants. Parenteral and enteral feeding are complementary strategies, particularly in the early stages when the dual clinical aims of importance are the satiation of high nutrient demands and the promotion of gastrointestinal adaptation in preparation for total enteral feeding. Human milk may have non-nutritional advantages at this stage of transition to complete dependence on enteral supply. Thereafter, when maternal milk is not available a preterm formula will support more rapid rates of growth than banked human milk and has advantages in having a known composition. Much important information remains to be established if the considerable obstacles to organization of comparative clinical studies in this group can be overcome. The potential of human milk constituents for the immunological protection of the immature gastrointestinal tract, potentially more vulnerable by virtue of its greater permeability, may be a particularly fruitful area of enquiry.

References

1. Ziegler, E. E., O'Donnell, A. M., Nelson, S. E. *et al.* (1976) Body composition of the reference fetus. *Growth*, **40**, 329
2. Reichman, B., Chessex, P., Verellen, G. *et al.* (1983) Dietary composition and macronutrient storage in preterm infants. *Pediatrics*, **72**, 322–327
3. Whyte, R. K., Haslam, R., Shannon, S. *et al.* (1983) Energy balance and nitrogen balance in growing low birthweight infants fed human milk or formula. *Pediatr. Res.*, **17**, 891–898
4. Lucas, A., Gore, S. M., Cole, T. J. *et al.* (1984) Multicentre trial on feeding low birth weight infants: effects of diet on early growth. *Arch. Dis. Child.*, **59**, 722–730
5. Tyson, J. E., Lasky, R. E., Mize, C. E. *et al.* (1983) Growth, metabolic response and development in VLBW infants fed banked human milk or enriched formula. I. Neonatal findings. *J. Pediatr.*, **103**, 95–104
6. Adamkin, D. H. (1986) Nutrition in very very low birth weight infants. *Clin. Perinatol.*, **13**, 419–443
7. Lucas, A., Cole, T. J. and Gandy, G. M. (1986) Birthweight centiles in preterm infants reappraised. *Early Hum. Dev.*, **13**, 313–322
8. Keen, D. V. and Pearse, R. G. (1985) Birthweight between 14 and 42 weeks gestation. *Arch. Dis. Child.*, **60**, 440–446
9. Brooke, O. G. and McIntosh, N. (1984) Birthweight of infants born before 30 weeks gestation. *Arch. Dis. Child.*, **59**, 1189–1190
10. Widdowson, E. M. and Spray, C. M. (1951) Chemical development *in utero*. *Arch. Dis. Child.*, **26**, 205–214
11. Reichman, B. L., Chessex, C. P., Putet, G. *et al.* (1981) Diet, fat accretion and growth in premature infants. *N. Engl. J. Med.*, **305**, 1495–1500
12. Lebenthal, E., Lee, P. C. and Heitlinger, L. A. (1983) Impact of development of the gastrointestinal tract on infant feeding. *J. Pediatr.*, **102**, 1–9
13. McLain, C. R. (1963) Amniography studies of the gastrointestinal motility of the human fetus. *Am. J. Obstet. Gynecol.*, **86**, 1079–1087
14. Milla, P. J. (1984) Development of intestinal structure and function. In *Neonatal Gastroenterology, Contemporary Issues* (eds M.S. Tanner and R.J. Stocks), Intercept Publications, Newcastle upon Tyne, pp. 1–19
15. Mayne, A., Hughes, C. A. Sule, D. *et al.* (1983) Development of intestinal disaccharidases in preterm infants. *Lancet*, **ii**, 622–623
16. Lucas, A., Bloom, S. R. and Aynsley-Green, A. (1986) Gut hormones and 'minimal enteral feeding'. *Acta Paediatr. Scand.*, **75**, 719–723
17. Heird, W. C., Schwartz, S. M. and Hansen, I. H. (1984) Colostrum induced enteric mucosal growth in beagle puppies. *Pediatr. Res.*, **18**, 512–515
18. Weaver, L. T., Laker, M. F. and Nelson, R. (1984) Intestinal permeability in the newborn. *Arch. Dis. Child.*, **59**, 236–241
19. Roberton, D. M., Paganelli, R., Dinwiddie, R. and Levinsky, R. J. (1982) Milk antigen absorption in the preterm and term neonate. *Arch. Dis. Child.*, **57**, 369–372

20. Lucas, A., McLaughlan, P. and Coombs, R. R. A. (1984) Latent anaphylactic sensitisation of infants of low birth weight to cows' milk proteins. *Br. Med. J.*, **289**, 1254–1256
21. Jakobsson, I., Lindberg, T., Benediktsson, B. and Hanson, B–G. (1985) Dietary β-lactoglobulin is transferred to human milk. *Acta Paediatr. Scand.*, **74**, 342–345
22. Heird, W. C., Driscoll, J. M., Schullinger, J. N. *et al.* (1972) Intravenous alimentation in pediatric patients. *J. Pediatr.*, **80**, 351
23. Pencharz, P. B., Steffee, W. P., Cochran, W. *et al.* (1977) Protein metabolism in human neonates: nitrogen-balance studies, estimated obligatory losses of nitrogen and whole-body turnover of nitrogen. *Clin. Sci. Mol. Med.*, **52**, 485–498
24. Nissam, I., Yudkoff, M., Pereira, G. and Segal, S. (1983) Effects of conceptual age and dietary intake on protein metabolism in premature infants. *J. Pediatr. Gastroenterol. Nutr.*, **2**, 507–516
25. Raiha, N. C. R. (1980) Protein in the nutrition of the preterm infant. Biochemical and nutritional considerations. In *Advances in Nutritional Research*, Volume 3 (ed. H.H. Draper), Plenum, New York, pp. 173–206
26. Churella, H. R., Bachhuber, B. S., MacLean, W. C. *et al.* (1985) Methods of feeding low birth weight infants. *Pediatrics*, **76**, 243–249
27. Whitfield, M. F. (1982) Poor weight gain of the infant fed nasojejunally. *Arch. Dis. Child.*, **57**, 597–601
28. Milner, R. D. G., Minoli, G., Moro, G. *et al.* (1981) Growth and metabolic and hormonal profiles during transpyloric and nasogastric feeding in preterm infants. *Acta Paediatr. Scand.*, **70**, 9–13
29. Hughes, C. A., Talbot, I. C., Ducker, D. A. and Harran, M. J. (1983) Total parenteral nutrition in infancy: effect on the liver and suggested pathogenesis. *Gut*, **24**, 241–248
30. Gross, S. J. (1983) Growth and biochemical response of preterm infants fed human milk or modified infant formula. *N. Engl. J. Med.*, **308**, 237–241
31. Raffles, A., Schiller, G., Erhardt, P. and Silverman, M. (1983) Glucose polymer supplementation of feeds for very low birth weight infants. *Br. Med. J.*, **286**, 935–936
32. Hagelberg, S., Lindblad, B. S., Lundsjo, A. *et al.* (1982) The protein tolerance of very low birth weight infants fed human milk protein enriched mother's milk. *Acta Paediatr. Scand.*, **71**, 597–601
33. Ronnholm, K. A. R., Simell, O. and Siimes, M. A. (1984) Human milk protein and medium chain triglyceride oil supplementation of human milk: plasma amino acids in very low birth weight infants. *Pediatrics*, **74**, 792–799
34. Lucas, A. and Hudson, G. J. (1984) Preterm milk as a source of protein for low birth weight infants. *Arch. Dis. Child.*, **59**, 831–836

Chapter 13

Intravenous nutrition

Victor Y. H. Yu

Extrauterine survival for ELBW babies depends on the maintenance of nutrition after birth and a successful transition to enteral feeding. Intravenous nutrition is indicated in all those whose gastrointestinal function is so immature that food cannot be provided via the gut. It is also indicated when there are severe respiratory problems.

Composition of solutions

Protein

Nitrogen requirements are supplied as amino acids. The source of amino acids used in intravenous nutrition has changed dramatically. Until the mid-1970s protein hydrolysates were used (generation 1) followed by early amino acid mixtures which contain two different optically active stereoisomers, designated D and L (generation 2). The amino acid mixtures used today contain only L isomers (generation 3) [1].

If an ELBW baby is to continue his intrauterine growth rate, he needs to retain nitrogen at the same rate as an equivalent fetus. The mean nitrogen accretion rate for a fetus is constant between 24 and 36 weeks gestation at 320 mg/kg/24 h (24 mmol/kg/24 h) [2]. The intravenous nitrogen required to achieve retention equal to the fetal accretion rate depends on its source. The low bioavailability of generation 1 amino acid solutions results in nitrogen retention rates from these formulae of below 40% of the amount infused [3]. Crystalline amino acid solutions have the advantage of better bioavailability. Generation 2 solutions are less efficient than generation 3 solutions because of excessive urinary nitrogen losses of D isomers. Examples of generation 3 amino acid solutions used in preterm babies are Vamin (KabiVitrum), Travasol (Travenol) and Aminosyn (Abbott). Nitrogen retention from Vamin is over 70% of the amount infused [2,3], a value which is significantly higher than that for Travasol which is 65% of the amount infused [4]. The nitrogen requirement of Vamin-fed preterm babies is 430 mg/kg/24 h (32 mmol/kg/24 h), equivalent to about 3.2 g/kg/24 h amino acids. A similar recommendation has been made for Aminosyn [5].

The optimal amino acid composition of an intravenous formula for ELBW babies is unknown. The oral requirements of normal babies cannot be extrapolated to intravenous intake, because the role of the gastrointestinal tract and liver in selective absorption, anabolism or catabolism of the ingested amino acid before systemic distribution has not been adequately studied. In addition, a formula appropriate for a term baby is not necessarily suitable for a preterm baby, especially one under 1000 g. The use of amino acid plasma concentrations to evalute the adequacy and safety of a number of formulae has been described. Abnormal plasma amino acid patterns were reported in babies receiving infusions of protein hydrolysates [6,7] and to a lesser extent, crystalline amino acid formulae, whether their composition is similar to egg albumin [8,9], mother's milk [10] or based on the transfer rates of individual amino acids [11]. Differences in plasma amino acid concentrations found in babies receiving different intravenous formulae were consistent with the composition of the amino acid solutions [4]. The interpretation of plasma aminograms during intravenous nutrition requires the arbitrary selection of 'normal values' for comparison. Control patients from whom these standards are derived vary from unfed term babies [12], breast-fed term babies [13], breast-fed preterm babies [9,14] to formula-fed preterm babies [5]. Plasma-free amino acids represent only 1% of the baby's total amino acid pool [15]. Furthermore, a discrepancy sometimes exists between theory and clinical outcome. Cysteine is thought to be an essential amino acid in babies, but nitrogen retention and growth are similar in those given cysteine-free and cysteine-supplemented solutions, even though the plasma cysteine level is significantly lower in the former group [16].

Improved solutions with tailor-made amino acids for optimal safety and growth in ELBW babies may be developed with the next generation of formulae. In the meantime, clinical studies have shown that normal intrauterine weight gain and nitrogen retention rate are achieved in intravenously fed babies with plasma amino acid values comparable to those measured on breast milk or formula feeding.

Carbohydrate

Non-protein energy sources contribute to improved nitrogen retention rates in intravenous nutrition [13,16]. The optimal calorie:nitrogen ratio is between 150 and 250 non-protein calories/g nitrogen. Fructose, sorbitol, ethanol and galactose have been used. Glucose is currently the predominant carbohydrate source in intravenous nutrition, together with a small amount of glycerol present in lipid solutions. Although most babies born at term can tolerate a glucose infusion rate of 14 mg/kg/min (20 g/kg/24 h) [17], preterm babies – especially those under stress from respiratory distress – would develop hyperglycaemia and its resultant complications of glycosuria, osmotic diuresis and dehydration [18,19]. Hyperglycaemia is thought to be due to persistent endogenous hepatic glucose production and decreased peripheral glucose utilization [20]. Insulin therapy is not recommended because of its unpredictable responses. Glucose tolerance improves with increasing postnatal age [21]. Therefore, in ELBW babies hyperglycaemia and its sequelae can be reduced by starting glucose infusion at a rate of 4–6 mg/kg/min (6–8 g/kg/24 h). This can then be increased with frequent measurements of blood glucose to determine tolerance limits. In some babies it is possible to establish an intravenous glucose intake of 11–13 mg/kg/min (16–18 g/kg/24 h) within 2–3 weeks after birth.

Fat

The source of the non-protein energy, whether carbohydrate or fat, makes no difference to its nitrogen-sparing effects in intravenously fed babies [22]. The use of intravenous fat solutions has been reviewed [23]. The requirement for essential fatty acid during intravenous nutrition in babies can be met by as little as 0.5 g/kg/24 h of

Intralipid (KabiVitrum) [24] although higher infusion rates are often used because it is a concentrated source of calories. However, ELBW babies have a diminished capacity to utilize exogenous fats; it has been shown that intravenous fat tolerance is poorer in preterm compared with term babies [25] and in small for gestational age (SGA) compared with appropriate for gestational age (AGA) babies [26]. Preterm babies have a delayed activation of lipoprotein lipase activity and a deficient cellular uptake and utilization of free fatty acids [27]. Heparin infused continuously at 150 IU/kg/24 h has no influence on fat clearance [28] and higher doses increase lipolytic activity only transiently [29]. Carnitine is a naturally occurring trimethylamine which plays a key role in the oxidation of fatty acids [30]. Babies have lower carnitine depots and limited capacity for carnitine biosynthesis [31]. None of the currently available amino acid solutions contain carnitine and intravenously fed preterm babies develop low blood and tissue carnitine concentrations [32,33]. Although one study had shown that carnitine supplementation improves fat utilization [34], other investigators have not confirmed that carnitine is rate-limiting for fat utilization in babies during intravenous nutrition [35,36].

In ELBW babies, Intralipid should be introduced in a dose of 1 g/kg/24 h. This should be gradually increased up to a maximum of 3 g/kg/24 h and the infusion should always be given continuously over a 24 h period [37,38]. Even smaller doses should be used in preterm babies suffering from sepsis as they have reduced utilization of infused fat [39]. Visual inspection of plasma turbidity and nephelometry have been used to determine lipid tolerance, but these do not correlate well with serum triglyceride and free fatty acid concentrations [40]. However, the latter measurements are not routinely available.

Fluid and energy intake

Aspects of fluid therapy have been reviewed in Chapter 9. In addition to the many factors which increase water loss in these babies, it has been shown that intravenous nutrition results in up to 60% increase in insensible water loss, probably due to an increase in thermogenesis and metabolic rate [41].

The basal metabolic rate in preterm babies is 40–47 mJ/kg/24 h and the energy cost of activity is 41 mJ/kg/24 h with minimal handling of the baby [42–44]. It has been shown that the specific dynamic action of intravenous nutrition is 13% of basal heat production of 10% of the calories infused [45]. An energy intake of 50–60 mJ/kg/24 h is adequate to match continuing expenditure, but it does not meet additional requirements of growth. Since the energy cost of gaining 1 g of new tissue is 5 kcal [44], an additional energy intake of 70–80 mJ/kg/24 h is required to achieve the equivalent intrauterine growth. Tables 13.1 and 13.2 show the fluid and nutrient intakes in a series of 42 ELBW babies receiving intravenous nutrition to supplement enteral feeding.

Minerals and trace elements

Fetal accretion rates for minerals and trace elements remain constant when expressed per kg body weight per day up to 36 weeks gestation [2]. Values are known for sodium (1.2 mmol), potassium (0.8 mmol), chloride (0.86 mmol), calcium (3.2 mmol), magnesium (0.16 mmol), phosphorus (2.45 mmol), iron (30.4 μmol), zinc (4.8 μmol), copper (1.3 μmol), manganese (132 nmol) and chromium (84 nmol). Balance studies carried out for these 11 elements in intravenously fed preterm babies form the basis for

Table 13.1 Mean (± s.d.) oral and intravenous nutrient intake (g/kg/24 h) in 42 ELBW babies

	Protein			*Carbohydrate*			*Fat*		
Week	*Oral*	*Intravenous*	*Total*	*Oral*	*Intravenous*	*Total*	*Oral*	*Intravenous*	*Total*
1	0.4	0.6	1.0 ± 1.2	1.2	9.3	10.5 ± 7.4	0.7	0.0	0.7 ± 1.6
2	1.2	1.6	2.8 ± 1.5	3.6	8.8	12.4 ± 3.5	2.3	0.6	2.9 ± 3.0
3	1.5	1.7	3.1 ± 1.0	4.4	8.3	12.8 ± 3.5	3.0	1.2	4.2 ± 2.8
4	1.5	1.7	3.2 ± 0.9	4.7	9.1	13.8 ± 3.5	3.1	1.2	4.3 ± 2.9
5	1.3	1.7	3.0 ± 1.0	2.7	9.2	11.9 ± 5.6	2.8	1.4	4.3 ± 2.5
6	1.6	1.4	3.0 ± 0.9	4.3	7.6	11.9 ± 5.3	3.4	1.2	4.6 ± 2.5
7	2.0	1.2	3.1 ± 0.8	5.7	6.7	12.4 ± 4.7	4.0	1.1	5.1 ± 2.5
8	2.0	1.2	3.2 ± 0.8	5.3	6.9	12.2 ± 5.4	4.3	1.0	5.3 ± 2.6

Table 13.2 Mean (± s.d.) oral and intravenous fluid and energy intake and weight gain in 42 ELBW babies

	Volume (ml/kg/24 h)			*Energy* (mJ/kg/24 h)			*Weight gain*	
Week	*Oral*	*Intra-venous*	*Total*	*Oral*	*Intra-venous*	*Total*	*Rate* (g/24 h)	*Weight* (g)
1	19	159	177 ± 143	13	40	52 ± 35	−8 ± 26	765 ± 33
2	53	121	174 ± 29	37	47	84 ± 29	12 ± 4	785 ± 32
3	66	100	166 ± 36	48	50	97 ± 27	13 ± 3	871 ± 31
4	68	95	162 ± 23	50	53	103 ± 22	12 ± 5	942 ± 30
5	66	91	158 ± 24	48	55	103 ± 24	20 ± 8	1041 ± 47
6	80	74	154 ± 22	60	45	105 ± 26	20 ± 7	1177 ± 61
7	94	65	159 ± 16	71	41	112 ± 21	21 ± 8	1281 ± 47
8	97	62	159 ± 17	74	40	114 ± 22	38 ± 25	1394 ± 62

arriving at intravenous requirements [46,47] with the exception of iron for which postnatal sources are derived from the breakdown of erythrocytes and repeated blood transfusions. Adequate amounts of most minerals and trace elements can be given during intravenous nutrition but it is not possible to provide the amount of calcium and phosphorus acquired transplacentally *in utero* because of precipitation problems in the intravenous preparation. Only half the estimated requirements can be delivered when given in a single solution.

Zinc [48–50] and copper [51,52] deficiencies have been reported in babies on prolonged intravenous nutrition without supplementation of trace elements. Zinc deficiency is associated with retarded growth, impaired wound healing, skin changes similar to those observed in acrodermatitis enteropathica, irritability and jitteriness. Copper deficiency is associated with anaemia, leukopenia and skeletal changes resembling those of scurvy. These deficiencies can be prevented by the addition of zinc and copper to intravenous solutions [53–55]. Although selenium levels are known to be low in preterm babies and haemolysis is associated with selenium deficiency, there is no evidence of deficient antioxidant systems in preterm babies on intravenous nutrition [56]. Trace elements in the fetus and young baby have been reviewed [57,58].

Vitamins

Current recommendations on intravenous vitamins are based on oral requirements and knowledge of enteral absorption. An intravenous preparation containing all the essential vitamins in recommended proportions is not yet available. What is currently used is determined by available preparations such as Multivitamin Infusion (S.A.S.). On a dose of 0.3 ml/kg/24 h, it provides (in μg/kg/24 h): vitamin A, 100; vitamin B_1, 1500; vitamin B_2, 300; nicotinamide, 3000; pyridoxine, 450; dexpanthenol, 750; vitamin C, 15 000; vitamin D, 2.5 and vitamin E, 150. Additional weekly supplements of vitamin K (0.5 mg), folic acid (0.5 mg) and vitamin B_{12} (100 μg) should also be given. Intravenous fat solutions are high in polyunsaturated fatty acid content which increases the risk of haemolysis and vitamin E deficiency in preterm babies. However, it has been shown that the addition of fat to intravenous nutrition leads to a rise in vitamin E levels and no deficiency in antioxidant systems [56]. An increased daily intake of 450 μg vitamin E is possible with the new Multivitamin Infusion Paediatric preparation currently available for intravenous use. Serum vitamin E levels using the latter preparation have been found to be in the range in which a reduction of severity of retinopathy of prematurity has been reported [59]. Further studies on this new product are required before it can be recommended for the baby under 1000 g[60,61].

Techniques

Preparation

The formulation and preparation of intravenous nutrition solutions can be simplified with the use of computers [62–64]. Computer programs allow convenient and accurate production of formulae based on prescriptions of individual nutrients expressed as quantities required per kg per 24 h. They also enable automatic physiological safety and precipitation checks. Ideally all dilutions and additions are carried out on commercially available stock solutions in the pharmacy under strict aseptic conditions utilizing a laminar flow hood prior to delivery to the ward.

Administration

A single 0.22 μm bacterial filter is recommended [65]. Calcium, magnesium and phosphorus concentrations have been shown to be stable across the in-line filter [66]. When lipid and amino acid solutions are infused simultaneously through the same vein, the use of a Y-connector distal to the filter to infuse lipids allows minimal mixing of the two solutions. The drip set, tubing and nutrient solutions are changed at least every 24 h.

Catheters

Intravenous nutrition can be maintained via peripheral veins using short 22 or 24 gauge catheters [67–69] or scalp vein needles [70–71]. Many neonatal units rely on nurses to insert intravenous drips [72]. The addition of heparin in the dose of 1 unit/ml to intravenous nutrition solutions has been shown to double the duration of patency of intravenous catheters and to reduce significantly the incidence of phlebitis [73]. In many neonatal units central venous catheters are relied on for long-term intravenous nutrition. The catheters are generally made of silicone rubber (Silastic), introduced subcutaneously into the subclavian vein, scalp vein or long saphenous vein, and threaded into the superior vena cava or right atrium. Sepsis complicating central catheter placement reduces dramatically with the use of the Broviac silastic catheter [74]. In a baby under 1000 g where intravenous access may be difficult or impossible, intravenous nutrition has been given via indwelling umbilical arterial catheters with no obvious increased risk [69,75,76].

Monitoring

Daily body weight and weekly length and head circumference measurements are required. Before full amino acid or glucose intake is achieved or during any period of metabolic instability, strict fluid balance, 6–12-hourly urine and blood glucose, and daily plasma and urine osmolality, haemoglobin, plasma sodium, potassium, calcium, urea and acid-base measurements are recommended. When a metabolic steady state is reached these investigations can be carried out once or twice weekly. In addition measurements of plasma magnesium, phosphorus, alkaline phosphatase, albumin, transaminases and bilirubin are recommended weekly.

Benefits

A number of randomized clinical trials have been conducted to assess the benefits and complications of intravenous nutrition in small preterm babies, though none of the study cohorts were exclusively under 1000 g. These reports did not show that total [69,71,77] or supplemental [75,78,79] intravenous nutrition improves survival. However, most did show that babies on intravenous nutrition had significantly earlier or faster weight gain [69,75,78,79]. It has been shown that the weight gain associated with intravenous nutrition is from tissue accretion rather than water retention [80,81]. Intrauterine growth rates can be achieved on intravenous nutrition in preterm babies, including those below 1000 g [82–84]. The long-term benefits of prompt restoration and maintenance of nutritional integrity are unproven. It is known, however, that in animals malnutrition during the period of rapid brain growth results in permanent reduction in brain size and cell number which cannot be corrected by a later period of liberal feeding [85]. Whether or not these findings can be extrapolated to humans is uncertain [86] although malnutrition in babies does result in reduced brain weight and DNA [87]. Satisfactory postnatal brain growth has been shown to occur during total intravenous nutrition [88].

In addition to achieving nutritional adequacy and satisfactory postnatal growth, intravenous nutrition contributes to a reduction in the morbidity and mortality from specific diseases. Enteral feeding increases the risk of aspiration pneumonia [69,89], cardiorespiratory disturbances [90] and necrotizing enterocolitis [69,77]. Intravenous nutrition allows the cautious and gradual establishment of enteral feeding, thus minimizing these risks.

Complications

Intravenous nutrition is contraindicated in babies with overwhelming sepsis such as necrotizing enterocolitis or septicaemia, prior to clinical stabilization with antibiotic therapy. It should be withheld in babies with acidosis, circulatory failure and uraemia (blood urea > 8 mmol/l). Intravenous fat is contraindicated in babies with severe oxygenation defect, a plasma bilirubin concentration above 200 μmol/l or thrombocytopenia.

Catheter-related bacterial infection rates of 9–15% have been reported in babies on intravenous nutrition [76,91]. In addition there is an increased risk of fungal sepsis which is generally related to central venous catheterization. Infections by *Candida albicans* [92] and *Malassezia furfur* [93] have been reported. Control trials have shown that the addition of heparin to the intravenous solution reduces the incidence of catheter-related sepsis [73,94]. The observation of fat deposition in the reticulo-endothelial system with Intralipid therapy [95] raised concerns that immune function may be impaired but both *in vitro* and *in vivo* studies have shown no evidence of this effect [96–98].

A complication rate of 4% has been reported to be associated with catheter insertion and migration [99]. Various reports have described superior vena cava thrombosis, pulmonary embolism, chylothorax, cardiac arrhythmia, intracardiac thrombi, hydrocephalus secondary to jugular vein thrombosis, localized necrosis, tissue ulceration and subcutaneous calcium deposition in babies receiving intravenous nutrition [100–106].

Metabolic complications

The problems of metabolic acidosis [107] and hyperammonaemia [108] have been ameliorated with generation 3 amino acid solutions currently in use. Disorders in water, nitrogen, glucose, minerals and trace element balance can either be prevented or recognized early by strict clinical and biochemical monitoring. In randomized clinical trials the incidence of metabolic complications was not different between the intravenously fed and control groups [8,69,71,75,78,79]. Osteopenia and rickets have been reported in babies receiving prolonged intravenous nutrition [109,110]. This is not surprising, given the data in Table 13.3, which shows that the calcium and phosphorus intakes in babies below 1000 g are well below intrauterine accretion rates.

Although fat accumulation in the lung has been found in association with Intralipid therapy [111,112], no impairment of oxygenation or pulmonary haemodynamics was detected unless the fat infusion rates exceeded 6–7 g/kg/24 h [113–115]. In babies with hyperbilirubinaemia it has been recommended that the molar ratio of free fatty acid to albumin in plasma should be kept below six [116]. Infants with plasma bilirubin concentration greater than 10 mg% (170 μmol/l) and serum albumin con-

Table 13.3 Mean (± s.d.) oral and intravenous sodium, calcium and phosphorus intake (mmol/kg/24 h) in 42 ELBW babies

	Sodium			*Calcium*			*Phosphorus*		
Week	*Oral*	*Intravenous*	*Total*	*Oral*	*Intravenous*	*Total*	*Oral*	*Intravenous*	*Total*
1	0.4	3.6	4.0 ± 4.0	0.2	1.3	1.5 ± 0.7	0.1	0.3	0.4 ± 0.6
2	1.5	4.9	6.4 ± 3.9	0.5	1.1	1.6 ± 0.7	0.4	0.8	1.2 ± 0.6
3	2.0	5.0	7.0 ± 6.1	0.6	0.9	1.6 ± 0.7	0.5	0.8	1.3 ± 0.6
4	2.1	4.7	6.8 ± 4.5	0.7	1.0	1.7 ± 0.9	0.5	0.9	1.4 ± 0.6
5	1.5	3.7	5.3 ± 3.6	0.8	0.9	1.7 ± 0.8	0.5	0.9	1.4 ± 0.7
6	1.7	3.6	5.3 ± 3.6	1.1	0.7	1.8 ± 0.8	0.8	0.7	1.5 ± 0.7
7	2.0	2.4	4.4 ± 2.7	1.5	0.6	2.1 ± 0.9	1.0	0.6	1.7 ± 0.7
8	2.0	2.2	4.1 ± 2.5	1.4	0.6	2.1 ± 1.0	1.0	0.6	1.6 ± 0.7

centration of 30 g/l should receive not more than 1 g/kg/24 h Intralipid [23]. It has been shown that lipaemia interferes with biochemical tests leading to spurious hyperbilirubinaemia, hypercalcaemia and hyponatraemia [117,118]. A fat infusion rate of 6 g/kg/24 h has been shown to result in hyperglycaemia [119].

Eosinophilia [71,120], thrombocytosis [71] and thrombocytopenia [121,122] have been reported during intravenous nutrition. Total leucocyte counts, absolute lymphocyte counts and T and B lymphocytes are unaffected [97].

Cholestatic jaundice [123–126], cholelithiasis [127] and hepatocellular carcinoma [128] have been reported in babies given intravenous nutrition. Possible mechanisms that have been suggested for cholestatic jaundice, which occurs in 10–40% of cases, are prolonged fasting, Intralipid, impaired bile secretion and bile salt formation, coexisting sepsis, hypotension and respiratory failure, and quality and quantity of the amino acids infused [129–135]. The cholestasis resolves promptly when intravenous nutrition ceases but progression to biliary cirrhosis and liver failure have been reported [124,126].

Conclusion

The use of intravenous nutrition has become a common paediatric practice [136] and is now routinely used in babies under 1000 g. In the majority of neonatal intensive care units where appropriate medical, nursing, pharmacy and laboratory expertise are available, its potential benefits outweigh the hazards. It allows the provision of adequate nutrition and the achievement of normal growth in many babies under 1000 g who cannot tolerate enteral feeding for many weeks after birth. As soon as the gastrointestinal tract is functional, transition to enteral feeding should nevertheless begin. The latter is believed to stimulate surges in circulating gut hormones which may facilitate physiological adaptation to extrauterine nutrition and promote gut growth and function [137]. The early initiation of enteral feeding in small subnutritional quantities is therefore of potential benefit, though supplemental intravenous nutrition should be continued until enteral feeding is adequate to fully meet the baby's nutritional requirements.

References

1. Stegink, L. D. (1983) Amino acids in pediatric parenteral nutrition. *Am. J. Dis. Child.*, **137**, 1008–1016
2. Shaw, J. C. L. (1973) Parenteral nutrition in the management of sick low birthweight infants. *Pediatr. Clin. North Am.*, **20**, 333–357
3. Duffy, B., Gunn, T., Collinge, J. and Pencharz, P. (1980) The effect of varying protein quality and energy intake on the nitrogen metabolism of parenterally fed low birthweight (< 1600 g) infants. *Pediatr. Res.*, **15**, 1040–1044
4. Chessex, P., Zebiche, H., Pineault, M., Lepage, D. and Dallaire, L. (1985) Effect of amino acid composition of parenteral solutions on nitrogen retention and metabolic response in very-low-birth weight infants. *J. Pediatr.*, **106**, 111–117
5. Zlotkin, S. H., Bryan, M. H. and Anderson, G. H. (1981) Intravenous nitrogen and energy intakes required to duplicate *in utero* nitrogen accretion in prematurely born human infants. *J. Pediatr.*, **99**, 115–120
6. Abitbol, C. L., Feldman, D. B., Ahmann, P. and Rudman, D. (1975) Plasma amino acid patterns during supplemental intravenous nutrition of low-birth-weight infants. *J. Pediatr.*, **86**, 766–772

7. Seashore, J. H. and Seashore, M.R. (1976) Protein requirements of infants receiving total parenteral nutrition. *J. Pediatr. Surg.*, **11**, 645–652
8. Anderson, T. L., Muttart, C. R., Bieber, M. A., Nicholson, J. F. and Heird, W. C. (1979) A controlled trial of glucose versus glucose and amino acids in premature infants. *J. Pediatr.*, **94**, 947–951
9. MacMahon, R. A., James, B., Shaw, P., Hendry, P., Yu, V. and Bornstein, J. (1981) Intravenous solutions in parenteral nutrition. *Acta Chir. Scand.* (*Suppl.*), **507**, 248–259
10. Burger, U., Fritsch, U., Bauer, M. and Peltner, H. U. (1980) Comparison of two amino acid mixture for total parenteral nutrition of premature infants receiving assisted ventilation. *J. Parenter. Enter. Nutr.*, **4**, 290–293
11. Hornchen, H. and Neubrand, W. (1980) Amino acids for parenteral nutrition in premature and newborn infants. Use of a mother's milk-adapted solution. *J. Parenter. Enter. Nutr.*, **4**, 294–299
12. Dickinson, J. C., Rosenblum, H. and Hamilton, P. B. (1965) Ion-exchange chromatography of the free amino acids in the plasma of the newborn infant. *Pediatrics*, **36**, 2–13
13. Pohlandt, F. (1978) Plasma amino acid concentrations in newborn infants breast fed *ad libitum*. *J. Pediatr.*, **92**, 614–616
14. Filer, L. F. Jr., Stegink, L. D. and Chandramouli, B. (1977) Effect of diet on plasma aminograms of low birth weight infants. *Am. J. Clin. Nutr.*, **30**, 1036–1043
15. Abumrad, N. N. and Miller, B. (1983) The physiologic and nutritional significance of plasma-free amino acid levels. *J. Parenter. Enter. Nutr.*, **7** 163–170
16. Zlotkin, S. H., Bryan, M. H. and Anderson, G. H. (1981) Cysteine supplementation to cysteine-free intravenous feeding regimens in newborn infants. *Am. J. Clin. Nutr.*, **34**, 914–923
17. Kerner, J. A. and Sunshine, P. (1979) Parenteral nutrition. *Semin. Perinatol.*, **3**, 417–434
18. Cowett, R. M. and Schwartz, R. (1979) The role of hepatic control of glucose homeostasis in the etiology of neonatal hypo and hyperglycaemia. *Semin. Perinatol.*, **3**, 327–340
19. Lilien, L. D., Rosenfield, R. L., Baccaro, M. M. and Pildes, R. S. (1979) Hyperglycemia in stressed small premature neonates. *J. Pediatr.*, **94**, 454–459
20. Pollak, A., Cowett, R. M., Schwartz, R. and Oh, W. (1978) Glucose disposal in low birth-weight-infants during steady state hyperglycaemia: effects of exogenous insulin administration. *Pediatrics*, **61**, 546–549
21. Yu, V. Y. H., James, B. E., Hendry, P. G. and MacMahon, R. A. (1979) Glucose tolerance in very low birthweight infants. *Aust. Paediatr. J.*, **15**, 147–151
22. Rubecz, I., Mestyan, J., Varga, P. and Klujber, L. (1981) Energy metabolism, substrate utilization, and nitrogen balance in parenterally fed postoperative neonates and infants. *J. Pediatr.*, **98**, 42–46
23. Heird, W. C. (1981) Use of intravenous fat emulsions in pediatric patients. Report of the American Academy of Pediatrics Committee on Nutrition. *Pediatrics*, **68**, 738–743
24. Tashiro, T., Ogato, H., Yokoyama, H., Mashima, Y. and Itoh, K. (1976) The effect of fat emulsion (Intralipid) on essential fatty acid deficiency in infants receiving intravenous alimentation. *J. Pediatr. Surg.*, **11**, 505–515
25. Shennan, A. T., Bryan, M. H. and Angel, A. (1977) The effects of gestational age on Intralipid tolerance in newborn infants. *J. Pediatr.*, **91**, 134–137
26. Andrew, G., Chan, G.and Schiff, D. (1978) Lipid metabolism in the neonate: III. The ketogenic effect of Intralipid infusion in the neonate. *J. Pediatr.*, **92**, 995–997
27. Andrew, G., Chan, G. and Schiff, D. (1976) Lipid metabolism in the neonate: I. The effects of Intralipid infusion on plasma triglyceride and free fatty acid concentrations in the neonate. *J. Pediatr.*, **88**, 273–278
28. Coran, A. G., Edwards, B. and Zaleska, R. (1974) The value of heparin in the hyperalimentation of infants and children with a fat emulsion. *J. Pediatr. Surg.*, **9**, 725–732
29. Dhanireddy, R., Hamosh, M., Sivasubramanian, K. N., Chowdhry, P., Scanlon, J. W. and Hamosh, P. (1981) Postheparin lipolytic activity and Intralipid clearance in very low-birth-weight infants. *J. Pediatr.*, **98**, 617–622
30. Schmidt-Sommerfeld, E., Penn, D. and Wolf, H. (1982) Carnitine blood concentrations and fat utilization in parenterally alimented premature newborn infants. *J. Pediatr.*, **100**, 260–264
31. Novak, M., Monkus, E. F., Chung, D. and Buch, M. (1981) Carnitine in the perinatal metabolism of lipids: I. Relationship between maternal and fetal plasma levels of carnitine and acylcarnitines. *Pediatrics*, **67**, 95–100

32. Schiff, D., Chan, G., Seacombe, D. and Hahn, P. (1979) Plasma carnitine levels during intravenous feeding of the neonate. *J. Pediatr.*, **95**, 1043–1046
33. Penn, D., Schmidt–Somerfeld, E. and Pascu, F. (1981) Decreased tissue carnitine concentrations in newborn infants receiving total parenteral nutrition. *J. Pediatr.*, **92**, 976–978
34. Schmidt–Sommerfeld, E., Penn, D. and Wolf, H. (1983) Carnitine deficiency in premature infants receiving total parenteral nutrition: effect of L-carnitine supplementation. *J. Pediatr.*, **102**, 921–935
35. Orzali, A., Maetzke, G., Donzelli, F. and Rubaltelli, F. F. (1984) Effect of carnitine on lipid metabolism in the neonate: II. Carnitine addition to lipid infusion during prolonged total parenteral nutrition. *J. Pediatr.*, **104**, 436–440
36. Rovamo, L. (1985) Postheparin plasma lipases and carnitine in infants during parenteral nutrition. *Pediatr. Res*,. **19**, 292–297
37. Hilliard, J. L., Shannon, D. L., Hunter, M. A. and Brans, Y. W. (1983) Plasma lipid levels in preterm neonates receiving parenteral fat emulsions. *Arch. Dis. Child.*, **58**, 29–33
38. Kao, L. C., Cherig, M. H. and Warburton, D. (1984) Triglycerides, free fatty acids, free fatty acid/ albumin molar ratio, and cholesterol levels in serum of neonates receiving long-term lipid infusions: controlled trial of continuous and intermittent regimens. *J. Pediatr.*, **104**, 429–435
39. Park, W., Paust, H. and Schroder, H. (1984) Lipid infusion in premature infants suffering from sepsis. *J. Parenter. Enter. Nutr.*, **8**, 290–292
40. Schreiner, R. L., Glick, M. R., Nordschow, C. D. and Gresham, E. L. (1978) An evaluation of methods to monitor infants receiving intravenous lipids. *J. Pediatr.*, **94**, 197–200
41. Marks, K. H., Farrell, T. P., Friedman, Z. and Maisels, M. J. (1979) Intravenous alimentation and insensible water loss in low-birth-weight infants. *Pediatrics*, **63**, 543–546
42. Mestyan, J., Jarai I. and Fekete, M. (1968) The total energy expenditure and its components in premature infants maintained under different nursing and environmental conditions. *Pediatr. Res.*, **2**, 161–171
43. Sinclair, J. C., Driscoll, J. M., Heird, W. C. and Winters, R. W. (1970) Supportive management of the sick neonate. *Pediatr. Clin. North Am.*, **17**, 863–893
44. Reichman, B. L., Chessex, P., Putet, G. *et al.* (1982) Partition of energy metabolism and energy cost of growth in the very low-birth-weight infant. *Pediatrics*, **69**, 446–451
45. Rubecz, I. and Mestyan, J. (1973) Energy metabolism and intravenous nutrition of premature infants. *Biol. Neonate*, **23**, 45–58
46. James, B.E., Hendry, P. G. and MacMahon, R. A. (1979) Total parenteral nutrition of premature infants. 1. Requirement for macronutrient elements. *Aust. Paediatr. J.*, **15**, 62–66
47. James, B. E., Hendry, P. G. and MacMahon, R. A. (1979) Total parenteral nutrition of premature infants. 2. Requirements for micronutrient elements. *Aust. Paediatr. J.*, **15**, 67–71
48. Michie, D. D. and Wirth, F. H. (1978) Plasma zinc levels in premature infants receiving parenteral nutrition. *J. Pediatr.*, **92**, 798–800
49. Sivasubramanian, K. N. and Henkin, R. I. (1978) Behavioural and dermatologic changes and low serum zinc and copper concentrations in two premature infants after parenteral alimentation. *J. Pediatr.*, **93**, 847–851
50. Herson, V. C., Philipps, A. F. and Zimmerman, A. (1981) Acute zinc deficiency in a premature infant after bowel resection and intravenous alimentation. *Am. J. Dis. Child.*, **135**, 968–969
51. Heller, R. M., Kirchner, S. G., O'Neill, J. A. *et al.* (1978) Skeletal changes of copper deficiency in infants receiving prolonged total parenteral nutrition. *J. Pediatr.*, **92**, 947–949
52. Sutton, A. M., Harvie, A., Cockburn, F., Farquharson, J. and Logan, R. W. Copper deficiency in the preterm infant of very low birthweight. *Arch. Dis. Child.*, **60**, 644–651
53. Friel, J. K., Gibson, R. S., Peliowski, A. and Watts, J. (1984) Serum zinc, copper, and selenium concentrations in preterm infants receiving enteral nutrition or parenteral nutrition supplemented with zinc and copper. *J. Pediatr.*, **104**, 763–768
54. Zlotkin, J. H. and Buchanan, B. E. (1983) Meeting zinc and copper intake requirements in the parenterally fed preterm and full-term infant. *J. Pediatr.*, **103**, 441–446
55. Lockitch, G., Godolphin, W., Pendray, M. R., Riddell, D. and Quigley, G. (1983) Serum zinc, copper, retinol-binding protein, prealbumin, and ceruloplasmin concentrations in infants receiving intravenous zinc and copper supplementation. *J. Pediatr.*, **102**, 303–308
56. Huston, R. K., Benda, G. I., Carlson, C. V., Sheerer, T. R., Reynolds, J. W. and Nerhout, R. C.

(1982) Selenium and vitamin E sufficiency in premature infants requiring total parenteral nutrition. *J. Parenter. Enter. Nutr.*, **6**, 507–510

57. Shaw, J. C. L. (1979) Trace elements in the fetus and young infant. I. Zinc. *Am. J. Dis. Child.*, **133**, 1260–1268
58. Shaw, J. C. L. (1980) Trace elements in the fetus and young infant. II. Copper, manganese, selenium and chromium. *Am. J. Dis. Child.*, **134**, 74–81
59. DeVito, V., Reynolds, J. W., Benda, G. I. and Carlson, C. (1986) Serum vitamin E levels in very low birth weight infants receiving vitamin E in parenteral nutrition solutions. *J. Parenter. Enter. Nutr.*, **10**, 63–65
60. Moore, M. C., Greene, H. L., Phillips, B. *et al.* (1986) Evaluation of a pediatric multiple vitamin preparation for total parenteral nutrition in infants and children. I. Blood levels of water-soluble vitamins. *Pediatrics*, **77**, 530–538
61. Greenett, L., Moore, M. E. C., Phillips, B. *et al.* (1986) Evaluation of a pediatric multiple vitamin preparation for total parenteral nutrition. II. Blood levels of vitamins A, D and E. *Pediatrics*, **77**, 534–547
62. May, F. and Robbins, G. (1978) A computer program for parenteral nutrition solution preparation. *J. Parenter. Enter. Nutr.*, **2**, 646–651
63. Giacoia, G. P. and Chopra, R. (1981) The use of a computer in parenteral alimentation of low birth weight infants. *J. Parenter. Enter. Nutr.*, **5**, 329–331
64. MacMahon, P. (1984) Prescribing and formulating neonatal intravenous feeding solutions by microcomputer. *Arch. Dis. Child.*, **59**, 548–552
65. Miller, R. C. and Grogan, J. B. (1975) Efficacy of inline bacterial filters in reducing contamination of intravenous nutritional solutions. *Am. J. Surg.*, **130**, 585–589
66. Koo, W. W. K., Hollis, B. W., Horn, J., Steiner, P., Tsang, R. C. and Steichen, J. J. (1986) Stability of vitamin D2, calcium, magnesium and phosphorus in parenteral nutrition solution: effect of in-line filter. *J. Pediatr.*, **108**, 478–480
67. Panter-Brick, M. (1976) Intravenous nutrition of babies and infants. *Eur. J. Int. Care Med.*, **2**, 45–51
68. Ikeda, K. and Suita, S. (1977) Total parenteral nutrition using peripheral veins in surgical neonates. *Arch. Surg.*, **112**, 1045–1049
69. Yu, V. Y. H., James, B., Hendry, P. and MacMahon, R. A. (1979) Total parenteral nutrition in very low birthweight infants: a controlled trial. *Arch. Dis. Child.*, **54**, 653–661
70. Filler, R. M. and Coran, A. G. (1976) Total parenteral nutrition in infants and children: central and peripheral approaches. *Surg. Clin. North Am.*, **56**, 395–412
71. Gunn, T., Reaman, G., Outerbridge, E. W. and Colle, E. (1978) Peripheral total parenteral nutrition for premature infants with the respiratory distress syndrome: a controlled trial. *J. Pediatr.*, **92**, 608–613
72. Babson, S. G., Benda, G. I. and Shenai, J. P. (1977) Role of the nurse in peripheral vein needle replacement. *Pediatrics*, **60**, 781
73. Alpan, G., Eyal, F., Springer, C., Glick, B., Goder, K. and Armon, J. (1984) Heparinization of alimentation solutions administered through peripheral veins in premature infants: a controlled study. *Pediatrics*, **74**, 375–378
74. Pollack, P. F., Kadden, M., Byrne, W. J., Fonkalsrud, E. W. and Ament, M. E. (1981) 100 patient years' experience with the Broviac silastic catheter for central venous nutrition. *J. Parenter. Enter. Nutr.*, **5**, 32–36
75. Brans, Y. W., Sumners, J. E., Dweck, H. S. and Cassady, G. (1974) Feeding the low birth weight infant: orally or parenterally? Preliminary results of a comparative study. *Pediatrics*, **54**, 15–22
76. Hall, R. T. and Rhodes, P. G. (1976) Total parenteral alimentation via indwelling umbilical catheters in the newborn period. *Arch. Dis. Child.*, **51**, 929–934
77. Glass, E. J., Hume, R., Lang, M. A. and Forfar, J. O. (1984) Parenteral nutrition compared with transpyloric feeding. *Arch. Dis. Child.*, **59**, 131–135
78. Bryan, M. H., Wei, P., Hamilton, J. R., Chance, G. W. and Swyer, P. R. (1973) Supplemental intravenous alimentation in low-birth-weight infants. *J. Pediatr.*, **82**, 940–944
79. Pildes, R. S., Ramamurthy, R. S., Cordero, G. V. and Wong, P. W. K. (1973) Intravenous supplementation of L-amino acids and dextrose in low-birth-weight infants. *J. Pediatr.*, **82**, 945–950

80. Rhodin, A. G. J., Coran, A. G., Weintraub, W. H. and Wesley, J. R. (1979) Total body water changes during high volume peripheral alimentation. *Surg. Gynecol. Obstet.*, **148**, 196–200
81. Polley, T. Z., Benner, J. W., Rhodin, A., Weintraub, W. H. and Coran, A. G. (1979) Changes in total body water in infants receiving total intravenous nutrition. *J. Surg. Res.*, **26**, 555–559
82. Cashore, W. J., Sedaghatian, M. R. and Usher, R. H. (1975) Nutritional supplements with intravenous administered lipid, protein hydrolysate and glucose in small premature infants. *Pediatrics*, **56**, 8–16
83. Wilson, F. E., Yu, V. Y. H., Hawgood, S., Adamson, T. M. and Wilkinson, M. H. (1983) Computerised nutritional data management in neonatal intensive care. *Arch. Dis. Child.*, **58**, 732–736
84. Gill, A., Yu, V. Y. H., Bajuk, B. and Astbury, J. (1986) Postnatal growth in infants born before 30 weeks gestation. *Arch. Dis. Child.*, **61**, 549–553
85. Winick, M. (1969) Malnutrition and brain development. *J. Pediatr.*, **74**, 667–679
86. Dobbing, J. (1974) The later growth of the brain and its vulnerability. *Pediatrics*, **53**, 2–6
87. Winick, M. and Rosso, P. (1969) The effect of severe malnutrition on cellular growth of the human brain. *Pediatr. Res.*, **3**, 181–184
88. Trompeter, R. S., Dobbing, J. Aynsley-Green, A. and Baum, J. D. (1976) Neonatal brain growth during prolonged intravenous feeding. *Arch. Dis. Child.*, **51**, 316–318
89. Wharton, B. A. and Bower, B. D. (1965) Immediate or later feeding for premature babies? A controlled trial. *Lancet*, 969–972
90. Yu, V. Y. H. (1976) Cardiorespiratory response to feeding in newborn infants. *Arch. Dis. Child.*, **51**, 305–309
91. Nelson, R. (1974) Minimising systemic infection during complete parenteral alimentation of small infants. *Arch. Dis. Child.*, **49**, 16–20
92. Baley, J. E., Kliegman, R. M. and Fanaroff, A. A. (1984) Disseminated fungal infections in very-low-birthweight infants: clinical manifestations and epidemiology. *Pediatrics*, **73**, 144–152
93. Powell, D. A., Aungst, J., Sneddon, S., Hansen, N. and Brady, M. (1984) Broviac catheter-related *Malassezia furfur* sepsis in five infants receiving intravenous fat emulsions. *J. Pediatr.*, **105**, 987–990
94. Bailey, M. J. (1979) Reduction of catheter-associated sepsis in parenteral nutrition using low-dose intravenous heparin. *Br. Med. J.*, **i**, 1671–1673
95. Friedman, Z., Marks, K. H., Maisels, M. J., Thorson, R. and Naeye, R. (1978) Effect of parenteral fat emulsion on the pulmonary and endothelial systems in the newborn infant. *Pediatrics*, **61**, 694–698
96. English, D., Roloff, J. S., Lukens, J. N., Parker, P., Greene, H. L. and Ghishan, F. K. (1981) Intravenous lipid emulsions and human neutrophil function. *J. Pediatr.*, **99**, 913–916
97. Puri, P., Reen, D. J., Browne, O. and Guiney, E. J. (1981) Immune status of the neonate maintained on total parenteral nutrition. *Arch. Dis. Child.*, **56**, 283–286
98. Strunk, R. C., Murrow, B. W., Thilo, E., Kunke, K. S. and Johnson E. G. (1985) Normal macrophage function in infants receiving Intralipid by low-dose intermittent administration. *J. Pediatr.*, **106**, 640–645
99. Ryan, J. A., Abel, R. M., Abbott, W. M. *et al.* (1974) Catheter complications in total parenteral nutrition. A prospective study of 200 consecutive patients. *N. Engl. J. Med.*, **290**, 757–761
100. Wiley, E. L. and Hutcins, G. M. (1977) Superior vena cava syndrome secondary to candid thrombophlebitis complicating parenteral alimentation. *J. Pediatr.*, **91**, 977–979
101. Wesley, J. R., Keens T. G., Miller, S. W. and Platzker, A. C. G. (1978) Pulmonary embolism in the neonate: occurrence during the course of total parenteral nutrition. *J. Pediatr.*, **93**, 113–115
102. Vain, N. E., Swarner, O. W. and Cha, C. C. (1980) Neonatal chylothorax: a report and discussion of nine consecutive cases. *J. Pediatr. Surg.*, **15**, 261–265
103. Brady, R. E. and Weinberg, P. M. (1976) Atrioventricular conduction disturbance during total parenteral nutrition. *J. Pediatr.*, **88**, 113–114
104. Mahoney, L., Snider, A. B. and Silverman, N. H. (1981) Echocardiographic diagnosis of intracardiac thrombi complicating total parenteral nutrition. *J. Pediatr.*, **98**, 469–471
105. Stewart, D. R., Johnson, D. G. and Myers, G. G. (1975) Hydrocephalus as a complication of jugular catheterization during total parenteral nutrition. *J. Pediatr. Surg.*, **10**, 771–777
106. Ramamurthy, R. S., Harris, V. and Pildes, R. S. (1975) Subcutaneous calcium deposition in the neonate associated with intravenous administration of calcium gluconate. *Pediatrics*, **55**, 802–806
107. Heird, W. C., Dell, R. B., Driscoll, J. M., Grebin, B. and Winters, R. W. (1972) Metabolic acidosis

resulting from intravenous alimentation mixtures containing synthetic amino acids. *N. Engl. J. Med.*, **287**, 943–948

108. Johnson, J. D., Albritton, W. L. and Sunshine, P. (1972) Hyperammonemia accompanying parenteral nutrition in newborn infants. *J. Pediatr.*, **81**, 154–161
109. Leape, L. L. and Valaes, T. (1976) Rickets in low birth weight infants receiving total parenteral nutrition. *J. Pediatr. Surg.*, **11**, 665–673
110. Klein, G. L., Cannon, R. A., Diament, M. *et al.* (1981) Infantile vitamin D-resistant rickets associated with total parenteral nutrition. *Am. J. Dis. Child.*, **136**, 74–75
111. Levene, M. I., Wigglesworth, J. S. and Desai, R. (1980) Pulmonary fat accumulation after Intralipid infusion in the preterm infant. *Lancet*, **ii**, 815–819
112. Dahms, B. B. and Halpin, T. C. (1980) Pulmonary arterial lipid deposit in newborn infants receiving intravenous lipid infusion. *J. Pediatr.*, **97**, 800–805
113. Adamkin, D. H., Gelke, K. N. and Wilkerson, S. A. (1985) Influence of intravenous fat therapy on tracheal effluent phospholipids and oxygenation in servere respiratory distress syndrome. *J. Pediatr.*, **106**, 122–124
114. Pereira, G. R., Fox, W. W., Stanley, C. A., Bakier, L. and Schwartz, J. G. (1980) Decreased oxygenation and hyperlipemia during intravenous fat emulsions in premature infants. *Pediatrics*, **66**, 26–30
115. Lloyd, T. R. and Boucek, M. M. (1986) Effect of Intralipid on the neonatal pulmonary bed: an echographic study. *J. Pediatr.*, **108**, 130–133
116. Andrew, G., Chan, G. and Schiff, D. (1976) Lipid metabolism in the neonate. II. The effect of Intralipid on bilirubin binding *in vitro* and *in vivo*. *J. Pediatr.*, **88**, 279–284
117. Shennan, A. T., Cherian, A. G., Angel, A. and Bryan, M. H. (1976) The effect of Intralipid on the estimation of serum bilirubin in the newborn infant. *J. Pediatr.*, **88**, 285–288
118. Giacoia, G. P. and Krasner, J. (1979) Interference of intravenous lipid emulsion with the determination of calcium in serum. *Am. J. Med. Technol.*, **45**, 767–768
119. Vileisis, R. A., Cowett, R. M. and Oh, W. (1982) Glycemic response to lipid infusion in the premature neonate. *J. Pediatr.*, **100**, 108–112
120. Bhat, A. M. and Scanlon, J. W. (1981) The pattern of eosinophilia in premature infants. *J. Pediatr.*, **98**, 612–616
121. Lipson, A. H., Pritchard, J. and Thomas, G. (1974) Thrombocytopenia after Intralipid infusion in a neonate. *Lancet*, **ii**, 1462–1463
122. Panter-Brick, M., Wagget, J. and Dale, G. (1975) Intralipid and thrombocytopenia. *Lancet*, **i**, 857–858
123. Touloukian, R. J. and Downing, S. E. (1973) Cholestasis associated with long-term parenteral hyperalimentation. *Arch. Surg.*, **106**, 58–62
124. Postuma, R. and Trevenen, C. L. (1979) Liver disease in infants receiving total parenteral nutrition. *Pediatrics*, **63**, 110–115
125. Beale, E. F., Nelson, R. M., Bucciarelli, R. L., Donnelly, W. H. and Eitzman, D. V. (1979) Intrahepatic cholestasis associated with parenteral nutrition in premature infants. *Pediatrics*, **64**, 342–347
126. Pereira, G. R., Sherman, M. S., DiGiacomo, J., Ziegler, M., Roth, K. and Jacobowski, D. (1981) Hyperalimentation-induced cholestasis. *Am. J. Dis Child.*, **135**, 842–845
127. Whitington, P. F. and Black, D. D. (1980) Cholelithiasis in premature infants treated with parenteral nutrition and furosemide. *J. Pediatr.*, **97**, 647–649
128. Vileisis, R. A., Sorensen, K., Gonzalez-Crussi, F. and Hunt, C. E. (1982) Liver malignancy after parenteral nutrition. *J. Pediatr.*, **100**, 88–90
129. Rager, R. and Finegold, M. J. (1975) Cholestasis in immature newborn infants: is parenteral alimentation responsible? *J. Pediatr.*, **86**, 264–269
130. Passwell, J., Katznelson, D. and Cohen, B. (1976) Pigment deposition in the reticuloendothelial system after fat emulsion. *Arch. Dis. Child.*, **51**, 366–368
131. Sondheimer, J. M., Bryan, H., Andrews, W. and Forster, G. G. (1978) Cholestatic tendencies in premature infants on and off parenteral nutrition. *Pediatrics*, **62**, 984–989
132. Manginello, F. P. and Javitt, N. B. (1979) Parenteral nutrition and neonatal cholestasis. *J. Pediatr.*, **94**, 296–298

133. Dosi, P. C., Raut, A. J., Chelliah, B. P. *et al.* (1985) Perinatal factors underlying neonatal cholestasis. *J. Pediatr.*, **106**, 471–474
134. Vileisis, R. A., Inwood, R. J. and Hunt, C. E. (1980) Prospective controlled study of parenteral nutrition-associated cholestatic jaundice: effect of protein intake. *J. Pediatr.*, **96**, 893–897
135. Sankaran, K., Berscheid, B., Verma, V., Zakhary, G. and Tan, L. (1985) An evaluation of total parenteral nutrition using Vamin and Aminosyn as protein base in critically ill preterm infants. *J. Parenter. Enter. Nutr.*, **9**, 439–442
136. American Academy of Pediatrics (1983) Commentary on parenteral nutrition. *Pediatrics*, **71**, 547–552
137. Lucas, A., Aynsley-Green, A. and Bloom, S. R. (1981) Gut hormones and the first meals. *Clin. Sci.*, **60**, 349–353

Chapter 14

Calcium and phosphorus metabolism and rickets

Neil McIntosh

Mineralization of the fetus occurs continuously and logarithmically and calcification of the skeleton is radiologically demonstrable from the eighth week of pregnancy [1]. Because of the logarithmic accumulation, infants born significantly early, e.g. at 28 weeks or less gestation, will have a considerable deficit in mineral compared to the full term baby. These very preterm infants now frequently survive and it is evident that provision of calcium and phosphorus is not only extremely inadequate postnatally but that the immaturity of the gastrointestinal tract further reduces the effective supply by relatively poor absorption mechanisms.

Maternal mineral supply in the last trimester

The skeleton of the newborn infant contains about 25 g calcium and 16 g phosphate and about 80% of this is transferred to the fetus during the last three months of pregnancy [2]. This represents a flux of 6.5 mmol/day of calcium and 4.6 mmol/day of phosphorus and is a considerable proportion of the maternal dietary intake. The fetal plasma calcium exceeds the maternal (as does the fetal phosphate) and it is thought that there is active transfer of calcium to the fetus across the placenta; 80% of the calcium transferred finds its way back to the mother [3].

However the neonatologist decides how to feed the ELBW infant and whatever the food he chooses, the calcium and phosphorus intake will be considerably less than the accumulation of these elements across the placenta during the last three months of pregnancy (Table 14.1). Most infants born at 28 weeks gestation or less will require a period – sometimes extended – of intravenous feeding. These regimens will supply usually between 50 and 70% of the bone mineral (calcium and phosphorus) required [4–7]. The solubility product of calcium and phosphate in intravenous feeding solutions restricts increasing the concentration further. Breast milk is extremely deficient in mineral content and, although the milk from the mothers of preterm infants may have higher concentrations of some minerals, Atkinson *et al.* [8] could show no significant difference in bone mineral, and the variable content of the constituents as a whole makes this food very inadequate [9]. The new preterm infant formulae acknowledge that the very immature infant requires a large amount of bone mineral and their concentrations have been increased very significantly. If the absorption of these formulae was complete, the small baby would receive an adequate supply for bone mineralization, but our own data on babies of less than 1000 g birth

Table 14.1 Calcium and phosphate intake and retention data in the perinatal period

	Calcium (mg)	*Phosphate* (mg)	*Calcium* (mmol)	*Phosphate* (mmol)
Transplacental intake/kg/24 h in the last three months of pregnancy[26]	140	70	3.5	2.3
Intake from typical intravenous feeding regime at 150 ml/kg/24 h[4]	45	23	1.1	0.8
Intake per day by breast-fed infant fed at 200 ml/kg/24 h	45–70	23–28	1.1–1.8	0.8–0.9
Retention per day by breast-fed infant fed at 200 ml/kg/24 h (day 30 data[10])	13.5–21	20–24	0.34–0.53	0.7–0.8
Intake per day by preterm formula-fed infant at 200 ml/kg/24 h (preterm SMA)	150	80	3.8	2.6
Retention per day by preterm formula-fed infant fed at 200 ml/kg/24 h (day 30 data[10])	75	56	1.9	1.8

weight show that although phosphorus absorption is good by the second week of life even in the most immature infants (70–80% of ingested), the calcium absorption is very poor for a long time. Thus these babies at 30 days of age are only retaining between 30 and 50% of their enteral calcium intake (depending on the food given) [10]. A full term formula with its low mineral content would be inappropriate now for the feeding of the ELBW infant.

Neonatal hypocalcaemia

Prematurity predisposes to early neonatal hypocalcaemia [11]. In our own unit, despite anticipating the fall in calcium and routinely using calcium gluconate in the first three days of life, 37% of 171 infants of less than 1000 g birth weight have over the last five years dropped their serum calcium levels to less than 1.65 mmol/l, though these infants have rarely been symptomatic. We have not seen any cases of late neonatal hypocalcaemia or neonatal tetany, probably because our routine feeding is with expressed breast milk and the serum biochemistry is closely monitored.

Early neonatal hypercalcaemia and hypophosphataemia

The inadequate supply of mineral to the extremely immature infant was postulated by Lyon *et al.* [12] to be the cause of hypercalcaemia seen in the second week of life. This hypercalcaemia, seen in ten infants of less than 1000 g birth weight, was always associated with extreme hypophosphataemia. It was suggested that even the immature infant, when faced with the need for phosphate for essential metabolic processes, will extract this mineral from bone. The extraction of phosphate will be accompanied by extraction of calcium which leads to both hypercalcaemia and hypercalciuria. The addition of extra phosphate to the diet (given as sodium dihydrogen phosphate to breast milk) reversed the hypophosphataemia, hypercalcaemia and hypercalciuria (Figure 14.1). It is suggested that all infants weighing less than 1000 g (and probably less than 1250 g) should receive phosphate supplements from the third day of life

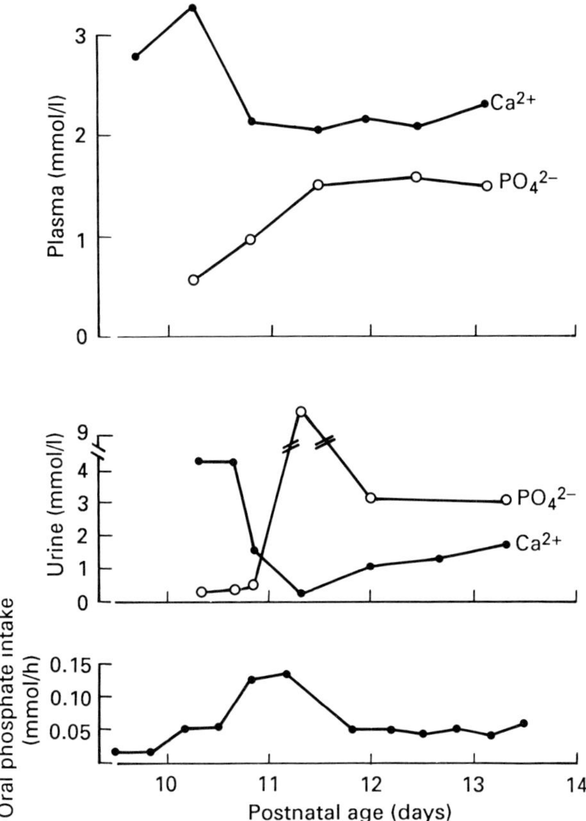

Figure 14.1 Hypercalcaemia, hypercalciuria and hypophosphataemia all normalized in an infant of 610 g given extra oral phosphate on the tenth and eleventh days of life

when early neonatal hypocalcaemia has resolved. Our own practice is to give 1 ml of buffered sodium phosphate (BP) daily even from the first day of life mixed with the breast milk that they receive in small quantities enterally, no matter how small and sick (our only contraindication is a congenital intestinal abnormality). This provides the baby with an intake of 0.83 mmol of phosphate in addition to that in the milk and the supplemental parenteral nutrition. The extra oral phosphate is given while the infant is on breast milk (but not formula) and is less than 1500 g in actual weight. We believe that radiological morphology is at least objective and the wrist should be X-rayed at two-week intervals beginning from the age of three weeks.

Rickets in ELBW infants

Incidence

At St. George's Hospital the incidence of radiological rickets in infants of less than 1000 g birth weight is more than 50% if they survive for more than 28 days (Table 14.2).

(a)

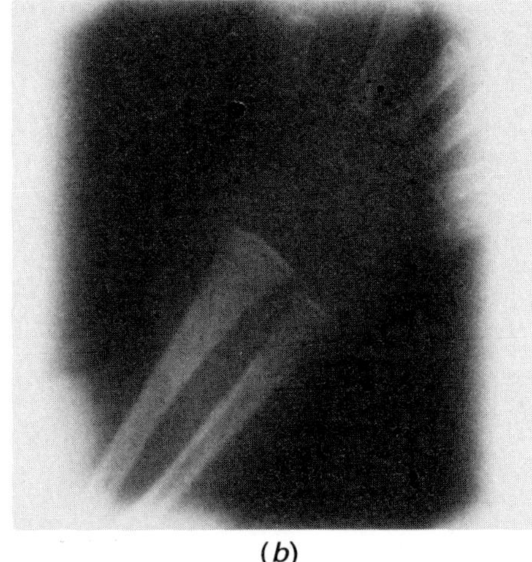

(b)

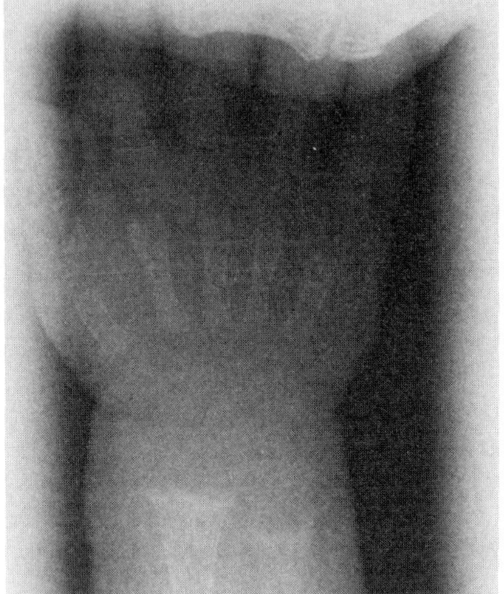

(c)

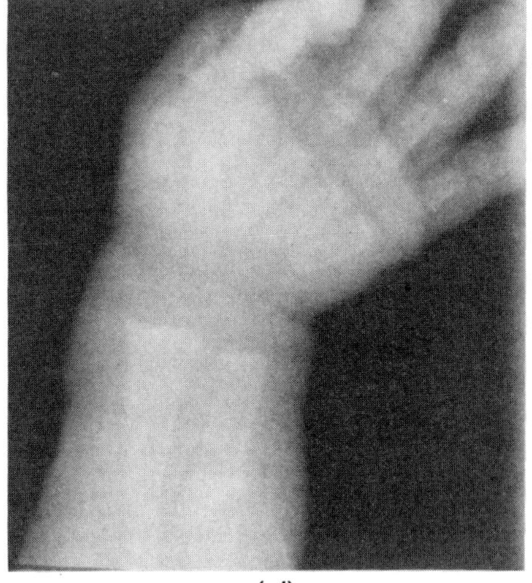

(d)

Figure 14.2 Radiological rickets: (*a*) grade 0, (*b*) grade 1, (*c*) grade 2, (*d*) grade 3 (see Table 14.3 for description)

Table 14.2 Incidence of rickets of prematurity (Koo grades 2 and 3) [28] in babies of < 1000 g birth weight managed at St. George's Hospital Neonatal Unit who survived for more than 28 days

	1981	*1982*	*1983*	*1984*	*1985*
No. of cases	7	8	11	13	12
Percentage incidence	47	44	50	42	56

Table 14.3 Radiological grading of rickets of prematurity described by Koo *et al.* [27]

Grade	*Description*
1	Loss of dense white line at the metaphysis, increased submetaphyseal lucency and thinning of the cortex
2	Irregularity and fraying, cupping and splaying, i.e. the changes of rickets
3	Changes of rickets with evidence of fractures

Diagnosis

The incidence depends on the method of diagnosis. All infants of this birth weight have a raised serum alkaline phosphatase and 75% have obvious radiological osteopenia [13]. The few studies available using photon absorptiometry invariably showed mineral deficiency [14,15]. However, although this technique allows considerable sophistication at quantifying the mineral deficit, it is not measuring or identifying classical changes. This, and the fact that most units do not have the method available, make it more likely that the diagnosis will be made on biochemical or radiological criteria. The alkaline phosphatase level in the serum has been suggested as a screening test for the diagnosis [16]. The levels are always high, being directly related to the gestation of the infant [17] and the type of food [10]. A comparison of maximum serum alkaline phosphatase concentrations with the radiological grading of rickets (shown in Figure 14.2 and described in Table 14.3) shows considerable overlap of levels in infants without radiological changes and in those with classical radiological signs (Figure 14.3).

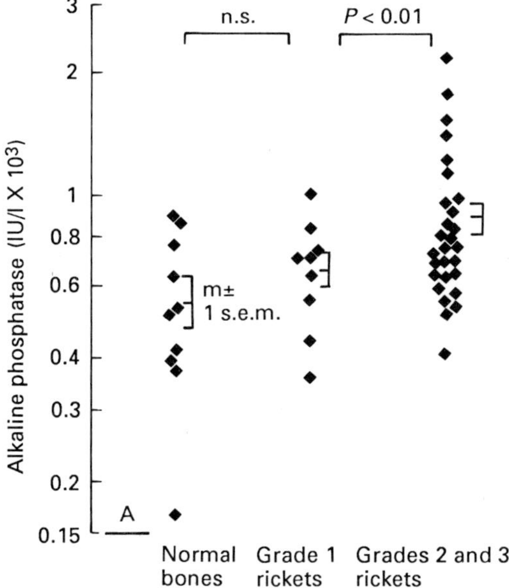

Figure 14.3 A comparison of serum alkaline phosphatase levels with the radiological grading of rickets described in Table 14.3. A = laboratory upper limit of normal for children

Aetiology

Although Von Sydow in 1946 suggested that rickets was due to calcium deficiency [18], most early workers assumed that it was a problem associated with the supply of or metabolism of vitamin D. Between 1981 and 1983 at St. George's Hospital, despite an intake of 2000 units of vitamin D daily from the seventh day of life, 54% of infants with a birth weight of less than 1000 g developed radiological rickets and at the time of diagnosis they had high circulating levels of 25-hydroxycholecalciferol [19]. In 1981 we treated half the cases with alphacalcidol in case there was a problem of 1α-hydroxylation by the kidney but these cases healed at the same rate as those untreated. Shortly afterwards, others demonstrated high levels of 1,25-dihydroxycholecalciferol [20,21] and although it is possible that there may be end organ insensitivity to the active hormone, it seems more likely that the major factor in the aetiology is a deficiency of mineral substrate [22]. The provision of adequate calcium and phosphorus in the diet is therefore an important goal in these infants. It should also be noted that the use of loop diuretics such as frusemide may lead to calcium loss in the urine which may exaggerate substrate deficiency.

It would appear that the osteopenia that is obvious radiologically in 75% of the babies in our unit with a birth weight of less than 1000 g and that is implied to be universally present by the few studies on preterm babies using photon absorptiometry [14,15], is not only a consequence of poor mineral supply in the weeks after birth but is likely to be particularly related to the demineralization process that goes on in the first two weeks as the infants try to maintain their serum phosphate concentration at an adequate level for essential metabolic processes (see p. 156).

Complications

If rickets of prematurity heals itself with time, should we worry about it? The development of spontaneous fractures cannot be pleasant for the baby and this complication was seen in 17% of our cases between 1981 and 1983. We have never knowingly seen the development of rachitic respiratory distress [23] but the undermineralization of the rib cage must reduce the efficiency of respiration.

Treatment

The prevention of rickets must be the goal but we have had remarkably little success. From 1981 to 1983 inclusive, 2000 units daily of vitamin D from the seventh day of life did not prevent rickets. In 1984, reduction of vitamin D to 1000 units daily from the first day and the addition of phosphate supplements (0.83 mmol/24 h) reduced the incidence but not significantly. In 1985, the addition of calcium 1.62 mmol/24h to this regime was associated with an increase, though again this was not significant [24]. The routine feeding of these ELBW infants has always been with expressed breast milk, and it is likely that the mineral intake is insufficient even with the added minerals. Seino *et al.* [25] suggested that the incidence could be reduced by the use of alphacalcidol but only three infants in their series had a birth weight of < 1000 g. Our own experience in a small number of cases suggests that once the radiological changes are apparent, the use of alpahacalcidol does not increase the natural rate of healing [19]. Since the study of this small series we have not used additional vitamin D therapy to heal the condition.

References

1. Hamilton, W. J. (ed.) (1976) *Textbook of Human Anatomy*, 2nd edn, Macmillan, London
2. McCance, R. A. and Widdowson, E. M. (1961) Mineral metabolism of the foetus and newborn. *Br. Med. Bull.*, **17**, 132–136
3. Ramberg, C. F., Delivoria-Papadopoulos, M., Crandell, E. D. and Kronfeld, D. S. (1973) Kinetic analysis of calcium transport across the placenta. *J. Appl. Physiol.*, **35**, 682–688
4. Shaw, J. C. L. (1973) Parenteral nutrition in the management of sick low birthweight infants. *Pediatr. Clin. North Am.*, **20**, 333–358
5. Cockburn, F. (1976) Complete intravenous feeding of the newborn. *Clin. Endocrinol. Metab.*, **5**, 191–219
6. Wretland, A. (1972) Complete intravenous nutrition. Theoretical and experimental background. *Nutr. Metab.*, **14** (Suppl. 1), 57
7. Fomon, S. J. (1974) *Infant Nutrition*, 2nd edn, W. B. Saunders, Philadelphia
8. Atkinson, S. A., Anderson, G. H. and Bryan, M. H. (1980) Human milk: comparison of the nitrogen composition in the milk from mothers of premature and full term infants. *Am. J. Clin. Nutr.*, **33**, 811–815
9. Hibberd, C. M., Brooke, O. G., Carter, N. D., Haug, M. and Harzas, G. (1982) Variation in the composition of breast milk during the first five weeks of lactation: implications for feeding of preterm infants. *Arch. Dis. Child.*, **57**, 658–662
10. Lyon, A. J. and McIntosh, N. (1984) Calcium and phosphorus balance in extremely low birthweight infants in the first six weeks of life. *Arch. Dis. Child.*, **59**, 1145–1150
11. Tsang, R. C. and Oh, W. (1970) Neonatal hypocalcaemia in low birthweight infants. *Pediatrics,* **45**, 773–781
12. Lyon, A. J., McIntosh N., Wheeler, K. and Brooke, O. G. (1984) Hypercalcaemia in extremely low birthweight infants. *Arch. Dis. Child.*, **59**, 1141–1144
13. McIntosh, N., Williams, J. E., Lyon, A. J. and Wheeler, K. A. (1984) Diagnosis of rickets of prematurity. *Lancet*, **ii**, 869
14. Steichen, J. J., Gratton, T. L. and Tsang, R. C. (1980) Osteopenia of prematurity: the cause and possible treatment. *J. Pediatr.*, **96**, 528–534
15. James, J. R., Congdon, P. J., Truscott, J., Horsman, A. and Arthur, R. (1986) Osteopenia of prematurity. *Arch. Dis. Child.*, **61**, 871–876
16. Kovar, I., Mayne, P. and Barltrop, D. (1982) Plasma alkaline phosphatase activity: a screening test for rickets in preterm neonates. *Lancet*, **i**, 308–310
17. Glass, E. J., Hume, R., Hendry G. M. A., Strange, R. C. and Forfar, J. O. (1982) Plasma alkaline phosphatase activity of prematurity. *Arch. Dis. Child.*, **57**, 373–376
18. Von Sydow, G. (1946) A study of the development of rickets in premature infants. *Acta Paediatr. Scand.*, **33** (Suppl. 2), 5–122
19. McIntosh, N., Livesey, A. and Brooke, O. G. (1982) Plasma 25-hydroxyvitamin D and rickets in infants of extremely low birthweight. *Arch. Dis. Child.*, **57**, 848–850
20. Rowe, J. C., Wood, D. H., Rowe, D. W. and Raisz, L. G. (1979) Nutritional hypophosphataemic rickets in a premature infant fed breast milk. *N. Engl. J. Med.*, **300**, 293–297
21. Steichen, J. J., Tsang, R. C., Greer, F. R., Ho, M. and Hug, G. (1981) Elevated serum 1,25-hydroxyvitamin D concentration in rickets of very low birthweight infants. *J. Pediatr.*, **99**, 293–298
22. Day, G. M., Chance, G. W., Radde, I. C. *et al.* (1975) Growth and mineral metabolism in very low birthweight infants. II. Effects of calcium supplementation on growth and divalent ions. *Pediatr. Res.*, **9**, 568
23. Glasgow, J. F. T. and Thomas, P. S. (1977) Rachitic respiratory distress in small preterm infants. *Arch. Dis. Child.*, **52**, 268–273
24. De Curtis, M., Nicholson, S., Fenton, T., Gibson, P. and McIntosh, N. (1986). Failure of mineral supplementation to reduce the incidence of rickets of prematurity in infants weighing less than 1000 g at birth. *Pediatr. Res.*, **20**, 98
25. Seino, Y., Ishii, T., Shimotsuji, T., Ishida, M. and Yabuuchi, H. (1981) Plasma active vitamin D concentration in low birthweight infants with rickets and its response to vitamin D treatment. *Arch. Dis. Child.*, **56**, 628–632

26. Shaw, J. C. L. (1976) Evidence for defective skeletal mineralization in low birthweight infants: the absorption of calcium and fat. *Pediatrics*, **57**, 16–25
27. Koo, W. W. I., Gupta, J. M., Nayanar, V. V., Wilkinson, M. and Posen, S. (1982) Skeletal changes in preterm infants. *Arch. Dis. Child.*, **57**, 447–552

Chapter 15

Haematology

Elizabeth Letsky

Normal haematological parameters and anaemia in babies under 1000 g

There are marked differences between fetal and adult red cells, and in the first few weeks of life many changes occur in the composition of the circulating blood. Only by six months of age has a stable population of red cells been established with characteristics which persist into adult life.

All newborn infants experience a fall in haemoglobin concentration in the first few weeks but this fall is greater and earlier in preterm infants. Sometimes this means that a transfusion must be considered. The indications for blood transfusion in small babies are not well defined. Some infants tolerate very low levels of haemoglobin with none of the accepted signs of tissue anoxia while others are clinically ill. Usually the anaemia results from several factors including repeated blood sampling.

To establish whether or not true anaemia is present and whether transfusion is indicated some knowledge of the normal physiology and potential of the adaptive processes in the very small preterm infant is required.

True anaemia at any time in life is present when the demand of tissues for oxygen, in order to maintain normal metabolism, exceeds the ability to deliver oxygen to the tissues.

Tissue oxygenation depends on cardiopulmonary function, concentration and composition of haemoglobin and the position of the haemoglobin-oxygen dissociation curve. Tissue oxygenation in the small preterm infant is suitably designed for intrauterine life and is ill adapted for postnatal existence [1].

The pathophysiology of anaemia of prematurity

Erythropoietin

Maternal erythropoietin does not cross the placenta. Fetal erythropoiesis is controlled by erythropoietin produced by the fetus; high concentrations have been observed in the amniotic fluid and fetal blood [2] in pregnancies complicated by severe erythroblastosis fetalis. Elevated levels of erythropoietin have also been found in cord blood of babies who have had stressful birth or have suffered hypoxia *in utero*. However the fetal production of erythropoietin in response to hypoxia or anaemia is poor compared with that of older infants or adults; this probably prevents accelerated erythropoiesis and hyperviscosity of the blood in the healthy fetus [3].

The preterm infant retains this poor response to hypoxic stimuli even though such infants tend to produce erythropoietin in response to a fall in haemoglobin concentration. The limited production of erythropoietin and the greatly shortened red cell life span appear to be the cause of the refractory anaemia of the preterm infant.

Prematurity is a major factor in erythropoietin response, the least mature babies having the lowest levels of erythropoietin [4] in spite of low haemoglobin concentration, high affinity of oxygen for haemoglobin and clinical hypoxia.

VLBW infants appear to have an inadequate haemopoietic response to anaemia related tissue hypoxia. This may be due to a shift in the site of erythropoietin production [3]. In many mammalian species, erythropoietin is produced in the liver in fetal life and there is a gradual shift to renal production of erythropoietin in the perinatal period. This fetal production of erythropoietin is much less sensitive to tissue hypoxia than that produced in the kidney, but this has not been confirmed in the human fetus. Human adult renal and hepatic erythropoietins have been shown to be structurally identical [5].

If the conclusion that the anaemia of prematurity results from inadequate erythropoietin production is correct, it raises the possibility of using erythropoietin in a clinical therapeutic trial [6]. Recombinant erythropoietin has been shown to stimulate erythroid proliferation *in vitro* [7] and has already been used to produce a reticulocyte response and to treat the anaemia of chronic renal failure [8].

Availability of oxygen and special problems of demand and supply

Tissue oxygen availability depends on arterial oxygen saturation, the concentration of haemoglobin and the position of the haemoglobin-oxygen dissociation curve. These are all different in VLBW infants. Arterial oxygen saturation is frequently low because of diseases of the lung and apnoeic attacks. The concentration and type of haemoglobin is different from a term baby.

Developmental changes in haemoglobins

There are embryonic, fetal and adult haemoglobins. The three embryonic haemoglobins – Hb Gower 1 and 2 and Hb Portland – disappear by 12 weeks gestation; they are probably restricted to the primitive red cells produced in the yolk sac (Table 15.1).

Table 15.1 Globin chain composition of human haemoglobins

Haemoglobin	*Globin composition*	*Site of production*	*Stage of development*
Gower 1	$\zeta_2\ \varepsilon_2$		Embryo
Gower 2	$\alpha_2\ \varepsilon_2$	Yolk sac	Embryo
Portland	$\zeta_2\ \gamma_2$		Embryo
Fetal	$\alpha_2\ \gamma_2$		Embryo
Fetal	$\alpha_2\ \gamma_2$	Liver	Fetus
Adult	$\alpha_2\ \beta_2$	Bone marrow	Fetus
Hb A_2	$\alpha_2\ \delta_2$		Fetus
Fetal	$\alpha_2\ \gamma_2$	Bone marrow	Adult
Adult	$\alpha_2\ \beta_2$		Adult
Hb A_2	$\alpha_2\ \delta_2$		Adult

Fetal haemoglobin, Hb F ($\alpha_2\gamma_2$) can be detected in the blood from embryos of 6–12 weeks gestation.

From the time when hepatic erythropoiesis is established Hb F ($\alpha_2\gamma_2$) forms the major respiratory pigment throughout intrauterine life, but from as early as 8–10 weeks gestation it is possible to detect about 5–10% of haemoglobin – Hb A ($\alpha_2\beta_2$). Between 32 and 36 weeks gestation the production of Hb A increases and there is a sharp decline in Hb F production (Figure 15.1). Hb F makes up less than 10% of haemoglobin at three months of age and has fallen to the adult level of less than 1% by six months to one year.

The decline of fetal haemoglobin in the newborn period appears to be strictly regulated. The switch from Hb F to Hb A synthesis occurs around 32 weeks gestation [9]; it is not related to birth, but it is based on postconceptional age. Thus the relative concentration of Hb F and Hb A in cord blood depends on gestation. Babies at 32–34 weeks have a mean of 90% Hb F; at term it is around 70–80%.

The efficiency of oxygen delivery to the tissues is directly related to the interactions of haemoglobin with 2,3-diphosphoglycerate (2,3-DPG). High concentrations of 2,3-DPG push the oxygen dissociation curve to the right and facilitate oxygen delivery to the tissues. The reduction in the oxygen affinity of Hb F by interaction with 2,3-DPG is only a fraction of that produced by the same concentration of 2,3-DPG with Hb A. The effect of this reduced reaction of Hb F with 2,3-DPG ensures that the oxygen affinity of fetal blood does not drop below that of its mother. This aids binding of oxygen from the maternal circulation in the placenta villi. More than half of the oxygen bound in the placenta by the fetal blood can be released to fetal tissue because the tissue oxygen levels in the fetus are much lower than those in the maternal tissues.

In the first few weeks of extrauterine life there is a progressive increase in the delivery of oxygen to the tissues. There is a gradual replacement of Hb F by Hb A, an increase in 2,3-DPG which shifts the oxygen dissociation curve to the right, and, of

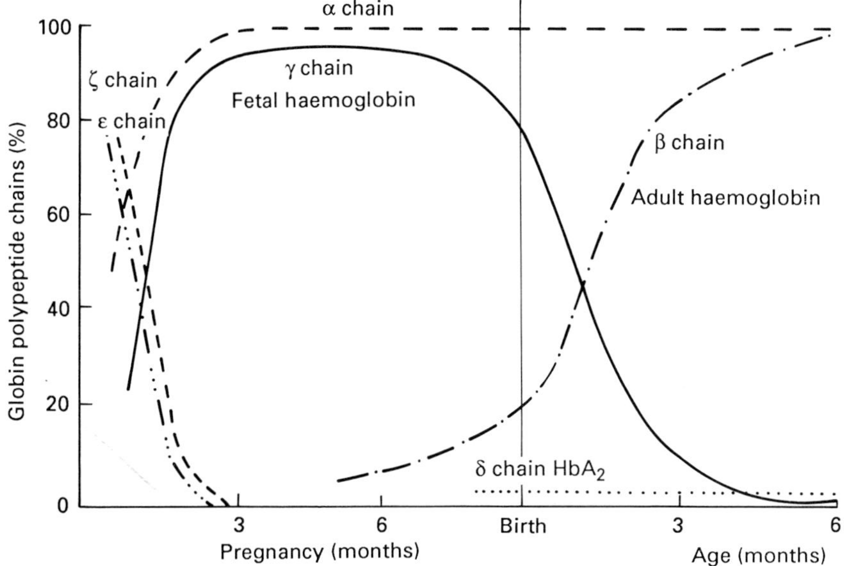

Figure 15.1 Developmental changes in human haemoglobins

course, increased availability of oxygen. The net result of these changes is that although the haemoglobin level in the term infant falls from 17 g/dl to 11 g/dl in the first 12 weeks of life, the oxygen delivery to the tissues at three months is greater than that in the newborn infant.

However, the infant under 1000 g is unlikely to have reached 32 weeks postconception and therefore the switch to predominant β globin chain production has not even begun and it may be some weeks later before significant amounts of Hb A are produced [10]. This compromises the delivery of oxygen to the tissues by preventing the shift of the oxygen dissociation curve to the right.

Haemoglobin concentration

Cord haemoglobin values for preterm infants (17.5 ± 1.6 g/dl) do not vary significantly from those observed at term.

Dependent upon the amount of placental transfusion and transient haemoconcentration due to poor oral fluid intake, a brief rise in haemoglobin is seen during the first 24 h of life. The haemoglobin returns to the original concentration of birth by the end of the first week, and there is then a progressive fall over 4–12 weeks. The rapidity of fall and the nadir of haemoglobin concentration vary inversely with gestational age; the fall results from a reduction in red cell mass and not from the haemodilutional effect of a greater plasma volume. The red cell life span is even shorter in the preterm infant than at term and there is a marked reticulocytopenia.

The supply of oxygen to the tissues of the healthy newborn is only just adequate. In the very preterm infant this marginal oxygen supply often fails. Superimposed on the multiple causes of anaemia in the baby under 1000 g are the sampling blood losses essential for the monitoring and intensive management of such small birth weight babies. Iatrogenic blood letting is probably the major cause of anaemia in such infants [11].

Haematinics

The VLBW infant is more prone to develop nutritional deficiencies than the term infant because of rapid growth and diminished resources. Factors that can accelerate the anaemia of prematurity are iron, folate and vitamin B_{12} and vitamin E deficiency.

Iron

Although iron transport to the fetus is unidirectional with ratio of maternal:fetal serum ferritin concentrations of 1:2 to 1:4 and there are adequate fetal iron stores even in cases of maternal iron deficiency, there is some evidence that there is a reduced red cell mass in the offspring of iron-deficient mothers; iron stores, although high by adult standards, are reduced in these infants compared to those born to iron-replete mothers [12]. The fetus normally recruits 75 mg iron/kg body weight; iron status will be related to birth weight and maturity [1].

The role of iron in the pathogenesis of the anaemia of prematurity has excited interest for almost 50 years. As a result of innumerable investigations a clearer picture has emerged from the initial confusion. Iron deficiency is not likely to play a part in the early anaemia of prematurity unless there has been perinatal blood loss or repeated blood sampling [13]. It follows that the administration of medicinal iron will not prevent the initial fall in haemoglobin. However, unless the premature infant is given iron supplements some time in the first 2–4 months of life, an anaemia – the so-called late anaemia of prematurity – inevitably develops from iron deficiency [14]. The time of the anaemia will depend on the initial haemoglobin level and the rate of growth. In general infants with normal haemoglobin levels at birth will have depleted their iron stores and therefore limit the rate of haemoglobin synthesis by the time they have doubled their birth weight [15]. Approximately 75% of the infant's total body iron is contained in the haemoglobin of the circulating and developing red cells; those who are anaemic at birth have reduced iron reserves [16].

There is now a consensus that all premature infants, and particularly those weighing less than 1500 g at birth, require supplemental iron to prevent the development of late anaemia due to iron deficiency. Cord blood haemoglobin level, birth weight and blood-letting in the first weeks of life will determine the timing of the development of iron deficiency.

Iron supplements in VLBW infants should be started on the fifteenth day of life in the following dosage regime [15]:

2 mg/kg/24 h for infants from 1500–2500 g birth weight
3 mg/kg/24 h for infants from 1000–1500 g birth weight
4 mg/kg/24 h for those less than 1000 g birth weight

and these supplements should be continued for at least 12–15 months after birth [17]. If the infant is receiving adequate vitamin E in relation to polyunsaturated fat in the diet then the early introduction of supplemental iron causes no adverse effects.

Copper

More than 90% of the copper normally present in plasma is bound to ceruloplasmin, which aids the absorption of iron and its release from body stores. Copper is also necessary for iron metabolism within erythroid precursors. Copper deficiency mimics iron deficiency by the production of the hypochromic microcytic anaemia, but also produces neutropenia. The term infant has abundant hepatic copper stores, sufficient to maintain him through the first six months of life; these are accumulated in the last 12 weeks of fetal life. Thus the preterm infant is born with poor copper stores [18] and severe symptomatic copper deficiency may develop in those fed cow's milk products with inadequate copper content. It is recommended that the infant receive 80 μg of copper/kg/24 h and most infant formulae have been supplemented appropriately.

The diagnosis of copper deficiency anaemia is made by the demonstration of low serum copper (< 40 μg/dl) or low ceruloplasmin values (< 15 mg/dl), together with vacuolated erythroid precursors and maturation arrest in the granulocyte series. Anaemia and neutropenia due to nutritional copper deficiency will respond promptly to the administration of 400–600 μg copper/24 h in a 1% copper sulphate solution [17].

Zinc

The role of zinc in haemopoiesis is still not established. Its deficiency is shown with diarrhoea, dermatitis with bullae on feet and hands, and crusts around the nose, mouth and perineum. Most zinc is acquired during the last trimester of pregnancy, therefore deficiency develops in the preterm infant if sufficient quantities are not given after birth. Intestinal interactions between copper and zinc may impair absorption of the former but a zinc concentration of 12.5 ng/l in artificial milk will prevent this [19].

The Committee on Nutrition of the American Academy of Pediatrics [20] recommends an intake of 0.5 mg zinc/100 kcal.

Vitamin E

Alpha-tocopherol (vitamin E) is a fat soluble dietary factor first shown to be required for successful reproduction in rats and now known to be an essential nutrient for man. Adults do not readily become deficient in vitamin E because there is α-tocopherol in foodstuffs. Vitamin E deficiency has been described in the newborn, especially the preterm [21]. This is because all newborn infants have relative tocopherol deficiency; the smaller the infant at birth the greater the lack of vitamin E.

A mother at term has a vitamin E level around 0.9 mg/100 ml whereas her baby's value is only 0.2 mg/100 ml. Term infants with a birth weight of 3500 g have vitamin E body stores of 20 mg while infants with a birth weight of 1000 g have only 3 mg. There is a relationship between the maternal level of vitamin E and that of her infant but a newborn infant never has a value in excess of 0.6 mg/100 ml, which is the lowest limit of normal for older children and adults.

Vitamin E is a potent antiperoxidant at the cellular level; its deficiency results in an increased rate of cell membrane lipid peroxidation which can lead to a shortening of the red cell life-span and a haemolytic anaemia.

The dietary requirement for vitamin E increases when the intake of polyunsaturated fatty acids (PUFA) increases. Although the breast-fed infant quickly attains normal adult levels, there is considerable variability in the vitamin E status in artificially fed infants. This results in part from the PUFA content of the artificial formulae. Most infant formulae contain quantities of linoleic acid, an 18-carbon fatty acid with two unsaturated double bonds, far in excess of the quantities found in breast milk.

The first reports of the association of vitamin E deficiency with haemolytic anaemia in the premature neonate came from the USA in the late 1960s [22,23]. These infants were aged 6–10 weeks and had been fed proprietary formulae with a high PUFA content. The administration of vitamin E to affected infants resulted in a prompt increase in the haemoglobin level and a fall in the reticulocyte count.

It is clear that the severity of the haemolysis in the premature infant was related to the level of vitamin E and the PUFA content of the diet (E:PUFA ratio). The lack of reports from the UK is probably a reflection of the lower PUFA content of our proprietary formulae at that time and hence a higher E:PUFA ratio.

It became evident through the passage of time that it was not just the high PUFA and low vitamin E content of the diet which were predisposing factors to haemolysis in the premature infant. Iron acts as a catalyst in the non-enzymatic auto-oxidation of unsaturated fatty acids and can result in the peroxidation of red cell membrane lipids. It has been shown that iron fortified formulae can trigger a haemolytic anaemia in the infant who receives large quantities of PUFA with inadequate amounts of vitamin E [24].

The incidence of vitamin E deficiency haemolytic anaemia varies from nursery to nursery and is rare in the UK. It should be appreciated that vitamin E deficiency may contribute to the magnitude of the physiological anaemia in all non-supplemented premature infants. The commercial formulae have, for the most part, corrected the potential problem by reducing the content of linoleic acid and increasing the concentration of vitamin E. Breast mik has a very low content of linoleic acid.

The problem of the triad of factors (iron, PUFA and vitamin E levels) contributing to anaemia in the premature infants is now well recognized and haemolysis can thus be prevented by:

(1) A delay in introduction of iron.
(2) Vitamin E can be administered to overcome the malabsorption of the natural vitamin.
(3) Formulae with a low PUFA content, or human milk, can be fed to small premature infants.

The removal or correction of just one of the contributing triad will prevent any significant haemolysis or anaemia in the premature neonate [25], but a recent study [26] showed no haematological difference between infants supplemented with 0.25 IU oral vitamin E daily and a control group.

It has been suggested that vitamin E supplements may also reduce the incidence of two serious complications of oxygen administration in the premature infant – retinopathy of prematurity (ROP) [27] and bronchopulmonary dysplasia (BPD) [21]. This is based on animal experiments which have demonstrated that vitamin E-deficient animals suffer more oxygen-induced damage to their lungs and brain as well as the red cells, than animals fed on a vitamin E-supplemented diet.

Reports of a reduction in incidence, severity and duration of ROP in the human neonate associated with vitamin E supplementation have appeared in recent years [21]. Preliminary studies suggesting that the intramuscular administration of a water-dispersible preparation of DL-α-tocopherol during the acute phase of therapy for respiratory distress syndrome prevented the development and modified the severity of BPD, still await confirmation from large combined studies.

Intraventricular haemorrhage and vitamin E About 40% of newborn babies under 32 weeks gestation develop ultrasound evidence of intra-ventricular haemorrhage within the first three days of life. This bleeding may be confined to the subependymal region where it originates or it may rupture into the ventricles or brain parenchyma.

It has been suggested by a group in Manchester that vitamin E given intravenously to preterm babies may protect against intraventricular haemorrhage in very preterm infants [28]. The situation is complicated by the different vitamin E preparations available, their route of administration, their ability to raise plasma vitamin E levels and their reported toxicity.

Oral vitamin E, 200 mg/kg daily has been associated with an increased incidence of necrotizing enterocolitis (NEC) in one report [29]. Although the intravenous route produces the most rapid response in vitamin E plasma levels, this method of administration cannot be recommended until concern about associated toxic effects has been resolved.

Folic acid

Serum and red cell folate levels are higher in the newborn than in the normal adult regardless of birth weight or gestation, but fall quickly to levels which are often below the normal adult levels within several weeks of birth. This fall occurs more rapidly in

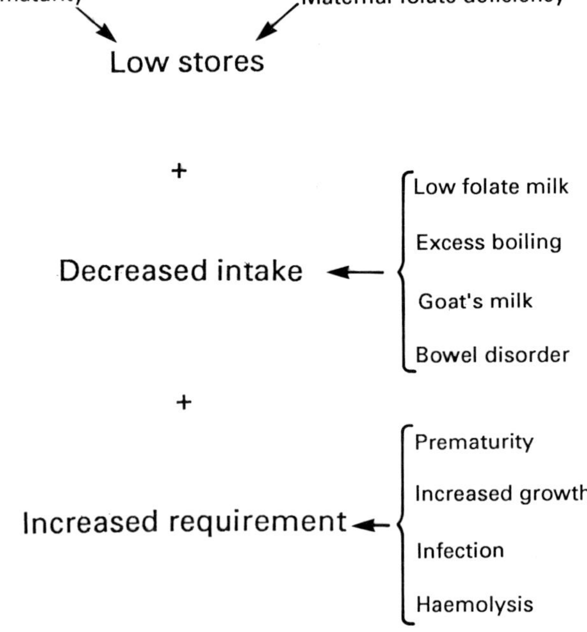

Figure 15.2 The factors which contribute to the development of megaloblastic anaemia due to folate deficiency in infancy

the preterm infant, subnormal levels being reached within the first few weeks of life, whereas low levels do not develop in the term infant until after six months of age. Controlled studies, however, have failed to demonstrate any alteration in the early anaemia of prematurity by giving routine folate supplementation. The normal premature infant absorbs folic acid easily and although there is no general recommendation for the prophylactic use of folic acid in the newborn [14], a dietary provision of 20–50 μg/24 h would ensure sufficiency.

There is an increased risk of megaloblastic anaemia occurring in the neonate of a folate-deficient mother, especially if delivery is preterm. The pathogenesis of the development of such an anaemia is shown in Figure 15.2. The young infant's requirement for folate has been estimated at 20–50 μg/24 h (4–10 times the adult requirement) on a weight basis. Serum and red cell folates are consistently higher in cord than in maternal blood, but the premature infant is in severe negative folate balance because of high growth rate and reduced intake. The usual fall in serum and red cell folate in the preterm neonate, and even in the absence of other complicating factors, may result in megaloblastic anaemia. This can be prevented by giving supplements of 50 μg/24 h [30].

In those infants whose dietary intake would be predictably poor, such as the very immature or those with chronic diarrhoea or recurrent infections, it would appear wise to give parenteral folic acid from time to time.

Vitamin B_{12}

Serum B_{12} levels in all neonates are generally higher than in maternal serum. This is the result of active transfer of vitamin B_{12} across the placenta to the fetus at the expense of maintaining maternal vitamin B_{12} serum levels. This makes little impact on the mother's own reserves because adult stores are of the order of 300 μg or more and vitamin B_{12} stores in the newborn infant are about 50 μg [31].

Because of these low storage reserves and because of poor dietary intake of vitamin B_{12} during the period of rapid growth, most premature infants will have lower than normal adult levels by the fourth or fifth month of life. A deficiency of vitamin B_{12} is not related to the early anaemia of prematurity.

The haemoglobin, red cell counts and haematocrit are similar in premature infants who are deficient or replete for vitamin B_{12}. Any supplements of these essential nutrients that are given to premature infants in the first few weeks of life are to prevent the late anaemia due to deficiencies which would inevitably develop by the fourth or fifth month of life.

Protein

Protein synthesis and turnover are increased in preterm infants because of their very high metabolic rates. Adequate protein is necessary for healthy haemopoiesis and therefore dietary requirements for protein must be increased in these immature infants.

It has been shown [32] that human milk proteins promote general growth and erythropoiesis in VLBW infants. The beneficial effect, particularly on erythropoiesis promoting higher haemoglobin concentration in the early weeks of life, appears to be dependent on the human origin of this protein, and an uptake of 4 g/kg daily which is double the usual intake.

Blood transfusion

All newborn infants, whether term or preterm, are more likely to be transfused than any other patient in hospital. In the majority of instances the need for transfusion in the premature infant arises from the loss of blood withdrawn for laboratory testing. The average daily blood loss per infant in newborn intensive care units, even those which use microtechniques, has been estimated to be in excess of 2.0 ml [33]. The indications for transfusion and the blood banking procedures to provide for the needs for sick neonates present major problems for the clinicians and blood transfusion serologists. There have been no firm guidelines which have been generally adopted, largely because the regulation of erythropoiesis in the perinatal period is more complex than at any other time in life. Transfusion policy for the anaemia of prematurity depends largely on how the clinician views this condition. Some believe that the fall in haemoglobin is a purely physiological process that is temporary and should never be interfered with and they emphasize the known hazards of transfusion. Raising the haemoglobin may prolong the suppression of marrow erythropoietin activity and delay reactivation. On the other hand, more severe anaemia of prematurity has been seen in recent years because of the improved survival and small babies seem to benefit from transfusions with improvement of general activity and weight gain.

The following discussion is an attempt to outline the indications for transfusion in the VLBW infant, to clarify the real risks of transfusion and to suggest the optimal utilization of blood and blood products.

Indications

The lack of firm guidelines as indication for the need for transfusion results largely from the inability to measure all the parameters determining oxygen availability and the need for oxygen in the preterm infant.

When considering the need for transfusion it is essential to compare the level of haemoglobin with the expected level in a premature infant of similar birth weight and age. Haemoglobin levels fall by 1 g/dl per week on average from the second to eighth week of life. A haemoglobin of 8.5 g/dl in an otherwise healthy premature infant at seven weeks may be within the normal range, but it would obviously be grossly abnormal in an infant of 2–3 weeks of age. Indeed the haemoglobin may fall naturally within the first eight weeks of life to 7.0 g/dl in an otherwise healthy premature infant weighing less than 1000 g at birth and may cause little concern [33].

However, in the more immature infant haemoglobin concentration as high as 10.5 g/dl may be associated with clinical manifestations of anaemia due to reduced tissue oxygen availability dependent on the high oxygen affinity of fetal haemoglobin [34]. In fact, as increasingly immature infants survive, *ex cathedra* statements are made about the necessity for transfusion at a certain haemoglobin level, e.g.

(1) 'As a general rule haemoglobin values in otherwise healthy low birth weight infants should be maintained above 12 g/dl during the first two weeks of life' [35].
(2) 'Sick babies of birth weight 1000 g or less who are being ventilated should have their haemoglobin concentration maintained at 14.0 g/dl or above' (London neonatal paediatrician).
(3) 'We believe it is logical to use normal values for Hb concentration, haematocrit and red cell mass for healthy term babies of the same postnatal age. However these *normal* values are likely to be the minimum desirable for preterm infants because of their proportionally greater lean metabolizing body tissue' [1].

Red cell mass in determining need for transfusion [36]

Assessment of severity of anaemia in the preterm infant and prediction of volume of red cells to be transfused are usually based on the level of haemoglobin or haematocrit. In the newborn period, the haemoglobin and haematocrit values correlate poorly with the mass of red cells/kg body weight (RCM). The proportion of adipose tissue in the VLBW baby is about 2.5% compared to 15% in a 3.5 kg term infant. This implies an optimal value for RCM in ml/kg about 15% higher in the leaner baby.

A new non-hazardous method for the rapid determination of RCM in infants requiring transfusion has been described [37]. The measured percentage of fetal haemoglobin (Hb F) in the infant's blood before and after a known volume of adult red cells (Hb A) is transfused allows estimation of the preterm RCM in ml/kg:

$$\text{RCM} = \frac{\text{V} \times \text{Post T\% Hb F}}{\text{Pre T\% Hb F} - \text{Post T\% Hb F}}$$

where T = transfusion. The frequency of transfusion may be reduced by giving red cells to correct the deficiency based on RCM estimation. If the RCM cannot be determined, the authors recommend transfusing enough red cells to bring the post-transfusion haematocrit to the upper limit of normal for a term baby of similar postnatal age.

Central venous oxygen tension

A fall in central venous oxygen tension would seem to be the most sensitive indicator of the presence of true anaemia [33]. This measurement represents the integration of all the variables that determine supply and demand of oxygen, and the values obtained correlate with erythropoietin levels. At values less than 30 torr (normal is greater than 38 torr) erythropoietin levels are uniformly increased above normal for gestation and postnatal age. This haemoglobin concentration is only one among many important variables determining oxygen availability and the need for red cell transfusion, but unfortunately most nurseries will not have access to investigations which determine RCM or central venous oxygen tissue, and for these reasons the clinical states and gestational age of the infant together with haemoglobin and haematocrit are the criteria used to determine the necessity for transfusion.

It should be remembered that a blood transfusion given solely on the basis of haemoglobin concentration is likely to be one of a series. The first transfusion will increase the concentration of Hb A, shift the oxygen dissociation curve, and thus lower the oxygen affinity of the circulating haemoglobin. This will then depress red cell production and the haemoglobin will fall to a lower level before erythropoiesis is reactivated.

A very important indication for the need for transfusion is a failure to achieve the expected daily weight gain. This is due to an increase in metabolic needs arising from an increase in oxygen consumption which appears to be an early response to anaemia. It has been shown that regular transfusion in the premature infant will result in improved weight gain in those babies who are lagging behind the expected average [38].

Until more precise guidelines are available concerning the expression of true anaemia in the premature infant, the physician caring for infants will have to make decisions based on clinical judgments about the need for blood transfusions. Certain simple measures should be instituted which will avoid unnecessary blood administration and result in essential transfusions only being given.

(1) All blood taken should be carefully recorded, and if 5–10% of the baby's blood volume should be removed over a short space of time, it should be replaced with packed red cells.
(2) The haemoglobin should be measured on entry to the nursery and at regular, at least weekly, intervals thereafter. The haemoglobin will drop about 1 g/dl per week. A transfusion should never be given based on the haemoglobin level alone; although haemoglobin values of 7.0 g/dl or less require explanation, they may not need correction.
(3) Evalution should include:
    (a) Weight gain;
    (b) Fatigue while feeding;
    (c) Tachypnoea and tachycardia;
    (d) Hypoxia, reflected by elevated levels of lactic and pyruvic acid.
(4) Infants with cardiac or pulmonary disease with a reduced arterial oxygen saturation may need to have the haemoglobin maintained in the range of 16–17 g/dl to ensure sufficient differential between arterial and venous oxygen tension.

Complications of blood transfusion

In principle, all of the hazards associated with blood transfusion apply to the newborn but in addition there are special complications and risks which arise from the unique blood banking needs in the nursery created by the small size of the recipient and the special vulnerability to transfusion of infections and metabolic disturbances because of the neonate's immaturity. These special complications have been well reviewed [39].

Metabolic problems

On storage of blood in the anticoagulant citrate-phosphate-dextrose (CPD), the pH will fall in the first week from 7.0 to 6.8 and to 6.7 on three weeks' storage. The serum potassium level may reach 10 mmol/l by the end of the first week, but the 2,3-DPG levels are maintained during this time. The adult recipient can quickly adjust these adverse metabolic changes on storage of blood which the immature neonate may find a problem. Massive transfusions as in exchange transfusions can result in systemic acidosis followed by rebound alkalosis. Occasionally citrate binding results in symptomatic hypocalcaemia and hypomagnesaemia.

Another complication seen after exchange transfusion is hyperglycaemia followed by rebound hypoglycaemia. Another potential source of problem is the fact that the serum sodium of CPD-stored blood is elevated. Because of these problems with CPD anticoagulation in the newborn, the use of heparin has been advocated since it does not result in any of these adverse metabolic changes. The major disadvantage is that it has a limited effect as an anticoagulant and in the UK blood taken into heparin has to be used within 12 h of donation. This necessitates tests for hepatitis and HIV being carried out on the donor before the blood is taken. It also results inevitably in much wastage of blood. Now that most blood banks separate components from a unit of blood such as red cells, platelets, fresh frozen plasma, and coagulant factor concentrates, they are not enthusiastic about the preparation of heparinized fresh blood which cannot be used for the preparation of component therapy. Therefore they encourage the use of CPD blood within 24–72 h of donation when the metabolic changes are at a minimum. This also allows blood to be safely screened for hepatitis B surface antigen, syphilis, cytomegalovirus (CMV), HIV and for the group to be checked before release from the centre.

Red cell injury

Haemolysis, due to physical injury of the erythrocyte, is the usual cause of what appears to be a haemolytic transfusion reaction in the newborn. This may be caused by forcing red cells through a fine bore needle or catheter or by excessive heating in a blood warmer. Rarely a true immuno-haemolytic transfusion reaction occurs; when this happens it is invariably the result of a clerical error.

Allo-immunization to red blood cell and white cell antigens

Recent studies have shown that neonates do not readily form allo-antibodies to either red cell or white cell antigens. It has been suggested that it is probably not necessary to continue red cell cross-matching for neonatal transfusion as this does not result in red cell allo-immunization. The cross-match is, however, a safeguard in recipient identification as long as rigorous adherence to established procedures are observed.

Graft versus host disease (GVHD)

GVHD has been described subsequent to red cell transfusion, white cell transfusion, plasma exchange and intrauterine transfusion. In the neonate the clinical picture is one of skin rash, hepatitis and marrow aplasia. GVHD may be an important cause of death following exchange transfusion and can be prevented by irradiation of blood prior to infusion into immunocompromised patients or preterm infants. Although there has been an increased frequency of reports in recent years, GVHD is a rare entity and routine irradiation of blood for simple transfusion to neonates is *not* indicated although a case can be made for irradiation of blood products for exchange transfusion [40,41].

In the last 12 years at Queen Charlotte's Maternity Hospital, which is a referral centre for severe haemolytic disease of newborn where frequent intrauterine and exchange transfusions are performed, irradiated blood has not been used and we have yet to see a case of GVHD as a result of blood transfusion.

Transmission of infection

Post-transfusion hepatitis is probably the most common and serious of all the problems associated with the transfusion of blood and blood products. In the neonate the risk is increased for a chronic carrier state and although blood can be fairly efficiently screened for hepatitis B there is an increasing problem of non-A non-B hepatitis.

CYTOMEGALOVIRUS INFECTION

It is known that massive transfusion of blood to an adult immune suppressed patient may result in infection with a variety of microbiological agents which would normally have little or no effect. Among these, cytomegalovirus which is widely spread in nature is one. Approximately 60% of all blood donors are CMV antibody positive. Unfortunately this does not mean that their blood confers passive immunity necessarily. Some carry live virus in their white cells which can be reactivated in a suitable milieu. In fact, congenital CMV infection has been reported in more than 3% of the offspring of sero-immune women, but it would appear that infants born to CMV negative mothers are more prone to morbidity induced by neonatal CMV infections. In the healthy immunocompetent child or adult, post-transfusion CMV infection results in sero-conversion with little or no morbidity – possibly only a transient atypical mononuclear cell syndrome.

In contrast, CMV infection in an immuno-incompetent individual such as premature newborns may be associated with significant morbidity and even mortality. Recently there has been an attempt to reduce the potential infectivity of donor blood from some blood banks in special situations, but blood transfusion is only one of many sources of CMV infection in the nursery and other environmental factors must also be taken into consideration.

The ways in which the infectivity of donor blood can be cut down is by selecting CMV negative donors or by transfusing frozen or leucocyte-depleted red cells. It would appear that it is difficult to identify the potentially dangerous carrier of live virus within the 60% of donors who are antibody positive, therefore they all have to be rejected if transfusion transmission is to be avoided. However blood which has been stored at 4 °C for 48 h is much less likely to transmit CMV infection than fresh blood, even if there is live virus in the blood when collected from the donor.

TRANSMISSION OF HUMAN IMMUNODEFICIENCY VIRUS (HIV) [42]

There are only two modes of transmission of HIV infection so far documented in the neonate:

(1) Parenteral contact with blood and blood products.
(2) Vertical transmission from an infected mother to her infant.

The first reported case of neonatally acquired AIDS came from California in 1982. A 20-month-old white boy, born preterm, who had received multiple top-up transfusions in the Special Care Baby Unit developed hepatosplenomegaly, neutropenia, autoimmune haemolytic anaemia, thrombocytopenia, *in vitro* evidence of T-cell dysfunction and opportunistic infection. One of the donors was a homosexual man who, although symptom-free at the time, subsequently developed AIDS and died.

There has not been one case of AIDS in a newborn baby resulting from blood transfusion received in the UK. A few cases of neonatal AIDS have been reported, some in the UK, related to transfusions received either by the mother or the baby itself, in other parts of the world, before testing of donors for antibody to the virus had become routine and before groups at risk voluntarily stopped donating blood.

The likelihood of a neonate acquiring AIDS from donor blood in the United Kingdom remains remote. The risk has been estimated as less than one in a million donations [43]. This is less than the risk of developing or dying from hepatitis, or being infected with cytomegalovirus from the donor blood. Perhaps the most important point to make is the fact that the risk of a 1000 g baby dying if the systolic blood pressure is allowed to remain below 40 mm and the haematocrit below 40% because of withholding transfusion far outweighs the remote risk of acquiring AIDS as a result of transfusion [44].

Problems associated with provision of small aliquots of blood

Unique difficulties for the blood transfusion service are created because procedures must be developed to provide unusually small quantities of reasonably fresh blood for transfusion to term and preterm infants with minimum wastage. Volumes of blood required in the nursery, other than for exchange transfusion, vary from 20 to 100 ml per transfusion. If the usual single unit of 450 ml of freshly donated blood was used for top-up transfusions, more than three-quarters would be wasted for each transfusion given. In the UK many large blood transfusion centres still do not provide smaller sub-units suitable for transfusion to infants.

WALKING DONOR SYSTEM

This is a controversial method which was developed because of the need for small quantities of blood for transfusion in the intensive care nursery. A pool of potential donors who work within the hospital where the nursery is situated are all grouped and screened for atypical antibodies. The donors are checked on registration for hepatitis antigen, syphilis and HIV antibody. When blood is thought to be clinically necessary for a neonate, compatibility, hepatitis, syphilis and AIDS testing are performed on the donor's blood. This can be done when 24 h warning is given that a transfusion is needed. This system should never be used in an emergency when suitably checked and processed blood should and can be obtained from the district blood bank at any time of day or night.

When the tests have been done, the donor is bled the exact amount to be transfused; the blood is taken into a syringe containing heparin.

The advantages of such a system are:

(1) Ease of administration with minimum delay.
(2) Elimination of wastage.
(3) Heparinized fresh blood can be used, so there are no metabolic problems.
(4) Ease of meticulous monitoring of the health of the donor.
(5) A single donor can be used for the same patient on a number of occasions, reducing exposure to infection.

The main disadvantages are:

(1) Removes quality control from blood bank.
(2) May increase risk of transmission of hepatitis (particularly non-A non-B) because hospital personnel are used.

In the USA where elaborate measures are taken by the blood banks to provide small aliquots of blood with a minimum of infective risk for use in the nursery, the Walking Donor System is largely frowned upon and the legal requirements for screening and compatibility testing have resulted in many hospitals finding little advantage in its use.

In the UK, in certain circumstances, a sensibly run Walking Donor Service can be justified. At Queen Charlotte's Maternity Hospital such a service was in operation for many years with no major adverse complications. Many donors also gave blood to the National Blood Transfusion Service; the small donations required for babies do not prevent the donors giving a larger donation at six-monthly intervals. In addition to the routine testing required for quality control, all donors were tested for CMV antibody. All mothers of babies who were admitted to the intensive care unit were tested for CMV antibody. If their serum was found to be positive, this was compared with the booking blood to ensure that sero-conversion had not taken place during the pregnancy. Babies of mothers who had been CMV antibody positive throughout pregnancy were transfused with compatible blood regardless of the CMV antibody status of the donor. CMV negative blood was transfused, if possible, to those babies whose mothers were not demonstrably immune to CMV infections. From 1985 onwards all donors were tested for HIV status at each donation.

In defence of this system, it should be pointed out that the blood bank which served Queen Charlotte's did not provide small sub-units and did not test potential donors for neonates for CMV status. It should be stressed, however, that this system was not for emergency use. It was administered and controlled strictly from the blood transfusion laboratory. The list of donors was not available to anyone except blood transfusion serology personnel. The Regional Transfusion Service now supply small packs of blood and CMV testing is done in addition to routine testing; the Walking Donor System has therefore been discontinued.

It is clear that there are special problems concerning the indications and complications of transfusion in the neonate.

Necrotizing enterocolitis and transfusion

The exact aetiology of necrotizing enterocolitis (NEC) is not defined as yet, but many now believe that the pathogenesis depends on the interaction of three factors:

(1) Disturbed intestinal mucosal integrity.
(2) Presence of pathogenic bacteria.
(3) Availability of substrate to promote growth of bacteria – enteral feeding [45].

Damage to the intestinal mucosa may be caused by a variety of events and procedures which occur regularly in the intensive care nursery. These include asphyxia, shock, umbilical vessel catheterization and exchange transfusion. The association of neonatal intestinal perforation and NEC with exchange transfusion was first reported from a number of independent centres in the UK in the late 1960s. Many argue that this association was a chance one concomitant with more aggressive and successful intensive care in the premature infant, but others suggested that the explanation may be in the increased use of plastic perfusion equipment and the widespread adoption of prepacked gamma-irradiated polyvinyl chloride (PVC) exchange transfusion kits in place of the rubber, glass and metal giving sets, at this time [46].

The plasticisers used in the treatment of PVC bags and catheters can be leached out and do accumulate in the blood during storage. The phthalate ester diethylhexyl phthalate (DEHP) may have toxic effects in the neonate. Perfused human umbilical arteries lose physiological responsiveness after perfusion using PVC apparatus. These responses can be restored after a return to the use of glass and silicone and rubber tubing [46]. DEHP has also been shown to inhibit mitosis and growth of lymphocytes *in vitro* [47]. There are at least two ways in which the use of PVC catheters during exchange may lead to NEC and intestinal perforations:

(1) The leached toxic substances could lead to direct chemical necrosis of the mucosa.
(2) The toxic substances may affect the responses of the portal vasculature exposing it to insults during the exchange.

Attempts to bring these possible potential dangers of the use of PVC catheters in the neonate to the attention of the medical profession, and paediatricians in particular, have not met with much response.

As little has been done to regulate the control of PVC equipment for the newborn, paediatricians should be alert for the possible complications and avoid precipitating factors as far as possible.

Many neonatologists feel that there may be an association between blood or component transfusion and NEC. However, this is hardly surprising as the sick infant is unlikely to avoid transfusion and NEC is a unique complication seen only in the preterm newborn. There are no objective studies which show a positive correlation between NEC and transfusion but there have been unexpected, albeit anecdotal, instances of NEC in babies who were beginning to thrive and who received transfusions. This gives one a nagging feeling that there might be a connection between transfusion and NEC.

Haemostasis and thrombosis in the baby under 1000 g

The haemostatic mechanism of the VLBW infant cannot be considered in isolation. A full account of haemostatic disorders in the pregnant woman and her offspring has recently been published by Hathaway and Bonnar [48].

Normal haemostasis is determined by the interaction between the vessel wall, platelets, procoagulation factors, naturally occurring anticoagulants and fibrinolysis.

Constant changes occur in the components of these systems in the healthy neonate over the first few weeks of life and the haemostatic mechanisms are not mature by adult standards until 6–9 months of age. To complicate matters further, these changes are dependent not only on the postnatal age of the infant, but also on the gestational age [49].

Although the healthy term infant can maintain haemostatic competence, profound physiological and pathological stimuli may tip the balance in the direction of either thrombosis or haemorrhage, particularly in the preterm infant.

The alterations in the haemostatic system in the sick premature infant can only be interpreted with a knowledge of normal physiology in the development and prenatal periods.

Developmental haemostasis

Platelets

Platelets are present in the circulation in fetuses from 11 weeks gestation onwards. There appears to be little difference between platelet counts in term and preterm infants as long as they are healthy. Sick preterm infants often develop moderate, and sometimes severe, thrombocytopenia depending on the cause. The normal neonatal platelet count lies in the adult range. Although platelet function tests *in vitro* are impaired due, it is thought, to a basic developmental defect in membrane, the bleeding time in normal term and preterm infants is the same or slightly shorter than in adults or older children (Table 15.2).

Clotting factors

Visible evidence of clotting of fetal blood has been observed as early as 12 weeks gestation [50]. Concentrations of clotting factors have been studied in cord blood of term and preterm infants at birth, but there are profound changes in the baby at and during birth and the levels obtained will be affected by these changes. Factor VIII:C levels are 30–50% higher in vaginally delivered infants as opposed to those delivered by caesarean section. Fibrinogen, factor V and factor VIII levels are within the normal range in term and preterm infants. Cord plasma shows a prolonged thrombin and reptilase time, suggesting an altered function of fibrinogen, but there is still controversy regarding the existence of a structurally distinct fetal fibrinogen.

Studies on the factor VIII:C–von Willebrand factor (VWF) complex show that the newborn factor VIII complex is elevated in both term and preterm infants. In addition VWF levels remain elevated until three months of age, suggesting that this elevation is not just a reaction to the process of delivery.

Concentrations of factors II, VII, IX and X, the vitamin K dependent procoagulants, are reduced in both term and preterm infants. Compared to adult levels the percentage increases from approximately 30% at 24 weeks gestation to 50% at term. There is also a defect of the γ carboxylation of the glutamic acid residues caused by the deficiency of vitamin K.

Factors, XI, XII – prekallikrein (PK) and high molecular weight kininogen (HMWK) – are the so-called contact factors. These are reduced by adult standards with concentrations of 20–30% in the preterm infant and 20–50% at term. These levels are not associated with significant haemorrhage in adults, but may be a major cause of prolonged *in vitro* partial thromboplastin time (PTT) in the normal newborn (Table 15.2).

Anticoagulants

The four major naturally occurring anticoagulants are α_2-macroglobulins, antithrombin III, protein C, protein S.

α_2-Macroglobulin depends upon reticuloendothelial clearance to exert its physiological role rather than inactivation. It complexes with serine proteases including the procoagulants thrombin Xa, IXa and kallikrein. Although there are normal levels by adult standards in the newborn, the effect may be reduced because of the immaturity of the reticuloendothelial system.

Antithrombin III levels are reduced in the newborn. They rise from levels of below 30% of adult values in preterm infants to 60% at term. However, these low levels, which can be associated with a thrombotic tendency in adults, are balanced by the lower levels of vitamin K dependent procoagulants which antithrombin III inhibits. The newborn is thought therefore not to be at thrombotic risk because of the low levels of antithrombin III. On the other hand the vitamin K dependent anticoagulants – protein C and its co-factor protein S – are reduced by adult standards in the newborn infant. The role of these factors is to inactivate factors V and VIII – two of the major rate-limiting steps in blood clotting. These factors are at normal adult or increased concentrations in both term and preterm infants. The physiological imbalance between factors V and VIII and protein C may be a cause for the thrombotic tendency in the newborn infant.

Fibrinolytic system

The newborn infant, whether mature or preterm, demonstrates an overall increased fibrinolytic activity which lasts for several hours, probably due to increased activator activity. This is in spite of levels of plasminogen ranging from 25% for preterm to 50% in term infants. Sick infants, with the additional stress of disseminated intravascular coagulation or RDS frequently deplete their fibrinolytic potential. In healthy infants plasminogen reaches normal adult levels by approximately two weeks of age. Because newborn plasminogen has been demonstrated to be defective in its function it has been suggested that infusions of plasminogen may help in reducing the severity of RDS. Normal infants do not show increased levels of fibrinogen degradation products if the blood is collected properly. Elevated levels of fibrinogen degradation products are seen frequently in sick infants.

In summary, pre-viable fetuses, less than 24 weeks gestation, do show a bleeding tendency which is associated with poor development of the entire mechanism of haemostasis including vessels, platelets and coagulation factors [50], but thriving, clinically stable preterm infants at 26–29 weeks appear to show no bleeding tendency even if subjected to major surgery. Screening tests for coagulation yield values for clotting factors and platelets within the currently accepted minimal haemostatic levels for older children and adults [51].

Thrombotic complications, in contrast, are frequently seen in association with low levels of coagulation inhibitors in both the healthy and ill preterm infant. The widely reported increased bleeding and clotting tendencies, together with significantly abnormal coagulation tests, are seen primarily in sick preterm infants.

In short, healthy preterm infants do not bleed excessively, but have extremely limited reserve to compensate for a decrease in procoagulants. Sick infants have an increased tendency to bleed due to the many pathological conditions often triggering disseminated intravascular coagulation which complicates their first few weeks of life.

Haemostasis, hepatic maturity and haemorrhagic disease of the newborn

The liver is the site of synthesis of plasminogen, antithrombin III, the contact factors (XII, XI, high molecular weight kininogen and prekallikrein) and the vitamin K dependent factors (II, VII, IX, X and protein C). The preterm infant shows moderate deficiencies of all of these factors which appear to be gestationally dependent; they increase in concentration as the infant matures. All preterm infants require parenteral vitamin K at birth to prevent the fall in prothrombin activity during the second and third day of life and to protect them against development of classic haemorrhagic disease of the newborn [52].

Disseminated intravascular coagulation (DIC)

This is always a secondary phenomenon. Laboratory evidence and clinical expression of DIC are frequent findings in the sick newborn infant because triggers of the process such as hypoxia, acidosis, hypothermia, poor tissue perfusion and hypotension quickly develop in the course of neonatal disease whatever its origin, particularly in the preterm infant. The severity of clinical expression is compounded by immaturity, limiting the ability to produce coagulation factors to replace those consumed and the fact that the poorly developed reticuloendothelial system is unable to clear efficiently the products of coagulation such as fibrinogen degradation products.

DIC in the neonate is frequently associated with maternal hypertension and shock, abruptio placentae, placentae praevia and also with a dead twin fetus. Post-delivery associations include both bacterial and viral infection, respiratory distress syndrome, erythroblastosis fetalis, necrotizing enterocolitis and hyperviscosity.

The most practical and useful tests for diagnosis and day to day management of DIC in the newborn are the platelet count, prothrombin and thrombin times (PT and TT) with fibrinogen titre and fibrinogen degradation products (Table 15.2). The management must depend on successful elimination of the trigger and will vary accordingly, but it is sometimes necessary to replace coagulation factors with fresh frozen plasma and occasionally exchange transfusion is indicated. Platelets are rarely severely depressed except in association with sepsis, and platelet transfusions are rarely required in this situation. Indeed their use may be harmful in providing free thromboplastin and a continuing trigger for DIC [53].

Table 15.2 Neonatal haemostasis – screening tests [61]

Bleeding time (min)	*Preterm infant* (≃27–30 weeks) *within normal range*	*Term infant* *within normal range*	*Adult* *2–10*
PTT (s)	70–110	40–60	35–45
PT (s)	17–29	12–20	12–14
TT (s)	20–28	18–24	15–19

Haematological manifestation in offspring of mothers with pre-eclampsia and intrauterine growth retardation (IUGR)

The haemostatic status of the fetus and newborn may be affected by the placental damage which occurs in association with severe pre-eclampsia and IUGR. Significant numbers of infants whose mothers have the HELLP (haemolysis elevated liver enzymes and low platelet count) syndrome and pre-eclampsia have been shown to have thrombocytopenia [54,55]. In addition to thrombocytopenia many infants show significant neutropenia at birth. However, it has also been observed [56] that although a proportion of infants of women with severe pre-eclampsia had thrombocytopenia and neutropenia, the same incidence of these abnormalities was observed in the gestationally matched preterm offspring of non-hypertensive women.

The reported coagulation factor changes in infants of hypertensive mothers are variable, although decreased platelets seem to be a constant finding [48]. These infants should be monitored closely for evidence of infection, DIC and thrombotic complications for which they appear to be at increased risk and managed appropriately.

Thrombocytopenia

There are many causes of neonatal thrombocytopenia (Table 15.3). The most usual mechanism for decreased platelets in the newborn is increased destruction and consumption as seen in DIC, particularly associated with infection and immunological disorders.

Immune thrombocytopenias in the neonate are relatively acute and transitory and depend on transplacental passage of maternal IgG anti-platelet antibodies and will therefore be dealt with a little more fully here.

The management of immune thrombocytopenia in the newborn is different for each type and therefore the pathogenesis must be clearly established so that the correct and optimum therapy can be instituted.

With Auto-immune Thrombocytopenia (AITP) the maternal platelet count can vary from normal to profound thrombocytopenia depending on activity of disease, response to therapy and whether or not the spleen has been removed.

Severity of thrombocytopenia in the fetus is difficult to assess, but a direct correlation has been shown between platelet associated IgG and affected infants. The hazard to the infant is that of intracerebral haemorrhage usually sustained during delivery and therefore management is aimed towards the most atraumatic delivery possible. In most units the obstetricians feel that Caesarean section is the delivery of choice. These babies are rarely delivered pre-term, usually weigh more than 1000 g and will not be discussed further.

Table 15.3 Causes of neonatal thrombocytopenia

Inherited	Absent radii (TAR syndrome) Megakaryocytic hypoplasia Fanconi's pancytopenia (occasionally in newborn period) Myeloproliferative disease (Down syndrome) Osteopetrosis Wiskott-Aldrich syndrome and variants Bernard-Soulier syndrome May-Hegglin anomaly
Immune disorders	Maternal idiopathic thrombocytopenia (ITP) Maternal systemic lupus erythematosus (SLE) Drug-induced Allo-immune
Consumption disorders	Disseminated intravascular coagulation (DIC) Large vessel thrombosis Necrotizing enterocolitis TTP Postmature and SGA infants (maternal eclampsia) Giant haemangioma Hyperviscosity syndrome
Infection	Bacterial: sepsis, congenital syphilis Viral: CMV, herpes simplex, rubella Other: toxoplasmosis
Drugs	Maternal: tolbutamide, thiazide diuretics Infant: Intralipid, tolazoline
Other	Congenital leukaemia Post-exchange transfusion Metabolic disorders Neonatal cold injury

Allo-immuno thrombocytopenia, on the other hand, may be associated with delivery of a very small infant. It is a much less common disorder and is due in the vast majority of cases to maternal antibodies directed against the platelet antigen PL^{A1} (also known as ZW^{a}), the mother being PL^{A1} negative and her fetus carrying paternally derived PL^{A1} antigens on its platelets. In this condition the mother's platelet count is normal but she has free identifiable specific antiplatelet antibodies in her serum. These IgG antibodies cross the placenta and fix to the glycoprotein receptor areas of the fetal platelets and seriously interfere with platelet function. It is probably for this reason that serious spontaneous intracranial haemorrhage may occur *in utero* before delivery and as early as 28–30 weeks gestation.

Allo-immune purpura can occur in the first pregnancy and recur in subsequent pregnancies. The first affected pregnancy cannot be predicted but it is important to identify the couple at risk if an otherwise healthy infant is born with thrombocytopenia so that future pregnancies can be managed optimally. Pre-delivery an affected fetus can be identified by finding the specific antibodies in the mother's serum and thrombocytopenia in a fetal cord blood sample. In this situation intravenous IgG immunoglobulin administration to the mother may have a beneficial effect although only one or two cases have been so treated. It is thought to block the passage across the placenta of specific IgG platelet antibodies.

Some fetuses have been treated by PL^{A1} negative platelet transfusions prior to delivery [57]. These should not be given unless it can be established that the fetus has not sustained any serious bleeding *in utero* before treatment. Sometimes, such fetal treatment provokes preterm labour.

Delivery should be by the most atraumatic route possible. There is a relatively high mortality rate in this condition compared with idiopathic thrombocytopenia purpura [58] and those who survive may have serious long-term morbidity if appropriate measures have not been taken. The treatment of neonatal allo-immune thrombocytopenia is with donor PL^{A1} negative platelet concentrates or washed maternal platelets. Occasionally other platelet specific antibodies are responsible, e.g. ZW^{b}, Ko^{A} Ko^{B} and PL^{E1} and either washed maternal platelets or platelets of the appropriate group should be administered. Some workers recommend the administration of intravenous immunoglobulin [59].

Paradoxically, immune thrombocytopenia may become worse in the first few days after birth in both allo-immune and auto-immune types, although the source of antibody has been cut off. This is probably due to the development of the reticuloendothelial circulation particularly in the spleen. The splenic circulation is not established at delivery, but after a few days it will more effectively remove coated platelets from the circulation. Mild thrombocytopenia may continue for several weeks although normal platelet counts are usually achieved by the end of the first month of life. Active treatment is rarely required after the first week or so of life. The greatest hazard is passed once delivery has been successfully negotiated.

Thrombosis

The preterm infant is particularly susceptible to acquired thrombotic lesions, both in the presence and absence of indwelling catheters [60]. It is difficult to know whether the apparent increasing incidence is due to the use of more searching and accurate diagnostic methods or due to changing modes of therapy and support in the special baby care unit.

Risk factors for neonatal thrombosis

Three major factors contribute to the formation of thrombin according to Virchow's postulates:

(1) Abnormalities of vessel wall.
(2) Disturbances of blood flow.
(3) Changes in blood coagulability.

Only those factors of particular significance in the newborn infant will be referred to.

ABNORMALITIES OF THE VESSEL WALL

Abnormal chorion vessels
A wide variety of maternal disorders, including hypertension, may result in thrombin formation in fetal placental veins. Chorion thrombi are of importance because they may embolize to fetal vessels.

Defective closure of the ductus arteriosus
If the ductus does not undergo its normal involutional change, thrombin may form

within the vessel and provide a source of emboli to both systemic and pulmonary circulations.

Intravascular catheters
Intravascular catheters both provide a foreign surface and may injure the vessel wall in which they are placed, exposing collagen and releasing thromboplastin. They are frequently associated with thromboembolism.

Shock and infection
Endothelial damage provoked by localized or generalized hypoxaemia may well initiate thrombosis as will the endothelial damage occurring in the course of septicaemia. These are well known triggers of DIC, but may also cause localized thrombosis.

DISTURBANCES OF BLOOD FLOW

The development of hyperviscosity in the neonate is due mainly to an abnormally high haematocrit. Hypotension and venous stasis will also contribute to the risk of developing venous thrombosis in the sick infant with or without pathological polycythaemia.

CHANGES IN BLOOD COAGULATION AND FIBRINOLYSIS

Normal physiological changes in neonatal haemostasis, as described above, do not seem to predispose the healthy infant to thrombotic complications. Low levels of antithrombin III are balanced by low levels of pro-coagulant factors against which antithrombin III is directed. However there is a discrepancy between the low levels of protein C in the neonate compared with the normal to high levels of factors V and VIII. Hereditary protein C deficiency in its heterozygous form is associated with a thrombotic tendency later in life. Severe or homozygous protein C deficiency is associated with massive thromboembolism and recurrent purpura fulminans in the neonate. Although successful management with fresh frozen plasma followed by warfarin therapy has been reported, this genetic condition is usually rapidly fatal.

It is not estimated whether or to what degree any of the special features of normal neonatal haemostasis contribute to the thrombotic tendency in the sick newborn infant. In contrast, convincing demonstrations of the role of vascular damage and disturbances of blood flow in the development of thrombosis have been made by several groups.

Thrombosis associated with the use of indwelling catheters

There is a potential risk of initiating thrombosis by the use of indwelling catheters in the neonate irrespective of the vessel catheterized.

UMBILICAL ARTERY CATHETERS

Umbilical artery catheterization is common in the sick newborn and has been associated with severe thromboembolic phenomena requiring aggressive intervention in 1% of cases. The incidence of subclinical thrombosis is much higher and can be detected by arteriography in 20–95% of infants with umbilical artery catheters.

Sequelae of clinically evident thrombosis include renal hypertension, necrotizing enterocolitis, peripheral gangrene, and even paraplegia. Follow-up studies in small groups of children up to the age of four years have not revealed any sequelae of clinically silent catheter-induced thrombosis.

Prevention of catheter-related thrombosis is an important but controversial issue. It is current practice to use heparin at a rate of 1–10 units or more/h in many SCBUs. Although catheter patency has been shown to improve when heparin is given in doses of 100–200 units/kg/day, the effect on incidence of catheter-related thrombosis is still not established. There is also the hazard of bleeding when heparin is given in doses of 5–10 units/kg/h in the VLBW infant.

UMBILICAL VEIN CATHETERS

It is generally believed that umbilical vein catheters carry a greater risk of thrombosis than arterial catheters but this has never been demonstrated in a prospective trial.

Misplacement of the catheter and rapid infusion of hyperosmolar solutions increase the incidence of thrombosis. The correct placement of the catheter in the portal or hepatic vein may lead to hepatic necrosis. Portal vein thrombosis resulting in portal hypertension has also been described.

Splenic vein thrombosis has been described as a late complication of umbilical catheterization. The patients present with splenomegaly and gastric and oesophageal varices.

Immediate clinical signs of thrombosis associated with umbilical vein catheterization are slight or absent in contrast to those associated with umbilical artery catheterization.

In order to reduce the risk of hepatic necrosis and portal vein thrombosis the tip of the catheter should be placed correctly in the inferior vena cava and its position checked by X-ray or possibly ultrasound before hyperosmolar fluids are infused.

Principles of treatment of neonatal thrombosis [48,50,60]

There is no generally accepted protocol for management of neonatal thrombosis. The actions will be influenced by the site and the size of the thrombus and the time elapsing between the occlusion of vessels and restoration of blood flow either by vessel recanalization or by establishment of efficient collaterals.

HEPARIN

Heparin in adult practice is used either in primary prevention of thrombosis or in the secondary prevention of thrombus extension. Objective evidence of the beneficial role of heparin in treatment of neonatal thrombosis is largely anecdotal. The haemostatic system of the newborn infant is unique and it is not certain whether the rules for efficient heparinization in adults can be applied. Laboratory monitoring is difficult because the *in vitro* coagulation times are already prolonged and rapidly become infinite with very small doses of heparin. The generally accepted guidelines are based on individual experience and have not been substantiated by controlled trials. The actual loading dose recommended is 50–100 units/kg. Maintenance levels of 0.3–0.5 units/ml are achieved by doses of 16–35 units/kg/h and this should be administered by continuing infusion. Duration of therapy depends on clinical state and may vary from a few days to several weeks.

Mild to moderate occlusion can probably be managed with heparin alone, but with extensive thrombosis with critical impairment of blood flow, many centres would attempt to lyse the clot with fibrinolytic agents and the drug of choice in the neonate is urokinase.

UROKINASE

Confirmation of large vessel thrombosis by angiography or ultrasound is a prerequisite for the use of fibrinolytic therapy. Absolute contraindications are pre-existing severe bleeding or previous major surgery up to ten days prior to the development of thrombosis. Arterial punctures and invasive procedures should be avoided during therapy.

Treatment is most likely to be successful if established within hours of signs and confirmation of major venous or arterial occlusion.

Considerably higher dosage may be tolerated and needed in the neonate compared with that in adults.

A loading dose of 4000 units/kg given intravenously over 10 min should be followed by a continuous infusion of 4000–6000 units/kg/h but should be increased if necessary within hours until improved perfusion of the affected part is achieved. It is obvious that such treatment should only be given in a fully equipped SCBU with ultrasound and Doppler facilities and appropriate laboratory back-up. The duration of useful therapy in newborns is as uncertain as the dosage, but may be continued for more than the usual 72 h. If the thrombin time is not prolonged by the generation of fibrinolytic degradation products then heparin may be added also to prevent extension of the thrombus. The degree of thrombolysis will be determined by the age of the thrombus, its location and plasminogen content.

Laboratory testing should be performed prior to administering urokinase to establish baselines. Thereafter regular monitoring is required. Suitable rapid tests are measurement of fibrinolytic degradation products and fibrinogen levels. Very low fibrinogen levels would indicate urgent readjustment of the dose.

SURGERY

In adult arterial thrombosis if the clot is not removed by end-arterectomy the thrombosis tends to recur. This is not so in smaller neonatal thrombosis. In addition the very small size of vessels in this age group makes surgical intervention difficult. Surgery is usually reserved for resection of non-viable tissue.

References

1. Holland, B. M. and Wardrop, C. A. J. (1988) In *Neonatal Pharmacology: Oxygen Transport by the Blood – Haematinics and Blood Cell Component Therapy* (ed. D. Harvey), Butterworths, London
2. Thomas, R. M., Channing, C. E., Cotes, P. M. *et al.* (1983) Erythropoietin and cord blood haemoglobin in the regulation of human fetal erythropoiesis. *Br. J. Obstet. Gynaecol.*, **90**, 795–800
3. Dallman, P. R. (1984) Erythropoietin and the anemia of prematurity. *J. Pediatr.*, **105**, 756–757
4. Brown, M. S., Garcia, J. F., Phibbs, R. H. and Dallman, P. R. (1984) Decreased response of plasma immunoreactive erythropoietin to 'available oxygen' in anemia of prematurity. *J. Pediatr.*, **105**, 793–798
5. Jacobs, K., Shoemaker, C., Rudersdorf, R. *et al.* (1985) Isolation and characterization of genomic and cDNA clones of human erythropoetin. *Nature*, **313**, 806–810

6. Shannon, K. M., Naylor, G. S., Torkildson, J. C. *et al.* (1987) Circulating erythroid progenitors in the anemia of prematurity. *N. Engl. J. Med.*, **317**, 728–733
7. Sieff, C. A., Emerson, S. G., Mufson, A., Gesner, T. G. and Nathan, D. G. (1986) Dependence of highly enriched human bone marrow progenitors on hemopoietic growth factors and their response to recombinant erythropoietin. *J. Clin. Invest.*, **77**, 74–81
8. Anon (1987) Erythropoietin. *Lancet*, **i**, 781–782
9. Stamatoyannopoulos, G. and Nienhuis, A. W. (1978) *Cellular and Molecular Regulation of Haemoglobin Switchings*, Grune and Stratton, New York
10. Bard, H. and Prosmanne, J. (1982) Postnatal fetal and adult hemoglobin synthesis in preterm infants whose birthweight was less than 1000 grams. *J. Clin. Invest.*, **70**, 50–52
11. Blanchette, V. S. and Zipursky, A. (1984) Assessment of anaemia in newborn infants. *Clin. Perinatol.*, **11**, 489
12. Fenton, V., Cavill, I. and Fisher, J. (1977) Iron stores in pregnancy. *Br. J. Haematol.*, **37**, 145–149
13. Lundstrom, U., Siimes, M. A. and Dallman, P. R. (1977) At what age does iron supplementation become necessary in low birthweight infants. *J. Pediatr.*, **91**, 878–883
14. Stockman, J. A. and Oski, F. A. (1978) Physiological anemia of infancy and the anemia of prematurity. *Clin. Hematol.*, **7**, 3–18
15. Siimes, M. A. (1981) Pathogenesis of iron deficiency in infancy. In *Iron Nutrition Revisited: Infancy, Childhood, Adolescence* (Report on the 82nd Conference on Pediatric Research), (eds F. A. Oski and H. A. Pearson), Ross Laboratories, Columbus, Ohio, pp. 96–108
16. Dallman, P. R. (1987) Iron deficiency and related nutritional anemias. In *Hematology of Infancy and Childhood* (eds D. Nathan and F. A. Oski), W. B. Saunders, Philadelphia, pp. 274–314
17. Oski, F. A. (1979) Nutritional anaemias. *Semin. Perinatol.*, **3**, 381–395
18. Sutton, A. M., Harvie, A., Cockburn, F. *et al.* (1985) Copper deficiency in the pre-term infant of very low birth weight. *Arch. Dis. Child.*, **60**, 644
19. Tyrala, E. E. (1986) Zinc and copper balances in preterm infants. *Pediatrics*, **77**, 513–517
20. Committee on Nutrition, American Academy of Pediatrics (1985) Nutritional needs of low birthweight infants. *Pediatrics*, **75**, 976
21. Ehrenkranz, R. A. (1980) Vitamin E and the neonate. *Am. J. Dis. Child.*, **134**, 1157–1166
22. Hassan, H., Hashim, S. A., Van Itallie, T. B. and Sebrell, W. H. (1966) Syndrome in premature infants associated with low plasma vitamin E levels and high polyunsaturated fatty acid diet. *Am. J. Clin. Nutr.*, **19**, 147–157
23. Oski, F. A. and Barness, L. A. (1967) Vitamin E deficiency: a previously unrecognised cause of hemolytic anemia in the premature infant. *J. Pediatr.*, **70**, 211–220
24. Melhorn, D. K., Gross, S. and Childers, G. (1971) Vitamin E-dependent anaemia in the premature infant. I. Effects of large doses of medicinal iron. *J. Pediatr.*, **79**, 569–580
25. Zipursky, A., Brown, R. T., Watts, J. *et al.* (1987) Oral vitamin E supplementation for the prevention of anemia in premature infants: a controlled trial. *Pediatrics*, **79**, 61
26. Zipursky, A. (1984) Vitamin E deficiency in newborn infants. *Clin. Perinatol.*, **11**, 393–402
27. Curran, J. S. and Cantolino, S. J. (1978) Vitamin E (injectable) administration in the prevention of retinopathy in prematurity: evaluation with fluorescein angiography and fundus photography. *Pediatr. Res.*, **12**, 404 (abstract)
28. Sinha, S., Toner, N., Chiswick, M. *et al.* (1987) Vitamin E supplementation reduces frequency of periventricular haemorrhage in very preterm babies. *Lancet*, **i**, 466
29. Finer, N. N., Peters, K. L., Hayek, K. and Merkel, C. L. (1984) Vitamin E and necrotizing enterocolitis. *Pediatrics*, **73**, 387–393
30. Haworth, C. and Evans, D. I. K. (1981) Nutritional aspects of blood disorders in the newborn. *J. Hum. Nutr.*, **35**, 323–334
31. Roberts, P. D., James, H., Petrie, A., Morgan, J. O. and Hoffbrand, A. V. (1973) Vitamin B_{12} status in pregnancy among immigrants to Britain. *Br. Med. J.*, **iii**, 67–72
32. Ronnholm, K. A. R. and Siimes, M. A. (1985) Haemoglobin concentration depends on protein intake in small preterm infants fed human milk. *Arch. Dis. Child.*, **60**, 99–104
33. Stockman, J. A. III (1986) The anemia of prematurity: current concepts in the issue of when to transfuse. *Pediatr. Clin. North Am.*, **33**, 111–128

34. Wardrop, C. A. J., Holland, B. M., Veale, K. E. A. *et al.* (1978) Nonphysiological anaemia of prematurity. *Arch. Dis. Child.*, **53**, 855–860
35. Oski, F. A. (1987) Neonatal hematology. The Erythrocyte and its Disorders. In *Hematology of Infancy and Childhood, 3rd Edition*, (eds D. Nathan and F. A. Oski) W. B. Saunders, Philadelphia. p. 40
36. Phillips, H., Holland, B. M., Jones, J. G. *et al.* (1986) Determination of red cell mass in the assessment and management of anaemia in babies needing blood transfusion. *Lancet*, **i**, 882
37. Phillips, H., Holland, B. M., Jones, J. G. *et al.* (1988) Definitive estimate of rate of haemoglobin switching: measurement of per cent Hb.F in neonatal reticulocytes. *Pediatr. Res.*, **23**, 595–597
38. Stockman, J. A. III and Clark, D. A. (1984) Weight gain: a response to transfusion in selected preterm infants. *Am. J. Dis. Child.*, **138**, 828
39. Blajchman, M. A., Sheridan, D. and Rawls, W. E. (1984) Risks associated with blood transfusions in newborn infants. *Clin. Perinatol.*, **11**, 403
40. Leitman, S. F. and Holland, P. V. (1985) Irradiation of blood products: indications and guidelines. *Transfusion*, **25**, 293
41. Luban, N. L. C. and Ness, P. M. (1985) Irradiation of blood products: indications and guidelines. *Transfusion*, **25**, 301
42. Connor, M. E., Minnefor, A-B. and Okeske, J. M. (1987) Human immunodeficiency virus infection in infants and children. In *Current Topics in AIDS*, Vol. 1 (eds M. S. Gottlieb *et al.*), John Wiley and Sons, Chichester, pp. 185–209
43. Acheson, D. (1987) Department of Health and Social Security, Press Release, 1 87/5
44. Roberton, N. R. C. (1987) Top-up transfusions in neonates. *Arch. Dis. Child.*, **62**, 984–986
45. Eyal, F., Sagi, E., Arad, I. and Avital, A. (1982) Necrotising enterocolitis in the very low birthweight infant: expressed breast milk feeding compared with parenteral feeding. *Arch. Dis. Child.*, **57**, 274–276
46. Rogers, A. F. and Dunn, P. M. (1969) Intestinal perforation, exchange transfusion and PVC. *Lancet*, **ii**, 1245
47. Turner, J. H., Petricciani, J. C., Crouch, M. L. and Wenger, A. (1974) An evaluation of the effects of diethyl hexyl phthalate (DEHP) on mitotically capable cells in blood packs. *Transfusion*, **14**, 560–566
48. Hathaway, W. E. and Bonnar, J. (1987) *Hemostatic Disorders of the Pregnant Woman and Newborn Infant*, John Wiley and Sons, Chichester
49. Andrew, M., Paes, B., Milner, R. *et al.* (1987) Development of the human coagulation system in the full-term infant. *Blood*, **70**, 165–172
50. Hathaway, W. E. (1987) Haemostatic disorders in the newborn. In *Haemostasis and Thrombosis*, 2nd edn, (eds A. L. Bloom and D. P. Thomas), Churchill Livingstone, Edinburgh
51. Barnard, D. R., Simmons, M. A. and Hathaway, W. E. (1979) Coagulation studies in extremely premature infants. *Pediatr. Res.*, **13**, 1330–1335
52. Lane, P. A. and Hathaway, W. E. (1985) Vitamin K in infancy. *J. Pediatr.*, **106**, 351–359
53. Sharp, A. A. (1977) Diagnosis and management of disseminated intravascular coagulation. *Br. Med. Bull.*, **33**, 265–272
54. Weinstein, L. (1982) Syndrome of hemolysis elevated liver enzyme and low platelet count. A severe consequence of hypertension in pregnancy. *Am. J. Obstet. Gynecol.*, **142**, 159–167
55. Thiagarajah, S., Bourgeois, F. J., Harbert, G. M. and Caudle, M. R. (1984) Thrombocytopenia in eclampsia: associated abnormalities and management principles. *Am. J. Obstet. Gynecol.*, **150**, 1–7
56. Sibai, B. M., Abdella, T. N., Hill, G. A. and Anderson, G. D. (1984) Hematologic findings in mothers and infants of patients with severe pre-eclampsia/eclampsia. *Clin. Exp. Hyper. Preg.*, **3**, 13–21
57. Daffos, F., Forestier, F., Muller, J. Y. *et al.* (1984) Prenatal treatment of allo-immune thrombocytopenia. *Lancet*, **ii**, 632
58. Andrew, M. and Kelton, J. (1984) Neonatal thrombocytopenia. *Clin. Perinatol.*, **11**, 359–391
59. Amato, M., Ruckstuhl, C. and Von Muralt, G. (1985) Treatment of neonatal thrombocytopenia. *J. Pediatr.*, **107**, 650
60. Schmidt, B. and Zipursky, A. (1984) Thrombotic disease in newborn infants. *Clin. Perinatol.*, **11**, 461–488
61. Stevens, R. F. (1987) Congenital and acquired coagulation defects. In *Practical Paediatric Haematology* (eds R. F. Hinchliffe and J. S. Lilleyman), John Wiley and Sons, Chichester, pp. 281–315

Chapter 16

Infection

John de Louvois

Introduction

Infection is one of the main problems that confront babies with a birth weight of less than 1000 g. La Gamma *et al.* [1] asserted that infection was the major contributing factor to death of ELBW babies who died after the fifth postnatal day. As with their more mature contemporaries, ELBW babies may be infected from the mother either as a result of intrauterine infection or from contamination and subsequent infection with bacteria from the genital tract, acquired during the birth process. Alternatively babies may become infected with bacteria from the neonatal environment in which they are being nursed. The wide range of invasive procedures to which these babies are subjected, prolonged periods of ventilation, the very long periods that many of them spend in the neonatal intensive care unit (NICU) and their susceptibility to infection by microorganisms passed on by older children visiting the unit, all contribute to the increased risk of infection among ELBW babies. In addition, because of their increased susceptibility to infection ELBW babies are prey to a wider range of bacteria than are more mature babies. Thus the viridans streptococci and *Branhamella catarrhalis*, for example, are both potential pathogens in this group of patients.

The increased risk of infection and the rapidly fatal outcome of any systemic infection which is not promptly and effectively treated dictates that virtually all ELBW babies receive at least one course of antibiotics and the majority receive antibiotics on repeated occasions and often for long periods. The widespread use of these drugs is due in part to the failure of conventional microbiological methods to diagnose infection rapidly in this group of patients and also to the difficulty of distinguishing between infected babies and those only colonized with potential pathogens. Given that, in common with all other systems, the immune system of babies under 1000 g is not competent, treatment of infection may on occasions need to be extended since there is currently no way of knowing whether a course of treatment has been effective or not.

Diagnosis of infection

The diagnosis of infection in very small premature babies poses special problems. Because of limited venous access it may only be possible to collect blood for culture through intravenous lines, many of which will be internally or externally contaminated with bacteria. Blood collected from a line used for the administration of antibiotics is useless for culture and may give dangerously misleading results. There is the added problem that the volume of blood that can be collected for culture from very small babies may be insufficient to give a reliable negative result. Blood culture methods using capillary samples have not proved successful. Samples of cerebrospinal fluid (CSF) may be heavily blood-stained either as the result of intraventricular haemorrhage or because of a 'bloody tap'. The literature contains a number of reports of meningitis developing as a consequence of bacteraemic blood contaminating the CSF at the time of lumbar tap. As with more mature neonates, aspirates from the respiratory tract are often less than helpful in the diagnosis of bacterial chest infections. Examination of gastric aspirates has been found also to be unrewarding. In addition to these problems, routine cultural methods for the recognition of sepsis take far too long to be of immediate use in the management of ELBW babies.

Non-cultural methods

In recent years new methods have been developed for the rapid diagnosis of infection. A number of research techniques have been applied to the problems of neonatal infection and with the development of commercial 'user friendly' kits these have become available for assessment as routine investigations.

The non-cultural methods available fall into two groups (Table 16.1), those designed to rapidly detect small amounts of a specific bacterial antigen and those that detect the physiological changes in the host which are consequent upon infection. It is largely these tests which require further investigation, for very little is known about the immune and other responses of the 1000 g baby to early infection.

Antigen detection methods

Counter immunoelectrophoresis (CIE) is performed in agar gels where the pH is controlled such that the antibody is positively charged while the antigen is negatively charged. Application of a voltage across the gel results in movement of the antigen and antibody towards each other. Precipitation occurs where they meet in optimum proportions.

Latex agglutination (LA) and coagglutination (COA) methods are slide agglutination techniques. In coagglutination a strain of *Staphylococcus pyogenes* with protein A in its cell wall is mixed with specific antibody such that the Fc portion of the immunoglobulin binds to the bacterial cell. When homologous antigen in a clinical specimen or bacterial culture is mixed with these cells it binds to the Fab portion of

Table 16.1 Non-cultural methods for the detection and diagnosis of infection

Microbiological	*Physiological*
Counter immunoelectrophoresis	C-reactive protein
Latex agglutination	Total neutrophil count
Coagglutination	Neutrophil band count
Limulus lysate coagulation	Micro ESR
	Thrombocyte count
	Nitroblue tetrazolium test

the antibody and results in visible agglutination. The principle of latex agglutination is the same but uses latex particles (0.81 μm diameter) instead of bacterial cells. Immunoglobulin types differ in their affinity for the various particles and cells used.

Although these methods have been applied to the diagnosis of infection in older neonates there are few reports of their use in premature babies. However antigen detection methods should be equally useful in the diagnosis of infection in ELBW babies.

The methods available for the detection of bacterial antigen or endotoxin have been dramatically improved with the advent of monoclonal antibodies and techniques now permit the detection of antigen in raw specimens rather than only in bacterial cultures. Antigens can easily be demonstrated in urine or CSF and rather less readily in serum. There are few reports of these methods being applied to clinical samples of gastric or tracheal aspirates from babies but they have been successfully used on adult sputum and on high vaginal swabs; 75–80% of swabs containing Lancefield group B streptococci give positive reactions with a two-minute latex agglutination test. The simplicity of the agglutination tests and their improved sensitivity has led to their widespread acceptance in clinical laboratories at the expense of CIE which is now rarely used routinely.

The range of commercial reagents available is still not sufficiently comprehensive to cover all the major bacteria responsible for infection in the newborn and at present there are no reagents for the recognition of coagulase negative staphylococci, *Listeria monocytogenes* or the Enterobacter/Citrobacter/Serratia group of Gram-negative rods. Nevertheless increasingly latex or coagglutination provide a means of rapidly diagnosing neonatal infection irrespective of birth weight. False negative 'prozone reactions' may occur if the sample contains excessive amounts of antigen. Samples giving negative results should therefore be retested at a 1 in 5 dilution.

Sensitivity of antigen detection methods

A variety of factors affect the sensitivity of antigen detection methods. These include the specificity and avidity of the antisera used, the specific bacterial antigen being sought and the clinical specimen being tested. The minimum amount of bacterial antigen that can be detected by various methods is shown in Table 16.2.

Comparison of methods

Direct scientific comparisons between CIE, COA and LA have in the past been

Table 16.2 Minimum concentration of bacterial antigen detected by CIE, coagglutination (COA) and latex agglutination (LA)

	Antigen detected (ng/ml)		
Bacteria	*CIE*	*COA*	*LA*
Group B streptococci	500–1400	–	62
H. influenzae	1–25	2–25	0.1–5
N. meningitidis	25–75	1.5	1–50
S. pneumoniae	25–1000	6	0.2–50

difficult because insufficient was known about the antibody being used and there was too much variation in reagents used by different workers. With the advent of commercial test kits comparisons between one product and another were possible, although such comparisons said more about the kits than the sensitivity of the methods used. The introduction of monoclonal antibodies has led to the production of fully characterized antibodies for use in these kits. Thus highly specific very sensitive reagents are becoming available for the detection of an increasing number of neonatal pathogens. There still remain some problems with cross reactions between bacteria with apparently identical antigens [2]. Major examples of this problem are the reactions between:

N. meningitidis type B and *E. coli* K1
S. pneumoniae type 14 and group B streptococci type III
Group B streptococci and *H. influenzae* type B
H. influenzae type B and *Staph. pyogenes*

These *in vitro* cross reactions do not, however, cause serious problems with clinical specimens. Non-specific false positive reactions occur with all three methods if crude antisera are used. In the majority of cases they can be easily recognized because the reactions occur with a number of antisera. Genuine false negative reactions may occur with CIE against some serotypes of *S. pneumoniae*, notably types 7 and 14, because the isoelectric point of the antigen is reached at the pH of the buffer usually used [3]. All these methods have the added advantage that they remain positive in cases of partially treated meningitis at a time when bacteria can no longer be cultured [4].

Evaluation of non-cultural methods

It is essential that any non-cultural method is assessed in comparison with positive culture results in untreated infections. Only in this way can the value of these new methods be measured. Data from the meningitis study of Roos, Daumling and Kreaft [4] comparing CIE and LA may be used as an example (Table 16.3). Given the

Table 16.3 CIE and LA: diagnostic yield in meningitis due to *H. influenzae, S. pneumoniae, N. meningitidis* and group B streptococci ($n = 225$)

	CIE		*LA*	
Culture	*Positive*	*Negative*	*Positive*	*Negative*
Positive	77	22	78	21
Negative	0	1026	8	1018
Sensitivity	$\frac{77}{77}+22=77\%$		$\frac{78}{78}+21=78\%$	
Specificity	$\frac{1026}{1026}+0=100\%$		$\frac{1018}{1018}+8=99\%$	
Prevalence	$\frac{99}{225}=44\%$		$\frac{99}{225}=44\%$	
Predictive value (+)		100%		98%
Predictive value (−)		84%		85%

results of culture and the results obtained by CIE and LA, the sensitivity and specificity of the non-cultural methods can be determined. From these the positive and negative predictive values of the tests can be calculated. It is essential that the prevalence of the condition being investigated is included in these calculations if misleading predictive values are to be avoided.

The sensitivity of the test refers to the percentage of positive test results in the population with the disease. Specificity is the percentage of negative results in the population who do not have the disease. Prevalence refers to the number of patients with the disease as a percentge of the number tested. The predictive value of a positive test is the probability of the disease in the study population if the test result is positive, and the predictive value of negative test means the probability of absence of the disease in the population with negative test results.

In the example cited (Table 16.3) the positive accuracy of CIE is 100% while that of the latex test is only 90% (78/86). The prevalence of meningitis in the population tested was 44% (99/225). The positive predictive value is determined from the formula:

$$\frac{\text{sensitivity} \times \text{prevalence}}{\text{sensitivity} \times \text{prevalence} + (100 - \text{specificity})\,(100 - \text{prevalence})}$$

$$\text{i.e. } \frac{44 \times 77}{44 \times 77 + (0)(56)} = 100\%$$

The negative predictive value is determined from the formula:

$$\frac{\text{specificity}\ (100 - \text{prevalence})}{\text{specificity}\ (100 - \text{prevalence}) + (100 - \text{sensitivity})\ \text{prevalence}}$$

$$\text{i.e. } \frac{100 \times 56}{(100 \times 56) + (23)(44)} = 84\%$$

The statistics associated with evaluating tests of this sort are discussed in detail by Feinstein [5].

The limulus lysate test

The limulus lysate test (LAL) is based on the observation that the amoebocyte lysate obtained from the horseshoe crab (*Limulus polyphemus*) forms a gel in the presence of pyrogens, including Gram-negative bacterial endotoxin [6,7]. The major problems with this test are the high incidence of false positive reactions [8] and that it will not detect infections due to Gram-positive bacteria.

The test is exquisitely sensitive and will detect antigen at picogram levels [9]. Unfortunately it is not specific for bacterial endotoxin and as a result false positive reactions due to insufficiently clean glassware or contamination during sample handling are a major problem. In addition 30% of VLBW babies may give a transient positive reaction due to circulating bacterial antigen in the absence of bacteraemia. These are not false positive reactions as resported by Schiefele, Melton and Whitchelo [10]. In patients with patent ductus arteriosus these positive reactions may persist because the toxin can bypass the liver and thus escape removal. False positive reactions occur also in samples from babies with hyperbilirubinaemia [11]. All positive reactions need to be checked by retesting the sample after it has been treated with polymixin. This specifically neutralizes reactions due to bacterial endotoxin but not those due to contamination. In babies more than five days old the limulus lysate test has a predictive value of 37% for bacteraemia and necrotizing enterocolitis due to Gram-negative rods. Two successive negative results have a 100% correlation with the absence of infection due to endotoxin-producing bacteria [12].

Physiological methods

C-reactive protein

Among the physiological indicators of infection (Table 16.1) C-reactive protein (CRP) is the best known and most widely studied. CRP is one of a group of acute phase proteins (Table 16.4) whose concentration increases or decreases in response to infection. CRP is produced in the liver by hepatocytes and has a molecular weight of 105 500 daltons. It consists of five identical covalently associated subunits forming a pentagonal structure. The function of CRP is not precisely understood. It has a calcium-dependent binding site for phosphorylcholine and galactosamine, hence C-reactive protein, and it interacts with complement factors of the classical pathway. The normal CRP level is 0.07–8.0 mg/l (median 0.8 mg/l) [13,14]. Of the various acute phase proteins CRP most closely parallels the clinical picture of infection in term babies increasing within hours of the start of cell necrosis or inflammation. It is not known whether the response is equally rapid in ELBW babies. CRP has a rapid turnover and is therefore of value in the diagnosis and monitoring of infection. The half-life of CRP in small babies is reported to be about 27 h [15]. During the first few days of life CRP levels may be non-specifically raised (15–20 mg/l or higher) with no clinical signs of infection [16]. Maternal pyrexia in the absence of infection, prolonged rupture of membranes, fetal distress following a traumatic delivery, birth asphyxia or aspiration may also result in elevated levels of CRP which may persist for a number of days [4]. Parenteral nutrition results in elevated CRP levels in adults [17]. It is not known whether intravenous feeding also stimulates CRP production in the newborn.

A number of authors have attempted to evaluate the value of CRP in the diagnosis of infection in the newborn [16,18–20] but there are very few references to ELBW babies. Aujard, Laudignon and Lebeau [21] studied the CRP response in 93 babies divided into three groups:

(1) Those with established bacteriologically proven infection.
(2) Those with clinically suspected but bacteriologically unproven infection.
(3) Those with no evidence of infection.

Table 16.4 Acute phase proteins

Coagulation proteins	C-reactive protein
Protease inhibitors	Orosomucoid
Transport proteins	Albumin and pre-albumin
Complement proteins	Serum amyloid A-related protein

Using a latex agglutination method to determine CRP (threshold value 5 mg/l) they found that all infected babies had serum CRP levels above 24 mg/l. The 41 babies with suspected infection, 18 of whom were premature, could be divided into two groups – 23 with normal levels and 18 with serum levels above 20 mg/l. Two of these were negative on retesting. Forty of 41 non-infected babies, 14 of whom were premature, had normal CRP levels on the first day of life. From these results the specificity of CRP was determined to be 97%. The sensitivity of the test was 64% on the first test and 73% when repeated 18–24 h later. This limited study suggests that premature and term babies show the same CRP response to infection. A negative result in babies less than 12 h old must be repeated after 18–24 h.

The sensitivity of CRP as an indicator of infection (60–70%) is similar to that reported for orosomucoid and fibrin and higher than the sensitivity for polymorphonuclear leucocyte band counts or thrombocyte counts (30–40%) [21]. Antibiotic treatment of the mother before delivery may lower fetal CRP levels although the infection may have been inadequately treated [21]. Both CRP and orosomucoid give a good guide to the efficacy of treatment. A number of authors have successfully monitored the treatment of meningitis by measuring CRP levels in serum [16,22]. They have demonstrated a fall in CRP accompanying therapeutic cure and persistence of elevated levels in association with relapse. CRP determinations in CSF are unhelpful in the diagnosis of neonatal meningitis [23,24] but serum levels have been used as a means of predicting sequelae following meningitis. Serum levels greater than 300 mg/l are strongly predictive of neurological sequelae [25]. Some infants who become infected fail to elicit an acute phase response; in these the prognosis is poor [12].

A further problem is the variation in CRP response to different microorganisms [22]. Coliforms elicit a good CRP response; with group B streptococci the response is less good.

Other physiological changes

There are problems with other physiological changes which have been used as indicators of infection (Table 16.1). ELBW babies exhibit a very wide range of 'normal' haematological values and dramatic changes occur during the early neonatal period. Neutrophil dynamics are not affected by gestational age, prolonged rupture of membranes, route of delivery or hyperbilirubinaemia [26]. However they are affected by intraventricular haemorrhage (IVH), birth asphyxia (Apgar < 5 at 5 min), a stressful labour, meconium aspiration, pneumothorax and hyaline membrane disease and as many as 70% of babies with these conditions will have an abnormal neutrophil picture. These abnormal effects usually only persist for 24 h. Following meconium aspiration they persist for 72 h and following an IVH for 120 h; 93% of babies without these complications and without infection will have a normal neutrophil picture, indicating the value of negative findings [27,28]. There is general agreement that differential white cell counts expressed as a percentage are unhelpful and that actual numbers reveal trends which are often not apparent from percentage figures. The non-segmented/total neutrophil ratio provides a very good indication of infection if it is greater than 0.2 and values above 0.15 are highly suggestive except in babies with hyperbilirubinaemia when the predictive value of a ratio of 0.15 falls to 50%. Toxic granulation within the neutrophils and thrombocytopenia increase the confidence limit.

Table 16.5 Physiological indicators of neonatal infection

Test	*Significant results*
Total white cell count	< 5000/cm
Band/total neutrophil	ratio > 0.2
C-reactive protein	> 8 mg/l
Micro ESR	> 15 mm in 1 h
Haptoglobin	> 250 mg/l
IgM	> 350 mg/l

Nitroblue tetrazolium test (NBT)

Phagocytically active polymorphonuclear leucocytes selectively take up the dye nitroblue tetrazolium. In healthy adults the number of NBT positive neutrophils is small. In acute systemic bacterial infection there is a dramatic increase in the percentage of NBT positive cells and this has been used as an indicator of infection. In the newborn the test has not proved useful, largely because of the high percentage of NBT positive cells in uninfected babies and the relatively small increase in the number of these cells associated with infection.

Micro ESR

An erythrocyte sedimentation rate (ESR) in excess of 15 mm in 1 h in the newborn is of value in recognizing infection. A rise occurs 12–24 h after clinical symptoms appear. The ESR is also raised in haemolytic disease of the newborn. A 75 mm heparinized tube of 1.1–1.2 mm diameter is used for this test. One end of the blood column is sealed with plasticine and the tube is taped to any vertical surface. The tube must be full and free from bubbles. After exactly 1 h the column of clear plasma is measured on a haematocrit scale. It has been suggested that if the tube is inclined at an angle of 45° the result can be read after only 15 min.

Recent studies [29,30] indicate that the best results are obtained by combining a number of rapid non-cultural investigations into an infection screen procedure. Philip and Hewitt [29] reported that significant results in two of the tests shown in Table 16.5 had a 39% predictive value for infection. If none of the findings were abnormal there was a 99% prediction that infection was not present. Such a system has yet to be applied to ELBW babies. The value of these tests will vary from one neonatal unit to another depending on the prevalence of infection.

Conclusion

There are four areas in which these non-cultural and haematological determinations might be of value in the management of ELBW babies:

(1) The more reliable early diagnosis of infection. This applies especially to infection

occurring *in utero*. In this context the antigen detection methods show most promise.

(2) The more reliable exclusion of infection either initially or at the end of 48 h antibiotic therapy. In VLBW babies it is probable that antibiotics would be used initially so these tests, coupled with negative cultural results, would help in the decision to stop treatment.

(3) A laboratory based assessment of the effectiveness of treatment. This would apply especially to the treatment of meningitis and septicaemia.

(4) In providing a means of distinguishing between colonization and infection in babies with respiratory problems.

The increasing availability of easy-to-use latex and coagglutination techniques for specific detection of neonatal pathogens offers the most immediate prospect of improving the rapid diagnosis of infection in ELBW babies. Less specifically the CRP and micro ESR are quick and easy to use but need further evaluation in very small babies, especially with regard to the clinical conditions which result in elevated readings in the absence of infection. Slight modification in the way in which routine white cell counts are reported and more frequent platelet and megathrombocyte counts would increase the value of haematology in the diagnosis of infection. Following careful evaluation it is probable that these investigations could increase the efficiency with which infection is recognized or excluded in babies weighing less than 1000 g.

References

1. La Gamma, E. F., Drusin, L. M., Macles, A. W., Machelek, S. and Auld, P. (1983) Neonatal infections. An important determinant of late NICU mortality in infants less than 1000 g at birth. *Am. J. Dis. Child.*, **137**, 838–841
2. Coonrod, J. D. and Rytel, M. W. (1971) Determination of the etiology of bacterial meningitis by counter immunoelectrophoresis. *Lancet*, **i**, 1154–1157
3. Friedman, A. D. and Ray, C. G. (1982) Rapid laboratory diagnosis of infections. *Pediatr. Infect. Dis.*, **1**, 366–372
4. Roos, R., Daumling, S. and Kreaft, H. (1986) Laboratory diagnosis of bacterial meningitis. In *Diagnosis of Infectious Diseases – New Aspects* (eds S. Simon and P. Wilkinson), Schattauer, Stuttgart, pp. 37–52
5. Fienstein, A. R. (1975) On the sensitivity, specificity and discrimination of diagnostic tests. *Clin. Pharamacol. Therap.*, **17**, 104–116
6. Nachum, R., Lipsey, A. and Seigel, S. E. (1973) Rapid detection of Gram-negative bacterial meningitis by the limulus lysate test. *N. Engl. J. Med.*, **289**, 931–934
7. Solum, N. O. (1973) The coagulogen of *Limulus polyphemus* hemocytes. *Thromb. Res.*, **2**, 55–58
8. D'Amato, R. F. (1982) Procedures for rapid diagnosis of perinatal infections. *Ann. Clin. Lab. Sci.*, **12**, 267–275
9. Sturk, A. and ten Cate, J. W. (1985) Endotoxin testing revisited. *Eur. J. Microbiol.*, **4**, 382–385
10. Scheifele, D. W., Melton, P. and Whitchelo, V. (1981) Evaluation of the limulus test for endotoxaemia in neonates with suspected sepsis. *J. Pediatr.*, **98**, 899–903
11. Goldberg, P. K., Kozinn, P. J., Kodis, B. *et al.* (1982) Endotoxemia and hyperbilirubinemia in the neonate. *Am. J. Dis. Child.*, **136**, 845–848
12. Mulhall, A. and de Louvois, J. (1986) Non-cultural methods in the diagnosis of infections in the newborn. In *Diagnosis of Infectious Diseases – New Aspects* (eds S. Simon and P. Wilkinson), Schattauer, Stuttgart, pp. 19–23
13. Pepys, M. B. (1981) C-reactive protein fifty years on. *Lancet*, **i**, 653–657

14. Pepys, M. B. (1982) Serum C-reactive protein, serum amyloid P component and serum amyloid A protein in autoimmune response. *Clin. Immunol. Allerg.*, **1**, 77–102
15. Boehm, T. J., Seeger, J., Loewenich, V. von and Solem, E. (1986) Determination of the half life of C-reactive protein in neonatal infection. In *Diagnosis of Infectious Diseases – New Aspects* (eds S. Simon and P. Wilkinson), Schattauer, Stuttgart, pp. 323–325
16. Sabel, K. G. and Hanson, L. A. (1974) The clinical usefulness of C-reactive protein (CRP) determinations in bacterial meningitis and septicaemia in infancy. *Acta Paediatr. Scand.*, **63**, 381–385
17. Coombes, E. J., Batstone, G. F., Moody, B. J. *et al.* (1986) Changes in the level of serum C-reactive protein during PN. *Br. J. Parenter. Ther.*, Jan/Feb, 6–10
18. Speer, C., Bruns, A. and Gahr, M. (1983) Sequential determination of CRP, alphatrypsin and haptoglobin in infancy. *Acta Paediatr. Scand.*, **72**, 679–683
19. Sann, L., Bienvenu, F., Bourgeois, J. and Bethenod, M. (1984) Evaluation of serum prealbumin, C-reactive protein and orosomucoid in neonates with bacterial infection. *J. Pediatr.* **105**, 977–981
20. Philip, A. G. S. (1984) Acute phase protein in neonatal infection. *J. Pediatr.*, **105**, 940–942
21. Aujard, Y., Laudignon, N. and Lebeau, R. (1986) Sensitivity and specificity of CRP for the diagnosis of neonatal infection. In *Diagnosis of Infectious Diseases – New Aspects* (eds S. Simon and P. Wilkinson), Schattauer, Stuttgart, pp. 221–223
22. Fasth, A. and Wadsworth, C. H. (1986) C-reactive protein as a diagnostic tool excluding infection and differentiating between bacterial and viral infections: clinician's opinion on the usefulness and reliability of the CRP assay. In *Diagnosis of Infectious Diseases – New Aspects* (eds S. Simon and P. Wilkinson), Schattauer, Stuttgart, pp. 327–333
23. Philip, A. G. S. and Baker, C. J. (1983) Cerebrospinal fluid CRP in neonatal meningitis *J. Pediatr.*, **5**, 715–717
24. Valmari, P. (1984) Towards earlier diagnosis in bacterial meningitis. In *CNS Infection in Children* (European Society for Paediatric Infectious Diseases, Interlaken), Abstract 7
25. Valmari, P., Peltola, H. and Ruuskanen, O. (1984) CRP and neurological prognosis in bacterial meningitis. In *CNS Infection in Children* (European Society for Paediatric Infectious Diseases, Interlaken), Abstract 33
26. Manroe, B. L., Weinberg, A. G., Rosenfeld, C. R. *et al.* (1979) The neonatal blood count in health and disease. *J. Pediatr.*, **95**, 89
27. Gregory, J. and Hey, E. (1972) Blood neutrophil response to bacterial infection in the first month of life. *Arch. Dis. Child.*, **47**, 747–753
28. Liu, C-H., Lehan, C., Speer, M. E., Fernbach, D. J. and Rudolph, A. J. (1984) Degenerative changes in neutrophils: an indicator of bacterial infection. *Pediatrics*, **74**, 823–827
29. Philip, A. G. S. and Hewitt, J. R. (1980) Early diagnosis of neonatal sepsis. *Pediatrics*, **65**, 1036–1042
30. Squire, E. N., Reich, H. M., Merenstein, G. B., Favara, B. E. and Todd, J. K. (1982) Criteria for discontinuation of antibiotic therapy during presumptive treatment of suspected neonatal infection. *Pediatr. Infect. Dis.*, **1**, 85–90

Chapter 17

Cardiac disorders including ductus arteriosus

James L. Wilkinson

Introduction

Cyanosis, respiratory distress and other manifestions of congestive cardiac failure are familiar and frequent phenomena in the VLBW infant. Such problems, however, are usually not related to primary cardiac disorders but are more often the consequences of respiratory disease, infection or other early postnatal problems common in this group of infants.

A variety of factors render the severely immature baby vulnerable to cardiac dysfunction. Immaturity of the ductus arteriosus coupled with high levels of endogenous prostaglandin E_2 predispose to prolonged ductal patency and the development of a left-to-right shunt [1]. The heart and lungs of the infant adapt poorly to the development of a significant ductal shunt with its associated high pulmonary blood flow [2,3]. Perinatal hypoxia, respiratory disease perpetuating pulmonary hypertension, metabolic disturbances such as hypoglycaemia or hypocalcaemia, and infection may also have a profoundly adverse effect on cardiac function.

Structural congenital heart disease (other than persistent ductus) does not present a common problem in the ELBW infant. However, such infants are not immune to any of the congenital defects which affect more mature infants and experience in Liverpool in recent years in small preterm babies has included a wide variety of cardiac malformations.

Infective endocarditis, though an uncommon problem in the infant age group generally, has been documented in the small preterm infant with long intravenous catheters (often used for parenteral nutrition) even if the heart is structurally normal.

Clinical examination

Assessment of cardiovascular signs in the ELBW infant is fraught with difficulty. This is related to the fact that observation is often impaired by the presence of monitoring equipment and multiple indwelling cannulae and various tubes and it is often difficult to gain satisfactory access to the infant for physical examination due to the various measures taken to reduce insensible fluid loss and to retain body heat in many Special Care Baby Units. Furthermore, such obvious signs as cyanosis and respiratory distress are frequently of pulmonary rather than cardiac origin. Pedal oedema – or oedema elsewhere – is a frequent finding in the premature nursery, is not cardiac in origin in most cases and may make assessment of peripheral pulses more difficult.

Palpation of peripheral pulses is extremely important and an assessment of peripheral tissue perfusion along with that of the radial and lower limb pulses is one of the most important initial observations. Bounding pulses are characteristic of the infant with a persistent ductus. Small peripheral pulses generally are common in very sick infants with a variety of non-cardiac problems – though the possibility of coarctation syndrome or hypoplastic left heart syndrome may need to be considered.

The significance of cyanosis is usually best assessed by measuring the arterial oxygen tension either directly or transcutaneously, repeating the measurement after a short period of 100% oxygen breathing (either spontaneous or on ventilator). For obvious reasons high concentrations of oxygen should not be continued beyond 15–20 min unless the arterial oxygen tension remains severely depressed. This test which is referred to as the 'hyperoxic' or 'nitrogen washout' test can be useful in distinguishing between cyanosis of cardiac origin and cyanosis due to other causes [4]. However, some infants with severe respiratory problems or with persistent pulmonary hypertension due to pulmonary disease may show depressed arterial oxygen tension despite high $F\text{io}_2$.

Palpation of the cardiac impulse is seldom very helpful in the VLBW infant but should be carried out as part of the routine. A forceful parasternal impulse may reflect pulmonary hypertension associated with pulmonary problems or the presence of a left-to-right shunt via a persistent ductus. Auscultation of the heart is mainly limited to the assessment and grading of any systolic or continuous murmur which is present. Such murmurs as are heard are usually ejection in timing and best heard over the mid or upper praecordium. These murmurs are essentially rather non-specific and it is usually difficult to reach a definite diagnosis of any specific cardiac pathology unless the co-existence of a murmur with bounding peripheral pulses with or without respiratory symptoms suggests that the murmur is due to a ductus.

Ancillary investigations

Chest X-ray

Radiography of the chest is carried out very frequently in the neonatal nursery, but unfortunately the radiographers involved are often lacking in expertise in handling tiny preterm infants and for a variety of reasons the quality of films produced is often poor. It is essential that the X-ray be taken with the help of nursing staff who can assist with positioning and holding the baby. Of necessity, the film will be taken antero-posteriorly with the infant lying supine and with a tube to film distances usually less than 1 m. Furthermore, the lungs are frequently incompletely inflated due to lung disease and the phase of respiration is uncontrolled. All these factors contribute to an exaggeration of heart size and a cardiothoracic ratio of 0.6 or even 0.65 is therefore quite frequent. Assessment of lung vascularity is complicated by the presence of lung disease.

Although chest radiography is clearly an essential part of the investigation of an infant with suspected cardiac problems, in practice clinical findings and echocardiography are usually much more helpful in deciding whether a significant cardiac problem is present.

Electrocardiogram

The ECG should include the standard 12 leads and a right-sided chest lead. Increased left ventricular forces may be found in the presence of a ductal shunt but are inconstant. The normal right ventricular preponderance which is seen in mature neonates may be rather less pronounced in the small preterm infant and can give way to left ventricular preponderance in the early weeks of life, even in the absence of a large ductal shunt.

Echocardiography

In skilled hands echocardiography is often extremely helpful in determining the presence and nature of cardiac defects in small infants. Examination of the heart can usually be accomplished simply and rapidly using a variety of standard views (long axis, four chambers, aortic arch, ductus). The left atrial diameter can be readily measured and the degree of dilatation of the left atrium in the presence of a persistent ductus is a helpful diagnostic clue. Simple M mode tracings can provide an accurate assessment of left atrial diameter but are of very limited value in the preterm infant in other respects.

Doppler echocardiography where available will often provide definite diagnostic evidence of a left-to-right ductal shunt even if the ductus itself cannot be imaged satisfactorily.

Limitations of echocardiography are related to the fact that hyperinflated lungs in a baby who is being ventilated may create considerable difficulties in gaining adequate imaging of the heart. Neonatal complications such as pneumothorax or interstitial emphysema in the mediastinum may provide a further barrier to echocardiography.

The largest single problem, however, relates to the degree of confidence which can be placed in the findings obtained from echocardiography relating to the fact that the technique is heavily operator-dependent. Many paediatricians, radiologists or technicians with a modest amount of training can acquire a clear idea of normal appearances in standard echocardiographic views and of the findings in premature infants with a persistent ductus. However, competence at examining infants with structural congenital heart disease depends on fairly advanced familiarity with a variety of congenital anomalies and the echocardiographic findings to be expected with them. It is unfortunate that some of the more important diagnostic problems which present in the newborn period due to structural cardiac defects, e.g. transposition of the great vessels, total anomalous pulmonary venous drainage, coarctation syndrome, tend to present quite substantial challenges even to an experienced echocardiographer and can easily be missed by the less experienced operator, as intracardiac anatomy may appear virtually normal.

Range of cardiac defects encountered in preterm infants

Whilst the entire range of structural congenital heart disease can occasionally be seen in premature infants, it is clear that persistent ductus arteriosus is the only lesion which presents with any frequency.

In Liverpool over the past ten years infants below 1500 g have been seen and treated with such lesions as ventricular septal defect, aortic stenosis, coarctation of the aorta, transposition of the great arteries, pulmonary atresia and total anomalous pulmonary venous drainage. Such malformations have not, however, presented in ELBW infants.

A variety of cardiac problems may arise secondarily in relation to other neonatal problems. These include congestive cardiac failure resulting from lung disease, fluid overload or sepsis. Cor pulmonale may result from bronchopulmonary dysplasia in infants who have required prolonged ventilation. Infective endocarditis in infants who have had long lines may also occur – even in infants without structural cardiac defects as a predisposing factor.

Management of congestive heart failure

Cardiac failure manifested by respiratory distress, hepatomegaly and oedema may require treatment regardless of its underlying cause. However, it is clearly important that the aetiological factors be identified and if possible treated actively.

Some degree of fluid restriction is desirable in the infant with evidence of congestive failure. This is especially important as fluid overload predisposes to ductal patency [5]. Fluid intake should be limited to 120–150 ml/kg depending on the severity of symptoms. In some cases fluid restriction alone may ameliorate the symptoms but if significant evidence of congestive failure persists diuretic therapy should be instituted. Traditionally in recent years frusemide (1 mg/kg once or twice daily orally) has been used as the first choice diuretic but there is some evidence that this drug may stimulate production of prostaglandin E_2 and may thus promote ductal patency [6]. As this would clearly be deleterious in the management of such infants it may be preferable to use chlorothiazide (15 mg/kg orally) which apparently does not produce the same effect on prostaglandin release. Thus far, however, there appears to be no conclusive evidence that morbidity or mortality are improved by the use of chlorothiazide in preference to frusemide.

Hyponatraemia or hypokalaemia may develop during diuretic therapy. Hypokalaemia can be prevented or corrected by the addition of potassium supplements or of a potassium-sparing diuretic such as amiloride (0.2 mg/kg given orally with frusemide or chlorothiazide).

The use of digitalis in the management of cardiac failure is controversial in premature infants. There is little evidence that digoxin has any useful therapeutic effect and its potential toxicity demands that it be used with considerable caution, if at all [7]. Most neonatologists prefer to avoid its use in the preterm infant.

Persistent ductus arteriosus

Failure of the ductus to close normally in the newborn period in the VLBW infant is related to a combination of factors. Immaturity of the ductus itself is associated with reduced responsiveness to the increased Po_2 of blood perfusing the ductus after birth. Secondly, high levels of endogenous prostaglandin E_2 further inhibit ductal constriction [1,8]. Thirdly, the presence of pulmonary problems such as hyaline membrane disease tend to result in reduced arterial Po_2 which itself prolongs ductal patency.

It has been suggested that delay in closure of the ductus is almost invariable in the VLBW infant and that it is possible to demonstrate a patent ductus on cross-sectional echocardiography in virtually all infants below 32 weeks gestation [9]. The incidence of clinically apparent persistent ductus in preterm babies has been reported as being 7–25% of all premature infants and 35% in those below 1500 g. In those below 1000 g the figure is probably greater than 70% [10].

Haemodynamics

The appearance of a left-to-right shunt through a persistent ductus arteriosus is dependent on a fall in the level of pulmonary artery pressure and resistance after birth. The presence of severe pulmonary problems and positive pressure ventilation may result in retention of high pulmonary resistance initially and hence a significant shunt may not become apparent for several days.

The development of a large shunt results in substantial volume loading on the left ventricle and, in the small preterm infant in whom left ventricular reserve is very limited, this rapidly results in the appearance of symptoms of left heart failure [2,3].

Symptoms and signs

The appearance of a praecordial murmur, often found in the course of routine examination, is usually the first manifestation of a ductal shunt. Such murmurs are usually systolic in timing and may be clearly heard along the left sternal border and up in the pulmonary area. In some cases the murmur is more obviously continuous. Commonly the murmur appears and increases in intensity in the latter part of the first week or the second week of life. Characteristically the murmur varies in timing and amplitude from day to day or even hour to hour – a source of considerable frustration to house doctors. Peripheral pulses are often bounding, and this feature in conjunction with murmur is very strongly suggestive of a persistent ductus.

Symptoms of pulmonary congestion include tachypnoea, dyspnoea and in more severe cases the development of respiratory failure with cyanosis and apnoeic attacks. Manifestions of right heart failure with hepatomegaly and oedema are inconstant.

The onset of respiratory symptoms in preterm infants with a persistent ductus often occurs at a time when the infant is beginning to improve after early respiratory difficulties related to hyaline membrane disease. The major indication of a significant ductal shunt may well be an exacerbation of respiratory symptoms in the latter part of the first week or the second week of life and it is often difficult to differentiate between symptomatology related to the initial respiratory disorder and that which results from ductal patency.

Diagnosis

Confirmation of the presence of a persistent ductus may best be achieved by cross-sectional echocardiography with or without Doppler examination. In the absence of echocardiography the diagnosis rests heavily on clinical findings. The chest X-ray (Figure 17.1) and ECG findings are frequently non-specific though radiological evidence of cardiomegaly and pulmonary plethora may be found and in some cases left ventricular hypertrophy may be apparent on the ECG after 2–3 weeks.

Cross-sectional echocardiography may show evidence of left atrial and left ventricular dilatation and the ductus arteriosus itself can often be visualized directly (Figure 17.2) [9]. Unfortunately it is not always possible to obtain good imaging of the ductus, especially in the ventilated infant, as the left lung if hyperinflated tends to intrude into the path of the ultrasound beam resulting in loss of image.

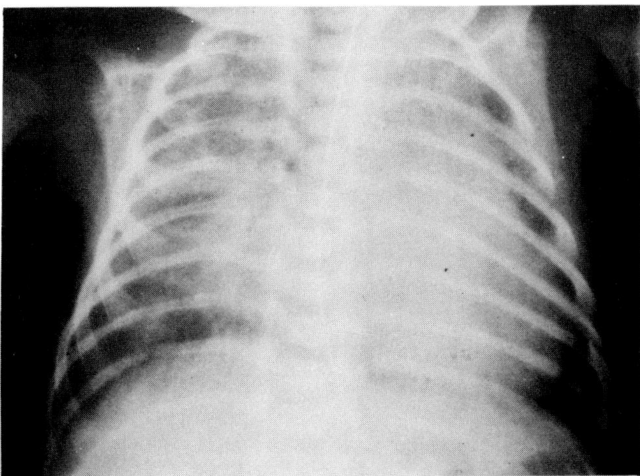

Figure 17.1 Chest radiograph from preterm infant with large patent ductus arteriosus. The cardiomegaly and pulmonary congestion are obvious but most of the features are non-specific in an infant of this age

Dilatation of the left atrium, as indicated by an increased ratio of left atrial diameter to aortic root dimension, has been regarded as a reliable indicator of a significant shunt [11]. This ratio is normally less than one but, in the presence of a ductus, values between 1.1 and 1.5 are usually obtained. These measurements may be made using M mode echocardiography or from cross-sectional images. Unfortunately a normal left atrial to aortic root ratio does not completely exclude a significant ductus.

Doppler examination can demonstrate high velocity flow through the ductus arteriosus from the aorta to the pulmonary artery and is the most precise non-invasive means of confirming the diagnosis. It is noteworthy that in some premature infants even when the ductus may appear still to be patent on cross-sectional imaging, no flow is demonstrable on Doppler examination – this being usually indicative that the ductus is functionally closed.

Cardiac catheterization is not usually regarded as being necessary to establish the diagnosis, and as it carries a significant morbidity and even mortality in small premature infants, it should be avoided.

Treatment

Initial treatment of infants with clinical signs of a persistent ductus follows the lines indicated for the management of congestive heart failure. In the infant who is only mildly symptomatic fluid restriction alone may be sufficient to tide him over until his ductus undergoes spontaneous closure. Those patients with more significant symptoms usually require institution of diuretic therapy.

Infants who remain severely symptomatic after 24 or 48 h of diuretic therapy combined with fluid restriction will usually benefit from treatment with prostaglandin synthetase inhibitors of which indomethacin is the drug which has been used clinically with significant effect [12]. This preparation may be administered orally, rectally or intravenously, and is usually given in a total dose of 0.6 mg/kg in divided doses. The

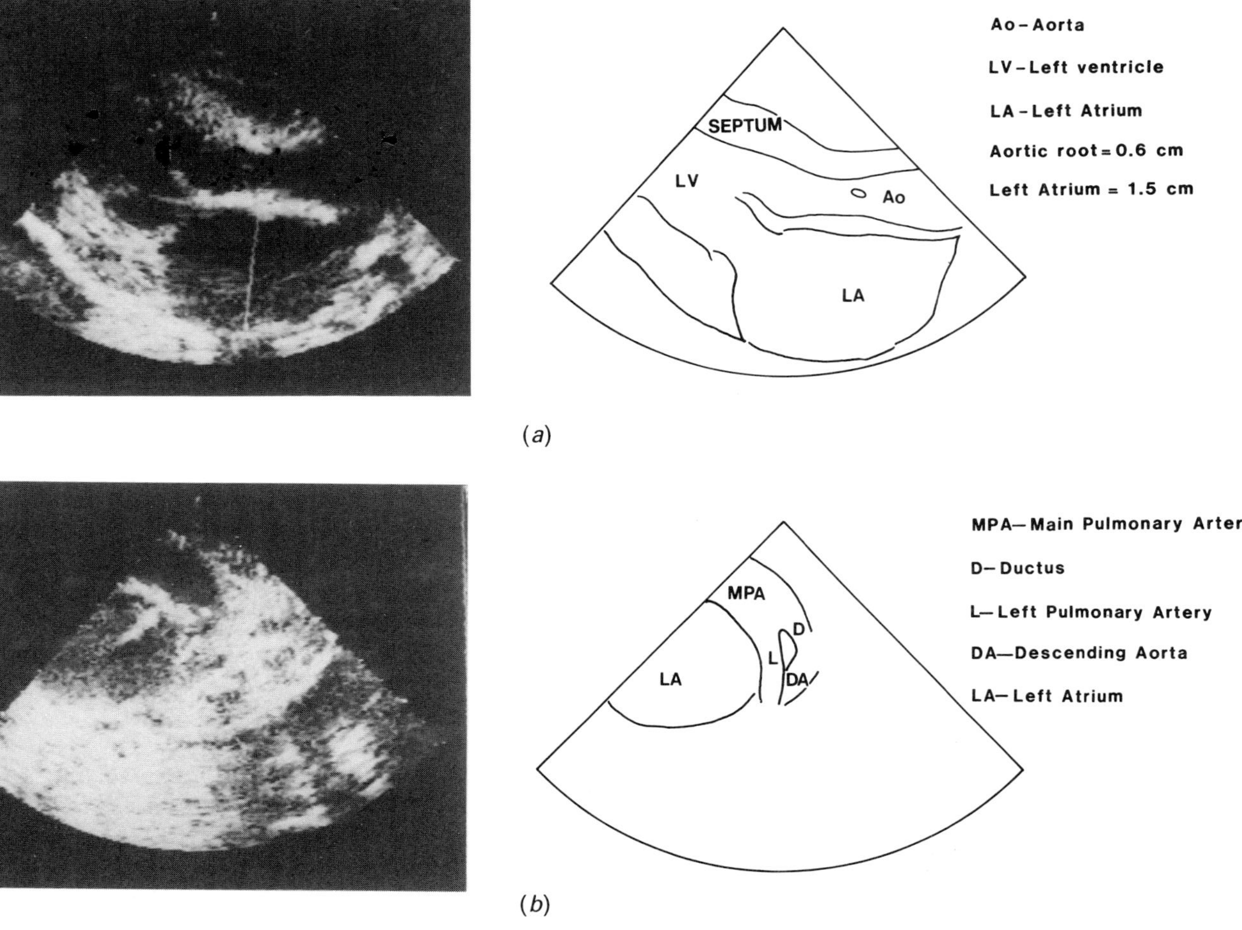

Figure 17.2 Echocardiograms from a preterm infant with a patent ductus arteriosus. (*a*) Long axis section illustrating dilatation of the left atrium and increased LA:aortic root ratio. (*b*) Semi long axis cut to show ductus. The image quality is relatively poor as it is very difficult to get good imaging of the ductus area especially in a ventilated infant with over-inflated lungs

course of treatment may be spread over 24 h using three doses of 0.2 mg/kg. An alternative is to spread the therapy over 5–6 days giving 0.1 mg/kg daily. Intravenous administration is simple and effective and is probably preferable to the oral or rectal routes [13].

The policy on the administration of indomethacin has varied widely between different neonatal units. In some centres a very low threshold for drug treatment has been maintained and a high proportion of preterm infants have been given indomethacin treatment in the early days of life [14]. This method of management of persistent ductus in the premature baby has some strong supporters who have reported high rates of spontaneous closure following such therapy. Many other centres have been more cautious in the use of indomethacin, being concerned about such side effects as gastrointestinal bleeding and renal impairment. In such neonatal units indomethacin treatment is usually withheld until the infant has had a prolonged trial of other conventional management. Only those infants who are very severely symptomatic and ventilator-dependent have been treated and often not until they are 2–3 weeks old or later. In general, results of such a highly selective approach to indomethacin therapy have been disappointing [15].

A large multicentre trial carried out in recent years has suggested that a more appropriate line to pursue is that those infants who have clear-cut manifestations of a ductus (murmur, bounding pulses, respiratory distress) should be managed vigorously with fluid restriction if necessary and subsequent diuretic therapy. If symptoms do not resolve satisfactorily within 48 h of the institution of such therapy, indomethacin treatment should be started [16].

The employment of prostaglandin synthetase inhibitors in the management of persistent ductus in the preterm neonate has certainly led to a significant increase in the spontaneous closure rate and a reduction in neonatal morbidity and mortality. The effectiveness of treatment can usually be judged by clinical evidence of a diminution in the ductal shunt. Respiratory symptoms improve and the murmur may well disappear, as also the bounding pulses. Echocardiography will often show a reduction in left atrial dilatation and actual closure of the ductus may be confirmed by cross-sectional imaging or Doppler interrogation.

Unfortunately a proportion of cases show subsequent re-opening of the ductus and if this leads to a recurrence of symptoms a second course of indomethacin may sometimes be worth considering after an interval of 3–4 days.

Infants who remain severaly symptomatic despite these measures and especially those who remain ventilator-dependent and cannot be weaned from respiratory support usually require surgical ligation of their ductus. This procedure can be carried out with low morbidity and mortality even in ELBW infants. In experienced surgical hands ductal ligation is remarkably safe and well tolerated [17]. In some centres surgery is performed in the special care baby unit, the surgeon and his team coming to the patient rather than vice versa. In other institutions the affected infant is transferred to the cardiac surgical department for operation in the cardiac theatre, but in general such infants are transferred back to the neonatal unit after surgery for postoperative care. The latter policy has been employed in Liverpool over many years, infants being transferred in some cases over long distances for surgery. The diagnosis is confirmed by echocardiography preoperatively but cardiac catheterization is avoided. Using this policy, and despite the potential for problems in regard to transportation to and from neonatal units, we have not had any surgical mortality in the past decade.

Other structural cardiac defects

Whilst a variety of congenital malformations have been seen in VLBW babies, it would not be appropriate in this chapter to discuss in any detail those problems which are not specific to this group of infants. As in the mature infant, the presentation of serious congenital heart disease in the newborn period is frequently related to ductal closure and its effects on the haemodynamic disturbance produced by the cardiac abnormality. Thus a substantial group of 'ductus-dependent defects' are characterized by presentation in the first week or ten days of life. Such defects include those in which the pulmonary circulation is largely or entirely ductus-dependent, e.g. pulmonary atresia, critical pulmonary stenosis, severe tetralogy of Fallot, tricuspid atresia. Defects of this kind are associated with increasing cyanosis as the ductus constricts. In the small premature infant ductal closure is often delayed for the reasons indicated earlier and infants with these conditions may therefore show little cyanosis in the early days of life, resulting in some cases in delay in diagnosis. It is also noteworthy that as the physical signs may be dominated by the murmur of a ductus and cyanosis may be minimal or absent in the immediate newborn period, therapy to bring about ductal constriction (indomethacin therapy or surgery) should not be instituted until the clinical diagnosis has been confirmed by echocardiography.

Another group of ductus-dependent defects are those in which part or all of the systemic circulation is ductus-dependent. Such defects include hypoplastic left heart syndrome, some examples of critical aortic stenosis and conditions in which the lower systemic segment is ductus-dependent postnatally as in aortic arch interruption and particularly infantile coarctation syndrome. Once again in the preterm infant where ductal closure is delayed the clinical signs and symptomatology associated with such defects may appear late and initially at any rate lower limb pulses may be easily palpable, resulting in diagnostic delay.

Cardiac problems secondary to non-cardiac disease in the premature

Cor pulmonale

The development of manifestations of heart failure in infants with chronic respiratory disease – notably bronchopulmonary dysplasia – is an increasingly frequent phenomenon as more tiny preterm infants survive following prolonged and vigorous intensive care.

In such infants manifestations of chronic respiratory disease including dyspnoea, tachypnoea and cyanosis with chronic oxygen dependence are often combined with signs of right heart failure including hepatomegaly and oedema.

The manifestations of cardiac failure tend to develop late, often after the first month of life. It is important to look for evidence of any structural cardiac problem – best excluded by cross-sectional echocardiography – but provided that no such abnormality is present, treatment of cardiac failure follows standard lines and the most important consideration is active management of the underlying lung disease with particular attention to nutrition and to chronic oxygen therapy where indicated. In treating congestive heart failure it is important to bear in mind that the respiratory symptoms are likely to be largely, if not entirely, unrelated to the presence of congestive failure (left heart failure usually being absent in such infants). Treatment should therefore only be aimed at controlling manifestations of right heart failure and diuretic doses should in general be kept to the minimum which will achieve this.

Endocarditis and sepsis

Whilst infective endocarditis is generally extremely rare, there are now a number of reports of endocarditis occurring in infants who have suffered from severe bacterial infections – especially septicaemia associated with parenteral nutrition [18,19]. Three infants have suffered this complication in Liverpool in recent years (two developing pulmonary valve endocarditis and one aortic valve involvement). In all these infants there was a clear history of severe sepsis associated with either *Staphylococcus aureus* or *Staphylococcus albus* on culture. Manifestations of congestive failure associated with the presence of a murmur were thought initially to be related to a ductus arteriosus and in one case surgical ligation of the ductus was carried out. Despite establishment of the diagnosis of endocarditis by echocardiography in two of the three cases and despite active therapy with intravenous antibiotics, all three infants died.

Reports from the literature suggest that tricuspid valve endocarditis is also an important site of infection and particularly in association with the use of central venous lines [18,19]. It is clear that the establishment of the diagnosis can be difficult and depends on a high index of suspicion coupled with careful echocardiography which will usually show evidence of vegetations.

The indications appear to be that most affected infants have no structural cardiac abnormality prior to the development of endocarditis and in this respect endocarditis in these infants clearly differs from the pattern seen in older children or adults.

Although successful treatment of neonatal endocarditis has been documented in term infants, it appears that the condition has proved almost universally lethal in the ELBW baby.

References

1. Clyman, R. I. (1986) Pharmacology of the fetal and neonatal ductus arteriosus. In *Pediatric Cardiology* (eds E. F. Doyle, M. A. Engle, W. M. Gersomy, W. J. Rashkind and N. J. Talner), Springer-Verlag, New York, pp. 871–875
2. Baylen, B., Meyer, R. A., Karfhagen, J., Benzig, G. III, Bubb, M. E. and Kaplan, S. (1977) Left ventricular performance in the critically ill premature infant with patent ductus arteriosus and pulmonary disease. *Circulation*, **55**, 182–188
3. Alverson, D. C., Marlowe, W. E., Johnson, J. D. *et al.* (1983) Effect of patent ductus arteriosus on left ventricular output in premature infants. *J. Pediatr.*, **102**, 754–757
4. Jones, R. W. A., Baumer, J. H., Joseph, M. C. and Shinebourne, E. A. (1976) Arterial oxygenation and response to oxygen breathing in differential diagnosis of congenital heart disease in infancy. *Arch. Dis. Child.*, **51**, 667–673
5. Stevenson, J. G. (1977) Fluid administration in the association of patent ductus arteriosus complicating respiratory distress syndrome. *J. Pediatr.*, **90**, 257–261
6. Green, T. P., Thompson, T. R., Johnson, D. E. and Lock, J. E. (1983) Frusemide promotes patent ductus arteriosus in premature infants with respiratory distress syndrome. *N. Engl. J. Med.*, **308**, 743–748
7. Berman, W., Dubynsky, O., Whitman, V., Friedman, Z. and Maisels, M. J. (1978) Digoxin therapy in low-birth-weight infants with patent ductus arteriosus. *J. Pediatr.*, **93**, 652–655
8. Olley, P. M. and Coceani, F. (1979) Mechanism of closure of the ductus arteriosus. In *Pediatric*

Cardiology, Vol. 2 (eds M. J. Godman and R. M. Marquis), Churchill Livingstone, Edinburgh, pp. 15–24

9. Rigby, M. L., Pickering, D. and Wilkinson, A. (1984) Cross sectional echocardiography in determining persistent patency of the ductus arteriosus in premature infants. *Arch. Dis. Child.*, **59**, 341–345
10. Siassi, B., Blanco, C., Cabal, L. A. and Coran, A. G. (1976) Incidence and clinical features of patent ductus arteriosus in low birth-weight infants. A prospective analysis of 150 consecutively born infants. *Pediatrics*, **57**, 347–351
11. Silverman, N. H., Lewis, A. B., Heymann, M. A. and Rudolph, A. M. (1974) Echocardiographic assessment of ductus arteriosus shunt in premature infants *Circulation*, **50**, 821–825
12. Heymann, M. A., Rudolph, A. M. and Silverman, N. H. (1976) Closure of the ductus arteriosus in premature infants by inhibition of prostaglandin synthesis. *N. Engl. J. Med.*, **295**, 530–533
13. Yeh, T. F., Luken, J. A., Thalji, A., Raval, D., Carr, I. and Pildes, R. C. (1981) Intravenous indomethacin therapy in premature infants with persistent ductus arteriosus, a double blind study. *J. Pediatr.*, **98**, 137–145
14. Mahony, L., Carnero, V., Brett, C., Heymann, M. A. and Clyman, R. I. (1982) Prophylactic indomethacin therapy for patent ductus arteriosus in very low birth-weight infants. *N. Engl. J. Med.*, **306**, 506–510
15. Cooke, R. W. I. and Pickering, D. (1979) Poor response to oral indomethacin therapy for persistent ductus arteriosus in very low birth weight babies. *Br. Heart J.*, **41**, 301–303
16. Gersony, W. M., Peckham, G. J., Ellison, R. C., Mieltinen, O. S. and Nadas, A. S. (1983) Effects of indomethacin in premature infants with patent ductus arteriosus: results of a national collaborative study. *J. Pediatr.*, **102**, 895–905
17. Edmunds, L. H. (1978) Surgical management. In *Report of the 75th Ross Conference on Pediatric Research* (eds M. A. Heymann and A. M. Rudolph), Ross Laboratories, Columbus, Ohio, p. 86
18. Delberg, D. G., Fisher, D. J., Gross, D. M., Denson, S. E. and Alcock, C. W. (1983) Endocarditis in high risk neonates. *Pediatrics*, **71**, 392–397
19. McGuiness, G. A., Schieken, R. M. and Maguire, G. F. (1980) Endocarditis in the newborn. *Am. J. Dis. Child.*, **134**, 577–580

Chapter 18

Renal function

Malcolm Coulthard

Good clinical practice has to be based on a sound understanding of physiology and pathophysiology, and there is no discipline where this is more true than renal medicine. Unfortunately few studies have been undertaken of renal function in babies weighing less than 1000 g, so that a great deal of our 'knowledge' is extrapolated from data on older and heavier subjects. There are dangers in this approach, and caution is needed to ensure that data from small babies are not misinterpreted by comparison with inappropriate standards, that investigation techniques for larger subjects really can be applied to these infants, and that what is often no more than extrapolation does not become regarded as fact. Furthermore, there is no ideal preterm animal model in which the various aspects of kidney function are known to mature in parallel with a human baby.

Standardizing measurements

To compare renal function between very small infants and larger subjects it is necessary to standardize the data by expressing them per unit body size. In older subjects the glomerular filtration rate (GFR) and the metabolic rate (which largely determines the need for the excretion of waste products) vary closely with body surface area, and this is the most commonly used standard to compare values between individuals. However, this has only been demonstrated to be appropriate over the age of two years when the relationship between body surface area and body weight alters only slowly. The relationship changes almost week by week in preterm babies (Figure 18.1) [1,2] so that the standard chosen makes a much greater difference.

Body weight is the best index for standardizing GFR in babies. Variations in GFR between infants of 27–40 weeks gestation are reduced more than two-fold by expressing the data as GFR/kg rather than GFR/m^2 [3], which is similar to previous findings for metabolic rate [4]. Furthermore, body weight can be accurately and directly measured, whereas values of body surface area can only be estimated from formulae which themselves have been constructed with relatively few actual measurements from very small infants. The proposal to relate function to the size of the pool over which the kidney exercises control [5] is similarly impractical because, like surface area, fluid volumes would be estimated rather than measured. Furthermore, no single fluid volume would be appropriate; total body water would be best for considering urea and water handling, whereas extracellular fluid volume would be best for creatinine or gentamicin handling. Clinical management decisions such as

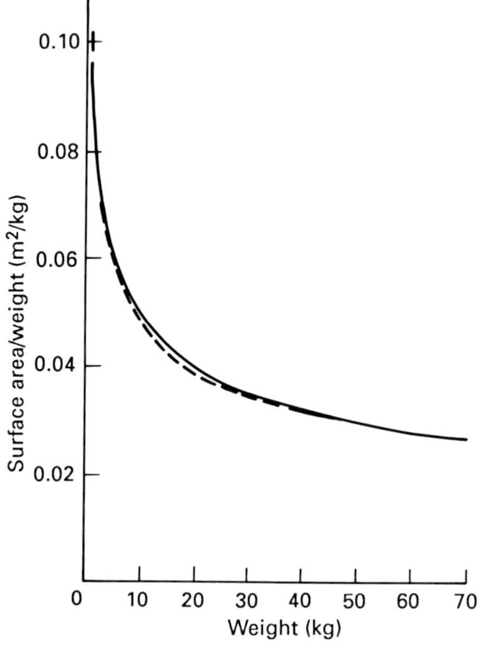

Figure 18.1 Relation between surface area:weight ratio and body weight, —— calculated from Boyd [1] and --- from Haycock *et al.* [2] using the 50th centile values from national height and weight standards and taken from Coulthard and Hey [3]

fluid and electrolyte requirements and drug dosages are all based on body weight, and the use of a different system to describe kidney function does nothing to help incorporate information derived from renal research into routine practice. Clearly body weight is the best practical standard, but as had been observed in the past [5], proposals to change established practice are likely to be opposed.

The role of the kidneys in babies under 1000 g

The kidneys of very preterm babies have a quantitatively different role from the kidneys of older children or adults with regard to both water and sodium handling.

Water

Because the proportionate growth rate of a 1000 g baby is extremely high and nutrition has to be provided in liquid form, the fluid intake has to be large. Thus, to maintain water balance the baby is obliged to have a high urine flow. Conversely, the GFR is relatively lower in a 1000 g baby than in an adult, and a combination of relatively less water being filtered, and more needing to appear as urine can only be achieved by a much greater fractional excretion of glomerular filtrate (Fe_{H_2O}). A mean value of 13.1% has been reported in babies with an average weight of 1600 g and a daily fluid intake of 200 ml/kg [6]. Similar Fe_{H_2O} values in adults would result in a daily urine volume of over 20 litres. Indeed, normal values of Fe_{H_2O} values in babies have previously been interpreted as evidence of a harmful osmotic diuresis because they were inappropriately compared to adult normal ranges [7].

Sodium

By contrast to its role in excreting water, the kidney of a preterm baby has to avidly conserve sodium for growth. If the *in utero* growth rate is to be matched 1 mmol/kg must be retained daily [8], and yet (mature) breast milk contains only about 0.65 mmol sodium/100 ml. A mature baby reabsorbs most of the filtered sodium load and thereby retains sufficient without supplements; a 1000 g baby usually does not manage this.

Glomerular filtration

The development of new glomeruli occurs only slowly in the last trimester and stops by about 36 weeks [9]; renal growth thereafter depends on an increase in the size and number of cells of the existing nephrons. The earliest glomeruli to mature are the deep (corticomedullary) ones which are associated with the longest loops of Henle and have the greatest role in sodium conservation [10]. The glomeruli are relatively larger than the tubules, with a glomerular surface area:proximal tubular volume ratio about ten times that seen in adults [11]. Despite this anatomical glomerulotubular imbalance, it is clear that glomerular and tubular functions must be linked and develop in parallel for physiological balance to be achieved.

Indeed, despite the relatively well developed glomeruli, GFR is low in very preterm babies. It has been described as increasing from 32 weeks [12] and 34 weeks [13] and even as slowing from 35 weeks gestation [14]. For some time it was thought that GFR was extremely low *in utero* while the baby was effectively dialysed through the placenta, and that it rose steeply 'in response to need' after birth [14] (Figure 18.2). However, more recently it has been shown that GFR rises logarithmically in a 'programmed' fashion with increasing conceptional age and is independent of

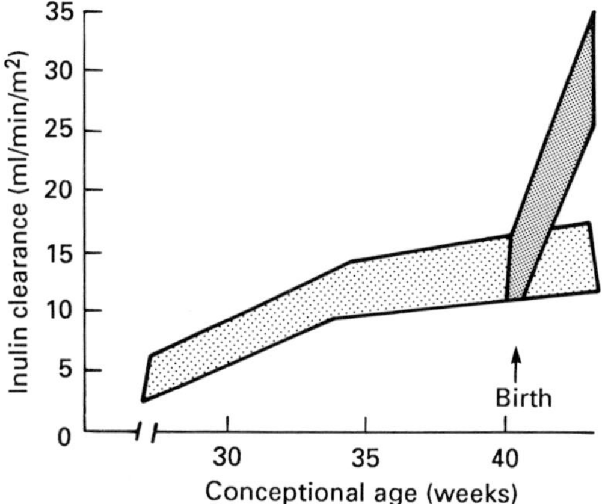

Figure 18.2 Diagram from Fawer *et al.* [14] showing how glomerular filtration rate/m^2 was considered to develop with conceptional age and illustrating how birth was considered to be 'the signal to a striking increase in glomerular filtration rate'

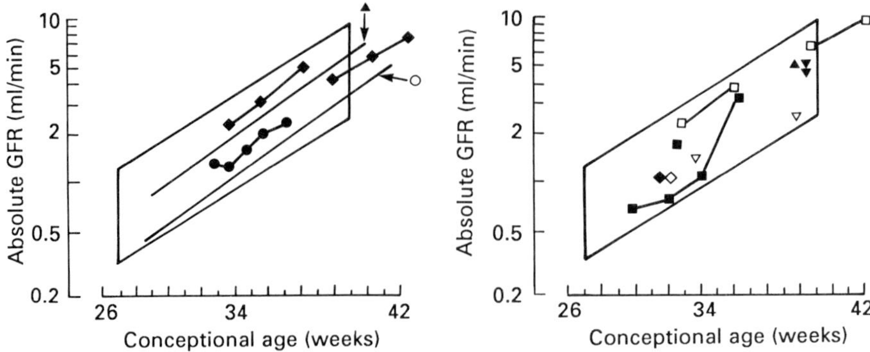

Figure 18.3 Graphs of the effects of absolute GFR (note the logarithmic scale) on conceptional age taken from Coulthard [15]. The boxes represent the confidence limits for data from that study and the other lines and symbols show the results in 12 other studies. Where necessary data were recalculated to be presented in this format. Note that (▲) is the regression line calculated from the data of Fawer *et al.* [14] (see Figure 18.2)

postnatal age [12,13,15]. Furthermore, apparent contradictions between these and previous studies have been shown to be the result of the way in which the data had been expressed, and on recalculation all studies show the same logarithmic rise of absolute GFR which is uninfluenced by the timing of birth, including the data from which Figure 18.2 was derived (Figure 18.3) [15]. It is almost universally assumed that GFR is especially low in the first two days after birth, but very few measurements have been made [15].

The efficiency of elimination of a substance that is removed mainly by glomerular filtration (such as gentamicin) is best defined by the half life ($T_{\frac{1}{2}}$); the time taken for its plasma concentration to fall to half of its original value. This is dependent on both the absolute GFR and the volume of the pool into which the substance is distributed, which in the case of gentamicin is the extracellular fluid (ECF). Thus for gentamicin clearance, $T_{\frac{1}{2}} = 0.693$ ECF/GFR, where 0.693 is the constant, $\log_e 2$.

Since GFR increases with conceptional age and ECF is determined primarily by body weight, it follows that the efficiency of the infant kidney to clear substances such as gentamicin depends upon the relationship between body weight and conceptional age. At 'normal' *in utero* growth rates the (exponential) rate of rise in GFR slightly exceeds the rate of rise in body weight, with the result that $T_{\frac{1}{2}}$ gradually falls and gentamicin clearance gradually increases with increasing maturity. However, the GFR of a baby with severe growth retardation will continue to rise with time while the ECF remains almost static, producing a much shorter $T_{\frac{1}{2}}$ and thus an enhanced ability to clear gentamicin. This phenomenon accounts [15] for the apparent acceleration of renal function seen in the weeks after birth [14] because GFR continues to increase but the *in utero* growth rate is not maintained. Body weight alone is therefore a poor predictor of a baby's renal clearance and decisions based on this, such as the correct dosage interval for aminoglycoside administration, also require a knowledge of maturity. For example, a newborn 1000 g baby of 26 weeks gestation will demonstrate much poorer gentamicin clearance than a baby born small for dates at 30 weeks and who still weighs only 1000 g a month later. We are presently validating a nomogram which will take this into account and will give the appropriate dosage interval from the baby's current position on a growth chart.

The estimation of GFR in very small infants is problematic [16] in the context of both research and clinical practice. It is difficult to obtain accurately timed and complete urine collections. It is possible to measure GFR by methods which do not rely on urine collection, such as the constant inulin infusion and single-shot inulin techniques. However, these must be greatly modified in babies because of the much slower equilibration of glomerular markers [17], or their application will lead to invalid results [18].

In clincial practice the plasma creatinine concentration is the most widely used measurement of GFR; urea is a very poor marker [19]. The published ranges for plasma creatinine concentrations in stable preterm infants in the first three months of life are wide, however, with more than a two-fold difference between the highest and lowest values in the first week after birth [19,20], increasing to about a five-fold difference later [20]. Thus, at best a plasma creatinine value alone provides a relatively crude estimate of renal function. Because it was predicted [21] and confirmed [21–24] that the accuracy of estimating GFR from plasma creatinine concentration in older children could be increased by factoring for body length, attempts have been made to apply this to babies. However, it was argued that because their GFR does not vary with surface area there would be no benefit for neonatal data [19,24], and little [25] or none [19] has been reported. Since the production of creatinine in babies varies closely with body weight [19,26], and its clearance depends on absolute GFR which varies with conceptional age, the normal range for plasma creatinine concentration for a particular baby would probably be best determined from his position on a growth chart in a similar way to that described for gentamicin clearance. Thus, the wide range of values seen for plasma creatinine against postnatal age [20] is probably due in part to the variation in weight for conceptional age in these babies.

Tubular function

Sodium

Term babies conserve the sodium they need for growth differently from older subjects. A smaller fraction of the filtered sodium is reabsorbed in the proximal tubule [27,28] where the net physical forces for reabsorption are less [29] and the cells are less developed for pumping sodium, with fewer basal interdigitations and lower Na-K-ATPase activity [30]. However the sodium delivered distally is avidly reabsorbed under the influence of very high renin-angiotensin-aldosterone system (RAAS) activity [31]. This high RAAS activity induces an increase in the Na-K-ATPase activity in rats [32], so that (unlike glomerular function) absolute tubular efficiency does improve after birth, and this is reflected by an increasingly positive sodium balance in babies during the first two weeks of life [33]. Acute sodium loading in neonates results in only a blunted fall in RAAS activity and limited natriuretic response [34] but there is no evidence that long-term sodium administration leads to sodium retention.

In very preterm babies the situation is similar, except Na-K-ATPase activity is even less developed [30], RAAS activity is even greater, and babies frequently develop hyponatraemia because they begin life in negative sodium balance and only very slowly achieve a positive balance [33]. The hyponatraemia can be largely abolished if babies of less than 34 weeks gestation are given about 5 mmol sodium/kg daily [35] (or more if they are administered theophyllines which are natriuretic [36]) from day 4 to 14. This amount of sodium is more than is provided by the currently available 'preterm humanized' milk formulae, or preterm human milk [37], and much more than that available in mature breast milk. Supplementing to this extent confers an improvement in growth which lasts beyond the period of supplementation and is not associated with any adverse effects, and in particular does not increase the incidence of patent ductus arteriosus, necrotizing enterocolitis or symptomatic intracranial haemorrhage [35].

It may be that very preterm babies can conserve sodium more avidly under conditions of stress: we have seen a 28 week gestation 960 g baby reduce its sodium excretion to only 1% of the filtered load under conditions of dehydration by three days after birth (unpublished observation). However, under conditions of very severe stress (e.g. prolonged profound acidosis) we have also seen preterm and mature babies maintain normal water balance, but lose huge amounts of sodium for between one and two days in an apparently uncontrolled way and become seriously hyponatraemic (unpublished observation).

Bicarbonate

The plasma bicarbonate concentrations in preterm babies are lower than in older children [38]. However, like fetal lambs [39], this appears to be due to the bicarbonate threshold being set lower [40,41] and not to an inability to reabsorb the filtered load. Babies of less than 1000 g reabsorb virtually all their filtered bicarbonate when the blood pH falls to 7.22 [42]. Presumably other factors such as a limited excretion of buffers and ammonia [40] must be responsible for the metabolic acidosis frequently described in these babies [43].

Water

Since the reabsorption of sodium and water by the proximal tubules is isotonic, a greater proportion of filtered water is also delivered distally in preterm babies compared to older subjects. To maintain fluid balance a much higher fraction of this water is then excreted as urine (see above). Healthy preterm babies have been shown to be able to adjust their water excretion appropriately from the second day of life when their daily intakes were varied between 95 and 200 ml/kg [6]. They achieved this by altering the Fe_{H_2O} from a mean of 7.4% to 13.1% of the filtered volume, and did so without causing any alteration to the amount of sodium lost in the urine. The widely held view that babies are unable to sustain a high urine flow without an increased loss of sodium [44–46] was suggested by a study [18] in which the design [6] and measurement techniques [17] have been questioned.

Neonates can achieve a maximum urine osmolality of about 500–600 mosmol/kg, compared to two or three times this in older subjects, a difference due in part to their lower urea concentrations and in part to their shorter loops of Henle. Fetal animals [47] and preterm babies are sensitive to antidiuretic hormone (arginine vasopressin, AVP) and can achieve these maximum osmolalities from birth. Some studies appear to contradict this by recording very high levels of AVP in babies whose urine is not maximally dilute, but this can be explained by the fact that in addition to its role in water homeostasis, AVP is a potent vasoconstrictor which is released in very large amounts (even in fetuses) in the face of hypotension [48], hypoxia [49], or hypovolaemia [50] and contributes to maintenance of the blood pressure [51–54]. Under these circumstances its release is paralleled by the release of prostaglandins which modulate its effects on the renal tubules [55,56] and allow the continued production of dilute urine. The 'syndrome of inappropriate antidiuretic hormone secretion' cannot therefore be diagnosed on the basis of high AVP levels alone, and is probably less common than is widely held [57–61]. So far the role of AVP in water homeostasis has not been properly defined by sequential studies in unstressed preterm babies.

Preterm babies are able to achieve similar minimal urine osmolalities to adults, with values of 50 mosmol/kg or less [6,62]. Using these values and the measured renal solute loads of about 10–15 mosmol/kg in healthy preterm infants [62], it is possible to estimate the approximate minimum and maximum urine flow rates that these infants can achieve and still remain in solute and water balance. Thus, a typical 1000 g baby who can produce urine with an osmolality of 600 would need to pass at least 22 ml urine in order to excrete 13 mmol solute daily. This compares closely to the 1 ml/kg/h widely used as a clinical indication of renal failure.

On the other hand, the largest daily volume of urine he could pass with a minimum osmolality of 50 and without passing more than 13 mosmol of solute would be 260 ml. This volume is probably greater than the amount available from glomerular filtration in many preterm babies, so that diluting ability is unlikely to limit water excretion. For example, a typical 26 week gestation baby weighing 700 g would have a GFR of 0.8 ml/kg/min [15], so that with 20% of the filtrate delivered distally, the maximum available for excretion would be 230 ml/kg daily.

Clinical implications of water handling

Attempts to produce clinical guidelines to predict the precise fluid requirements for any particular baby are complicated by not knowing the exact renal solute load for that individual, and by the number of factors that can influence non-renal water losses [63]. These include gestation and postnatal age, ambient humidity and the use of radiant heaters and phototherapy lamps, as well as pathology such as diarrhoea and some skin disorders. Rather than adhere to such guidelines, it would seem more appropriate to use them as a starting point, and then to adjust the fluid intake according to the urine osmolality achieved. A check that this lay between 70 and 400 mosmol/kg would confirm that the kidneys were working within their homeostatic range without stressing either their diluting or concentrating capacities. Although urine specific gravity is easy to measure and will generally parallel the osmolality, the presence of proteinuria would significantly alter this relationship and render the specific gravity measurement unreliable.

Because mature babies ingest relatively small volumes of milk initially, and preterm babies are usually intolerant of full volume feeds soon after birth, it has been traditional to increase fluid volumes slowly, even when much or all of the volume is administered parenterally. Since healthy preterm babies have been shown to be capable of excreting large volumes of water from the third day [6] there seems to be no logic behind this gradualistic approach, and we have practised parenteral supplementation to provide a total volume of 200 ml/kg from day 3 for many years without problem.

It seems reasonable, however, to slightly restrict water on the first two days while the babies undergo their physiological diuresis [64]. A high fluid intake may make heart failure due to a patent ductus arteriosus clinically apparent, but fears that liberal intakes might thereby cause an increase in morbidity or mortality [65] or of necrotizing enterocolitis [66] have not been substantiated [64].

Respiratory distress and renal function

It is widely assumed that babies with respiratory distress syndrome (RDS) or requiring ventilation have an impaired GFR, but evidence for this is far from definite. While it is not surprising that babies who are extremely ill and dying of respiratory distress studied before [67] or since the advent of artificial ventilation [68] are likely to have a reduced GFR, there is no evidence that this is true for those infants whose clinical and biochemical status has been stabilized by therapy [69]. Furthermore, reports that continuous positive airway pressure causes a fall in GFR [70] or that intermittent positive pressure ventilation alters intrarenal blood flow [71] should be considered with caution. These observations were made in newborn animals with normal lungs, capable of transmitting inflation pressures to the rest of the intrathoracic contents and thereby altering factors such as venous return; the situation is probably very different in the baby with RDS and an almost non-compliant lung.

It is also held [72] that preterm infants with respiratory distress may develop a diuresis from about the second day which leads to an improvement in the alveolar oxygen gradient and heralds recovery [73,74]. However, there is no evidence that the diuresis has a causal relationship to the improvement in respiratory symptoms as a diuresis also occurs at a similar time in healthy preterm infants [6,64]. Attempts have been made to improve RDS by inducing a diuresis with frusemide. In one study there was no clinical improvement, but an increased incidence of patent ductus arteriosus was noted, probably due to the stimulation of prostaglandin E synthesis by frusemide [75]. Another group demonstrated that frusemide increased pulmonary compliance but without causing a diuresis, and have postulated a direct pulmonary effect [76]. A detailed review of the role of frusemide in respiratory distress has suggested that it is negligible [77].

Indomethacin and renal function

Indomethacin is a prostaglandin synthetase inhibitor which is commonly used to facilitate the closure of a symptomatic patent ductus arteriosus. In older subjects it is known to reduce sodium excretion and urine flow by enhancing tubular reabsorption, but in addition to this there have been anxieties that it may lower GFR in preterm infants. This difference may reflect the dependence of these subjects on renal prostaglandins to maintain an adequate renal blood flow in the face of high RAAS acivity; a parallel can be seen in the study of dogs where indomethacin was shown to induce a fall in GFR only when the RAAS activity was increased by sodium depletion [78].

Although a temporary reduction of sodium and water excretion is described in all reports of babies given indomethacin for duct closure, a fall in GFR is not always seen [79]. When it is reported, the fall averages about 30% and lasts less than a day [80,81] even when the indomethacin is continued for a week [82]. There do not appear to be any long-term renal sequelae [83]. The simultaneous administration of 1 mg/kg of frusemide has been shown to eliminate the renal side effects of 0.3 mg indomethacin without reducing its efficacy in duct closure [84]. Differences in the effects of indomethacin on GFR between other studies could be due to whether or not frusemide was administered during the previous days [85].

Management of acute renal failure

The majority of babies who weigh less than 1000 g and have renal failure will not have a primary kidney disease but will have developed pre-renal failure or progressed to established renal failure secondary to factors such as hypotension, hypoxia, acidosis and cardiac failure. Degrees of renal failure are common in very small infants because all those that die slowly on ventilators will develop measurable impairment.

It is, nevertheless, important to exclude congenital abnormalities of the kidneys such as agenesis, dysplasia and infantile-type polycystic disease, and to diagnose renal vein thrombosis or treatable obstructive lesions such as posterior urethral valves. These can all be identified using ultrasound; the intravenous urogram produces poor images in normal preterm babies and has no role in those with renal impairment. As in older patients, the best indicator to distinguish pre-renal from established renal failure is the fractional excretion of sodium (Fe_{Na}). This is readily calculated from the sodium and creatinine concentrations of plasma (P) and a spot urine (U) sample:

$$Fe_{Na} = (U/P) \text{ sodium} \times (P/U) \text{ creatinine} \times 100\%$$

If the tubules are still functioning and the infant is in oliguric pre-renal failure then the Fe_{Na} will certainly be less than 2.5% [86] or 3% [87] and, in our experience, even as low as 1%. Once tubular necrosis has occurred the Fe_{Na} is usually considerably higher, and often about 10% [86,87].

The management of a baby with pre-renal failure is to ensure that the vascular compartment is adequately filled, usually by the administration of up to 20 ml/kg saline or plasma, and then to administer frusemide. The latter not only increases the flow of tubular fluid, but also stimulates prostaglandin release and reduces renal metabolic requirements by inhibiting the sodium pump. Doses of 1 mg/kg [88] or up to 3 mg/kg [87] have been recommended. Because frusemide exerts its effects on the loop of Henle only after glomerular filtration, high plasma levels are necessary when the GFR is low, and we use 5 mg/kg. However, because the half life of frusemide clearance is almost 24 h in healthy preterm infants that are not in renal failure [85], clearance will almost certainly be several days in babies remaining in renal failure, and there is no rationale for repeating the dose; this would only lead to accumulation. If this therapy does not produce a diuresis then the baby needs to be managed like an infant in established renal failure. Although dopamine has been reported to enhance the action of frusemide in this situation [88], the diuresis produced may equally have been due to the simultaneous administration of a second 1 mg/kg dose of frusemide. Others have concluded that neither mannitol nor dopamine are of benefit [89].

The management of the VLBW infant who is in established renal failure or has failed to respond to volume repletion and frusemide is difficult. All efforts should be continued to try to reverse the conditions which caused the renal failure (e.g. treatment of heart failure and RDS) and the prognosis for the baby should be carefully assessed. To help determine the prognosis in an anuric baby, radionuclide scans such as ^{99}Tc-DTPA may be used to assess whether the kidneys are still perfused, but a false negative has been reported [90]. If it is felt that the baby would be likely to survive but for its renal failure then dialysis could be considered; if not, then conservative management consists of a 10% glucose intravenous infusion to replace fluid losses and the cautious use of sodium bicarbonate to correct the inevitable acidosis.

Peritoneal dialysis

Babies weighing less than 1000 g who need dialysis have a very poor prognosis. At the moment peritoneal dialysis is the only practical technique, and haemodialysis and continuous arteriovenous ultrafiltration cannot be considered. The standard peritoneal dialysis catheters are unsuitable for such small babies; they are too rigid and the side holes extend too far. We use very soft chest drain tubes with side holes inserted in the left upper quadrant so that they can curl up in the peritoneal space. Hourly cycles of up to 35 ml/kg are used initially provided they do not cause respiratory difficulty, and the cycle times are lengthened as dictated by the biochemical response. Because we have been anxious whether such unwell small infants would adequately metabolize the lactate present in commercially available dialysis fluids, we have made up bicarbonate-containing fluids from intravenous fluid preparations as shown in Table 18.1. The fluids are usually mixed in the administration burette to produce a bicarbonate concentration of 40 mmol/l, and the contribution of solutions **B** and C can be varied to alter the glucose concentration and adjust ultrafiltration. Because these fluids cannot have calcium added, intravenous calcium supplements are used starting at 1 mmol/kg daily and then adjusted according to the plasma concentrations. In some cases very high plasma glucose concentrations have been noted in dialysed babies, presumably because they have received their normal carbohydrate intake and have absorbed glucose from the dialysis fluid. As the plasma glucose rises the plasma:dialysis fluid osmotic gradient falls and ultrafiltration slows or ceases, so

Table 18.1 Bicarbonate-based peritoneal dialysis solutions made up from intravenous fluids

Solution	*Procedure*	*Final concentrations*		
		Sodium (mmol/l)	*Bicarbonate* (mmol/l)	*Glucose* (%)
A	500 ml 5% Dextrose Remove 60 ml Add 60 ml 8.4% $NaHCO_3$	120	120	4.4
B	500 ml Normal saline	150	0	0
C	500 ml Normal saline Remove 50 ml Add 50 ml 50% glucose Add 1.5 ml 30% (strong) saline	150	0	5.0
Example mixtures				
$\frac{1}{3}A+\frac{2}{3}B$		140	40	1.47
$\frac{1}{3}A+\frac{1}{2}B+\frac{1}{6}C$		140	40	2.30
$\frac{1}{3}A+\frac{1}{3}B+\frac{1}{3}C$		140	40	3.13
$\frac{1}{3}A+\frac{2}{3}C$		140	40	4.80

control must be maintained by the use of a very low dose insulin infusion, beginning with 0.02 units/kg/h. Heparin (1 unit/ml) may be added to the dialysis fluid initially if it is blood-stained to prevent clots forming in the catheter holes. If an aminoglycoside is indicated this may be added to the dialysis fluid at the appropriate concentration to be achieved in the plasma (10 mg/l for gentamicin) and one loading dose given parenterally if it had not previously been started. The dose of systemically administered penicillins should be halved during dialysis, and other renally excreted drugs individually adjusted; digoxin should be prescribed according to plasma concentrations.

Peritonitis is a major hazard of peritoneal dialysis at all ages. The risks can be minimized by using a complete neonatal administration set rather than making one up from separate components, and by obsessional nursing care. We microscope and culture the effluent fluid daily and add antibiotics to the dialysis fluid at the earliest suspicion of an infection.

Conclusion

Much of our understanding of the renal function of babies weighing less than 1000 g is extrapolated from studies involving heavier subjects; great care is necessary to avoid misinterpretation. The kidneys of such small infants have very different physiological demands put upon them from those of larger babies, children and adults. In order to maintain salt and water balance and allow growth to occur they have to excrete very large volumes of water indeed, and to conserve sodium avidly.

Anatomically the glomeruli of preterm babies are much more highly developed than the tubules, but physiologically the difference is not so great. The absolute GFR is very low and increases logarithmically with increasing conceptional age. Thus, if body weight increases 'normally' the GFR per unit body size gradually rises with greater maturity, but if growth arrest occurs (such as after preterm delivery) the GFR per unit body size rises rapidly and gives the impression of sudden renal maturation. The tubules, however, do undergo a rapid maturation in function after birth under the influence of high circulating aldosterone levels, and can conserve sodium much more avidly within two weeks of delivery.

Well preterm babies given a supplemented sodium intake can maintain salt and water balance over a wide range of water intakes. There is no need to increase fluids gradually after the first two days, nor to use complex formulae to adjust the water intake if the urine osmolality is maintained well within physiological limits, nor to further increase the sodium intake if the water intake is increased. Data for babies with respiratory distress are not so clear, and a slight reduction in fluid intake might be helpful. Although the use of indomethacin can be shown to alter urine flow and GFR, the effects are transient and probably have little clinical importance.

Acute renal failure in babies weighing less than 1000 g carries a poor prognosis and is usually the result of multisystem disease. The best indicator of pre-renal failure is a low fractional excretion of sodium which is readily calculated from a sample of plasma and a random urine. The treatment of pre-renal failure is to ensure an adequate circulating volume and to administer one substantial dose of frusemide, and is frequently successful. The treatment of established renal failure is difficult. Peritoneal dialysis is possible, although technically demanding, and is justified particularly when the cause of the renal failure can be identified and reversed.

References

1. Boyd, E. (1935) *The Growth of the Surface Area of the Human Body*, University of Minnesota Press, Minneapolis
2. Haycock, G. B., Schwartz, G. J. and Wisotsky, D. H. (1978) Geometric method for measuring body surface area: a height-weight formula validated in infants, children, and adults. *J. Pediatr.*, **93**, 62–66
3. Coulthard, M. G. and Hey, E. N. (1984) Weight as the best standard for glomerular filtration in the newborn. *Arch. Dis. Child.*, **59**, 373–375
4. Hey E. N. (1969) The relation between environmental temperature and oxygen consumption in the new-born baby. *J. Physiol.*, **200**, 589–603
5. McCance, R. A. and Widdowson, E. M. (1952) The correct physiological basis on which to compare infant and adult renal function. *Lancet*, **ii**, 860–862
6. Coulthard, M. G. and Hey, E. N. (1985) Effect of varying water intake on renal function in healthy preterm babies. *Arch. Dis. Child.*, **60**, 614–620
7. Stonestreet, B. S., Rubin, L., Pollak, A., Cowett, R. M. and Oh, W. (1980) Renal functions of low birth weight infants with hyperglycaemia and glucosuria produced by glucose infusions. *Pediatrics*, **66**, 561–567
8. Widdowson, E. M. (1968) Growth and composition of the fetus and newborn. In *Biology of Gestation*, Vol. 2 (ed. N. S. Assali), Academic Press, New York and London, pp. 1–49
9. MacDonald, M. S. and Emery, J. L. (1959) The late intrauterine and postnatal development of human renal glomeruli. *J. Anat.*, **93**, 331
10. Aschinberg, L. G., Goldsmith, D. I., Olbing, H., Spitzer, A., Edelmann, C. M. Jr and Blaufox, M. D. (1975) Neonatal changes in renal blood flow distribution in puppies. *Am. J. Physiol.*, **228**, 1453
11. Fetterman, G. F., Shuplock, N. A., Philipp, F. G. and Gregg, H. S. (1965) The growth and maturation of human glomeruli and proximal convolutions from term to adulthood. Studies by microdissection. *Pediatrics*, **35**, 601
12. Al-Dahhan, J., Haycock, G. B., Chantler, C. and Stimmler, L. (1983) Sodium homeostasis in term and preterm neonates: 1. Renal aspects. *Arch. Dis. Child.*, **58**, 335–345
13. Arant, B. S. Jr (1978) Developmental patterns of renal function maturation compared in the human neonate. *J. Pediatr.*, **92**, 705–712
14. Fawer, C. L., Torrado, A. and Guignard, J. P. (1979) Maturation of renal function in full-term and premature neonates. *Helv. Paediatr. Acta*, **34**, 11–21
15. Coulthard, M. G. (1985) Maturation of glomerular filtration in preterm and mature babies. *Early Hum. Dev.*, **11**, 281–292
16. Arant, B. S. Jr (1984) Estimating glomerular filtration rate in infants. *J. Pediatr.*, **104**, 890–893
17. Coulthard, M. G. (1983) Comparison of methods of measuring renal function in preterm babies using inulin. *J. Pediatr.*, **102**, 923–930
18. Leake, R. D., Zakauddin, S., Trygstad, C. W., Fu, P. and Oh, W. (1976) The effects of large volume intravenous fluid infusion on neonatal renal function. *J. Pediatr.*, **89**, 968–972
19. Coulthard, M. G., Hey, E. N. and Ruddock, V. (1985) Creatinine and urea clearances compared to inulin clearance in preterm and mature babies. *Early Hum. Dev.*, **11**, 11–19
20. Stonestreet, B. S. and Oh, W. (1978) Plasma creatinine levels in low-birth-weight infants during the first three months of life. *Pediatrics*, **61**, 788–789
21. Counahan, R., Chantler, C., Ghazali, S., Kirkwood, B., Rose, F. and Barratt, T. M. (1976) Estimation of glomerular filtration rate from plasma creatinine concentration in children. *Arch. Dis. Child.*, **51**, 875–878
22. Davies, J. G., Taylor, C. M., White, R. H. R. and Marshall, T. (1982) Clinical limitations of the estimation of glomerular filtration rate from height/plasma creatinine ratio: a comparison with simultaneous ^{51}Cr-edetic acid slope clearance. *Arch. Dis. Child.*, **57**, 607–610
23. Morris, M. C., Allanby, C. W., Toseland, P., Haycock, G. B. and Chantler, C. (1982) Evaluation of height/plasma creatinine formula in the measurement of glomerular filtration rate. *Arch. Dis. Child.*, **57**, 611–615
24. Schwartz, G. J., Haycock, G. B., Edelmann, C. M. Jr and Spitzer, A. (1976) A simple estimate of glomerular filtration rate in children derived from body length and plasma creatinine. *Pediatrics*, **58**, 259–263

25. Zacchello, G., Bondio, M., Saia, O. S., Largaiolli, G., Vedaldi, R. and Rubaltelli, F. F. (1982) Simple estimate of creatinine clearance from plasma creatinine in neonates. *Arch. Dis. Child.*, **57**, 297–300
26. Sutphen, J. L. (1982) Anthropometric determinants of creatinine excretion in preterm infants. *Pediatrics*, **69**, 719–723
27. Horster, M. and Valtin, H. (1971) Postnatal development of renal function: micropuncture and clearance studies in the dog. *J. Clin. Invest.*, **50**, 799
28. Spitzer, A. and Brandis, M. (1974) Functional and morphologic maturation of the superficial nephrons. Relationship to total kidney function. *J. Clin. Invest.*, **53**, 279
29. Spitzer, A. (1982) The role of the kidney in sodium homeostasis during maturation. *Kidney Int.*, **21**, 539–545
30. Aperia, A. and Larsson, L. (1979) Correlation between fluid reabsorption and proximal tubule ultrastructure during development of the rat kidney. *Acta Physiol. Scand.*, **105**, 11–22
31. Kotchen, T. A., Strickland, A. L., Rice, T. W. and Walters, D. R. (1972) A study of the renin-angiotensin system in the newborn infant. *J. Pediatr.*, **80**, 938
32. Aperia, A., Larsson, L. and Zetterstrom, R. (1981) Hormonal induction of Na-K-ATPase in developing proximal tubular cells. *Am. J. Physiol.*, **241**, F356–360
33. Al-Dahhan, J., Haycock, G. B., Chantler, C. and Stimmler, L. (1983) Sodium homeostasis in term and preterm neonates. Part I. Renal aspects. *Arch. Dis. Child*, **58**, 335–342
34. Drukker, A., Goldsmith, D. I., Spitzer, A., Edelmann, C. M. Jr and Blaufox, M. D. (1980) The renin angiotensin system in newborn dogs: developmental patterns and response to acute saline loading. *Pediatr. Res.*, **14**, 304
35. Al-Dahhan, J., Haycock, G. B., Nichol, B., Chantler, C. and Stimmler, L. (1984) Sodium homeostasis in term and preterm neonates. Part III. Effect of salt supplementation. *Arch. Dis. Child.*, **59**, 945–950
36. Harkavy, K. L., Scanlon, J. W. and Jose, P. (1979) The effects of theophylline on renal function in the premature newborn. *Biol. Neonate*, **35**, 126–130
37. Schanler, R. J. and Oh, W. (1980) Composition of breast milk obtained from mothers of premature infants as compared to breast milk obtained from donors. *J. Pediatr.*, **96**, 676–681
38. Sulyok, E., Heim, T., Soltesz, G. and Jaszai, V. (1972) The influence of maturity on renal control of acidosis in newborn infants. *Biol. Neonate*, **21**, 418–435
39. Robillard, J. E., Sessious, C., Burmeister, L. and Smith, F. G. Jr (1977) Influence of fetal extracellular volume contraction on renal reabsorption of bicarbonate in fetal lambs. *Pediatr. Res.*, **11**, 649–655
40. Svenningsen, N. W. (1974) Renal acid-base titration studies in infants with and without metabolic acidosis in the postneonatal period. *Pediatr. Res.*, **8**, 659–672
41. Schwartz, G. J., Haycock, G. B., Edelmann, C. M. Jr and Spitzer, A. (1979) Late metabolic acidosis: a reassessment of the definition. *J. Pediatr.*, **95**, 102–107
42. Zilleruelo, G., Sultan, S., Bancalari, E., Steele, B. and Strauss J. (1986) Renal bicarbonate handling in low-birth-weight infants during metabolic acidosis. *Biol. Neonate.*, **49**, 132–139
43. Kerpel-Fronius, E., Heim, T. and Sulyok, E. (1970) The development of renal acidifying processes and their relation to acidosis in low birth weight infants. *Biol. Neonate*, **15**, 156–168
44. Anon. (1982) Fluid therapy in the neonate – concepts in transition. *J. Pediatr.*, **101**, 387–389
45. Leake, R. D. (1977) Perinatal nephrobiology: a developmental perspective. *Clin. Perinatol.*, **4**, 321–349
46. Engle, W. D. (1986) Evaluation of renal function and acute renal failure in the neonate. *Pediatr. Clin. North Am.*, **33**, 129–151
47. Alexander, D. P., Bashore, R. A., Britton, H. G. and Forsling, M. L. (1976) Antidiuretic hormone and oxytocin release and antidiuretic hormone turnover in the fetus, lamb and ewe. *Biol. Neonate*, **30**, 80–87
48. Daniel, S. S., Stark, R. I., Zubrow, A. B., Tropper, P. J. and James, L. S. (1985) Vasopressin and plasma renin activity following disturbances in blood pressure, osmolality and/or blood volume in the fetus. In *The Physiological Development of the Fetus and Newborn* (eds C. T. Jones and P. W. Natrianidez), Academic Press, London, pp. 331–334
49. Alexander, D. P., Forsling, M. L., Martin, M. J. *et al.* (1972) The effect of maternal hypoxia on fetal pituitary hormone release in the sheep. *Biol. Neonate*, **21**, 219–228
50. Alexander, D. P., Britton, H. G., Forsling, M. L., Nixon, D. A. and Ratcliffe, J. G. (1974) Pituitary and plasma concentrations of adrenocorticotrophin, growth hormone, vasopressin and oxytocin in

fetal and maternal sheep during the latter half of gestation and the response to haemorrhage. *Biol. Neonate*, **24**, 206–219
51. Aisenbrey, G. A., Handelman, W. A., Arnold, P., Manning, M. and Schrier, R. W. (1981) Vascular effects of arginine vasopressin during fluid deprivation in the rat. *J. Clin. Invest.*, **67**, 961–968
52. Gardiner, S. M. and Bennett, T. (1985) Interactions between neural mechanisms, the renin-angiotensin system and vasopressin in the maintenance of blood pressure during water deprivation: studies in Long Evans and Brattleboro rats. *Clin. Sci.*, **68**, 647–657
53. Cowley, A. W. Jr, Switzer, S. J. and Guinn, M. M. (1980) Evidence and quantification of the vasopressin arterial pressure control system in the dog. *Circ. Res.*, **46**, 58–67
54. Gardiner, S. M. and Bennett, T. (1983) Effects of haemorrhage in rats lacking vasopressin (Brattleboro strain): influence of naloxone. *Clin. Sci.*, **65**, 19–25
55. Joppich, R., Haberle, D. A. and Webber, P. C. (1981) Studies on the immaturity of the ADH-dependent cAMP system in conscious newborn piglets – possible impairing effects of renal prostaglandins. *Pediatr. Res.*, **15**, 278–281
56. Ertl, T., Sulyok, E., Nemeth, M., Tenyi, I., Csaba, I. F. and Varga, F. (1982) The effect of sodium chloride supplementation on the postnatal development of plasma prostaglandin E and $F_{2\alpha}$ values in premature infants. *J. Pediatr.*, **101**, 761–763
57. Wiriyathian S., Rosenfeld, C. R., Arant, B. S. Jr, Porter, J. C., Faucher, D. J. and Engle, W. D. (1986) Urinary arginine vasopressin; pattern of excretion in the neonatal period. *Pediatr. Res.*, **20**, 103–108
58. Rees, L., Brook, C. G. D., Shaw, J. C. L. and Forsling, M. L. (1984) Hyponatraemia in the first week of life in preterm infants. Part I. Arginine vasopressin secretion. *Arch. Dis. Child.*, **59**, 414–422
59. Rees, L., Shaw, J. C. L., Brook, C. G. D. and Forsling, M. L. (1984) Hyponatraemia in the first week of life in preterm infants. Part II. Sodium and water secretion. *Arch. Dis. Child.*, **59**, 423–429
60. McIntosh, N. and Smith, A. (1985) Serial measurement of plasma arginine vasopressin in the newborn. *Arch. Dis Child.*, **60**, 1031–1035
61. Stern, P., LaRochelle, F. T. Jr and Little, G. A. (1981) Vasopressin and pneumothorax in the neonate. *Pediatrics*, **68**, 499–503
62. Ekhard, E., Ziegler, M. D. and Ryu, J. E. (1976) Renal solute load and diet in growing premature infants. *J. Pediatr.*, **89**, 609–611
63. Thompson, M. H., Stothers, J. K. and McLellan, N. J. (1984) Weight and water loss in the neonate in natural and forced convection. *Arch. Dis. Child.*, **59**, 951–956
64. Lorenz, J. M., Kleinman, L. I., Kotagal, U. R. and Reller, M. D. (1982) Water balance in very-low-birth-weight infants: relationship to water and sodium intake and effect on outcome. *J. Pediatr.*, **101**, 423–432
65. Bell, E. F., Warburton, D., Stonestreet, B. S. and Oh, W. (1980) Effect of fluid administration on the development of symptomatic patent ductus arteriosus and congestive heart failure in premature infants. *N. Engl. J. Med.*, **302**, 598–604
66. Bell, E. F., Warburton, D., Stonestreet, B. S. and Oh, W. (1979) High volume fluid intake predisposes premature infants to necrotising enterocolitis. *Lancet*, **ii**, 90
67. Cort, R. L. (1962) Renal function in the respiratory distress syndrome. *Acta Paediatr.*, **51**, 313–323
68. Tulassay, T., Ritvay, J., Bors, Z. and Buky, B. (1979) Alterations in creatinine clearance during respiratory distress syndrome. *Biol. Neonate*, **35**, 258–263
69. Siegel, S. R., Fisher, D. A. and Oh, W. (1973) Renal function and serum aldosterone levels in infants with respiratory distress syndrome. *J. Pediatr.*, **83**, 854–858
70. Fewell, J. E. and Norton, J. B. (1980) Continuous positive airway pressure impairs renal function in newborn goats. *Pediatr. Res.*, **14**, 1132–1134
71. Moore, E. S., Galvez, M. B., Paton, J. B., Fisher, D. E. and Behrman, R. E. (1974) Effects of positive pressure ventilation on intrarenal blood flow in infant primates. *Pediatr. Res.*, **8**, 792–796
72. Guignard, J-P and John, E. G. (1986) Renal function in the tiny, premature infant. *Clin. Perinatol.*, **13**, 377–401
73. Heaf, D. P., Belik, J., Spitzer, A. R., Gewitz, M. H. and Fox, W. W. (1982) Changes in pulmonary function during the diuretic phase of respiratory distress syndrome. *J. Pediatr.*, **101**, 103–107
74. Langman, C. B., Engle, W. D., Baumgart, S., Fox, W. W. and Polin, R. A. (1981) The diuretic phase of respiratory distress syndrome and its relationship to oxygenation. *J. Pediatr.*, **98**, 462–466
75. Green, T. P., Thompson, T. R., Johnson, D. E. and Lock, J. E. (1983) Furosemide promotes patent

ductus arteriosus in premature infants with the respiratory-distress syndrome. *N. Engl. J. Med.*, **308**, 743–748

76. Najak, Z. D., Harris, E. M., Lazzara, A. Jr and Pruitt, A. W. (1983) Pulmonary effects of furosemide in preterm infants with lung disease. *J. Pediatr.*, **102**, 758–763
77. Aranda, J. V., Chemtob, S., Laudignon, N. and Sasyniuk, B. I. (1986) Furosemide and vitamin E: two problem drugs in neonatology. *Pediatr. Clin. North Am.*, **33**, 583–599
78. Oliver, J. A., Pinto, J., Sciacca, R. R. and Cannon, P. J. (1980) Increased renal secretion of norepinephrine and prostaglandin E_2 during sodium depletion in the dog. *J. Clin. Invest.*, **66**, 748–756
79. Betkerur, M. V., Yeh, T. F., Miller, K., Glasser, R. J. and Pildes, R. S. (1981) Indomethacin and its effect on renal function and urinary kallikrein excretion in premature infants with patent ductus arteriosus. *Pediatrics*, **68**, 99–102
80. Catterton, Z., Sellers, B. and Gray, B. (1980) Inulin clearance in the premature infant receiving indomethacin. *J. Pediatr.*, **96**, 737–739
81. Cifuentes, R. F., Olley, P. M., Balfe, J. W., Radde, I. C. and Soldin, S. J. (1979) Indomethacin and renal function in premature infants with persistent patent ductus arteriosus. *J. Pediatr.*, **95**, 583–587
82. Seyberth, H. W., Rascher, W., Hackenthal, R. and Willie, L. (1983) Effect of prolonged indomethacin therapy on renal function and selected vasoactive hormones in very-low-birth-weight infants with symptomatic patent ductus arteriosus. *J. Pediatr.*, **103**, 979–984
83. Peckham, G. J., Miettinen, O. S., Ellison, R. C. *et al.* (1984) Clinical course to 1 year of age in premature infants with patent ductus arteriosus: results of a multicentre randomized trial of indomethacin. *J. Pediatr.*, **105**, 285–291
84. Yeh, T. F., Wilks, A., Singh, J., Bethkerur, M., Lilien, L. and Pildes, R. S. (1982) Furosemide prevents the renal side effects of indomethacin therapy in premature infants with patent ductus arteriosus. *J. Pediatr.*, **101**, 433–437
85. Peterson, R. G., Simmons, M. A., Rumack, B. H., Levine, R. L. and Brooks, J. G. (1980) Pharmacology of furosemide in the premature newborn infant. *J. Pediatr.*, **97**, 139–143
86. Mathew, O. P., Jones, A. S., James, E., Bland, H. and Groshong, T. (1980) Neonatal renal failure: usefulness of diagnostic indices. *Pediatrics*, **65**, 57–60
87. Norman, M. E. and Asadi, F. K. (1979) A prospective study of acute renal failure in the newborn infant. *Pediatrics*, **63**, 475–479
88. Tulassay, T. and Seri, I. (1986) Acute oliguria in preterm infants with hyaline membrane disease: interaction of dopamine and furosemide. *Acta Paediatr. Scand.*, **75**, 420–424
89. Gouyon, J-B. and Guignard, J-P (1986) Drugs and acute renal insufficiency in the neonate. *Biol. Neonate*, **50**, 177–181
90. Chevalier, R. L., Campbell, F. and Brenbridge, A. N. A. G. (1984) Prognostic factors in neonatal acute renal failure. *Pediatrics*, **74**, 265–272

Chapter 19

Neurological abnormalities

Richard W. I. Cooke, Lilly M. S. Dubowitz, Janet Eyre, Andrew Whitelaw

I. AETIOLOGY

Richard W. I. Cooke

Introduction

The human brain is exceptionally vulnerable to a variety of insults in the perinatal period which may have lifelong consequences in survivors. The ELBW infant is more vulnerable than most as shown by the highest incidence of neurological sequelae of any weight group. Although the disease processes involving the ELBW brain are similar to those in larger infants, the frequency of systemic disturbances from illnesses such as hyaline membrane disease and birth asphyxia is higher, and the size and maturity of the brain very different even from that of a larger preterm infant.

Most ELBW infants will be of 28 weeks gestation or less, although a few will be up to 34 weeks or more. The maturity determines which parts of the brain have developed and which are yet to form, the distribution and responsiveness of the cerebral circulation, the state of calcification and resilience of the skull and capillary function, especially permeability. Irrespective of maturity, the relative size of the brain to body weight is a major problem for the ELBW infant. The brain will be 16–20% of the body weight [1], and will require a very large proportion of the total cardiac output for its functioning. While the infant is well this supply will be achieved, but in the face of any major illness resulting in a fall in cardiac output, there is no spare capacity to allow blood to be directed from other tissues, and the cerebral blood flow must fall too, irrespective of the ability or otherwise of the cerebral vasculature to autoregulate. Such problems account for the frequency with which ischaemic and haemorrhagic injury is seen in the ELBW brain.

Development of the cerebral circulation

In the early embryo the arterial supply to the developing brain consists of two systems, one ventriculopetal and the other ventriculofugal [2]. Both systems originate on the surface of the brain, but the latter on reaching the periventricular area recurves to flow outwards. The arterial supply does not extensively anastomose and thus acts as an end arterial system with a series of vulnerable boundary zones between ventriculopetal arteries in the cortex, and between the ventriculopetal and ventriculofugal arteries in the periventricular area. The arterial system supplying the brain is established at least externally by about seven weeks of embryonic life, although there is extensive branching later as the cerebrum greatly increases in size during fetal life [3]. Penetration of the cerebrum and internal vascularization proceeds from seven weeks with the development of a superficial capillary network and later deep branches to the subependymal rete at 12 weeks of age [4]. For a period between the sixth and seventh months of gestation the basal branches of the anterior and middle cerebral arteries which supply the basal ganglia are relatively larger reflecting their phylogenetic importance [5].

The subependymal layer or germinal matrix is the source of 80% of intraventricular haemorrhages, and consists of a mass of glioblastic cells supplied by a primitive vascular rete. The germinal matrix thins out after 30 weeks and becomes vestigial in the more mature brain. The arterial supply is by Heubner's artery, branches of the lateral striate arteries and the anterior choroidal artery. The capillary network in the germinal matrix supplies the superficial and deep parts leaving the centre relatively avascular [6]. The developing cortex is supplied at 24 weeks by spiral perforating medullary arteries. By 28 weeks cell migration to the cortex has largely ceased and dendritic proliferation begins [7]. The short cortical arteries increase in number and the longer perforating arteries increase in calibre to meet the increasing metabolic demands of the expanding cerebrum. By 32 weeks differentiation of white matter from the cortex begins.

The cerebral venous system develops from a number of venous plexuses which extensively communicate and are remodelled greatly during fetal development. Eventually the thin walled dural sinuses and the deep or Galenic system remain. The cortex is drained by regularly branching veins which develop in parallel to the cortical arteries but are fewer in number. The white matter of the cerebral hemispheres is drained almost entirely by the thalamostriate or terminal veins, the septal veins, and the basal veins into the Galenic system. Although anastomoses do exist between the deep and superficial venous systems, obstruction of the deep venous system frequently leads to venous infarction of the white matter suggesting that in the immature brain these alternative pathways are unable to cope, as a much greater proportion of the brain is drained by the deep system than later in development [8].

The maturation of the capillary at an ultrastructural level is poorly documented. Animal studies are difficult to extrapolate to the human fetus and newborn. Human studies seem to indicate that a wide variety of stages of development of capillaries may be seen in the same embryo or fetus, and that the appearance of structures such as the basement membrane, important for the function of the 'blood-brain barrier', is more related to the age of the capillary than the age of the fetus, at least in the first half of gestation [9]. Another study suggests that the structure of the capillaries is mature at 22 weeks, although no functional information is available [10]

Capillary permeability in newborn rabbits as measured by fluorescein-labelled dextran of differing molecular weights was increased in preterm offspring, but more markedly so in rabbits at all gestational ages when exposed to hypoxia or an increase in venous pressure [11]. Grontoft showed in the human fetus that the blood-brain barrier was impermeable to Trypan blue dye in fetuses of 5–30 cm in length, but that hypoxia readily increased the permeability [12]. The resistance to hypoxia appeared to increase with the maturity of the fetus. Increased capillary permeability is usually considered in relation to hypoxia or venous pressure but a variety of other variables such as hypercarbia, acidosis, arterial hypertension and hyperosmolality of the plasma may equally be of importance. Various prostaglandins, in particular prostacyclin, increase capillary leakage. High circulating levels of prostacyclin have been demonstrated in preterm infants suffering from hyaline membrane disease, and especially those going on to show evidence of cerebral haemorrhage [13]. The source of these prostanoids is likely to be the lungs, and their release to be associated with mechanical ventilation [14]. There seems to be little evidence that the capillaries of the extremely preterm infant are functionally immature, but that perhaps they are more vulnerable to the frequent insults to which they are liable.

Causes of perinatal brain injury

Although it is generally agreed that the cerebral blood supply is critical for the support of cerebral function, the lack of reliable methods for measurement in the preterm infant makes much of our knowledge of the role of the cerebral circulation in the aetiology of perinatal brain injury speculative. Such attempts as have been made to measure cerebral blood flow in the preterm infant suggest that in health it is not dissimilar from older infants when related to brain weight. It is, however, more labile and may be severely reduced in sick infants [15,16]. Unstable flow has been shown to increase the likelihood of later haemorrhage and to be related to unstable systemic blood pressure, assumed in turn to be the result of the infant struggling against mechanical ventilation [17,18].

The cerebral circulation is likely to be affected by the birth process. Both a fall and a rise in cerebral blood flow after birth in the first two days of life have been reported by different investigators. Most recently, using volumetric Doppler techniques, the flow to the brain has been shown to be relatively stable following birth, but with the velocity in the cerebral arteries increasing over the first three days [19]. These findings, more marked in preterm subjects, imply that cerebral artery reactivity and thus autoregulatory control develop over this period. They also suggest that for this early period in preterm infants there may be a period of increased vulnerability of the cerebral circulation to exposure to surges in flow related to the unstable systemic circulation. This idea is supported by the known high incidence of haemorrhagic lesions in the periventricular region at this time.

Hypotension in ELBW infants has been shown to relate closely to periventricular haemorrhage when present in the first 48 h of life [20,21]. The cause of the hypotension is not certain, but likely to be related to poor cardiac output or to hypovolaemia. Hypovolaemia may be related to fluid losses from the vascular space due to capillary permeability, or to cord clamping at birth before lung expansion occurs. The perinatal circulation may also be affected by maternal factors such as antepartum haemorrhage. This has often been cited as preceding major parenchymal lesions, and has its effect through a reduction in placental perfusion leading to fetal ischaemia or hypovolaemia [22].

Major clinical factors such as birth asphyxia and hyaline membrane disease are clearly related to an increase in cerebral injury [23], and both these factors are commonest in infants below 1000 g. The influence of these factors is likely to be through their action in causing changes in capillary permeability, hypotension and circulatory instability.

Other physical factors which may be relevant include the properties of the skull in the infant under 1000 g. It is very soft and may allow considerable deformation to occur during delivery. In a few cases this may cause direct brain trauma from fracture and displacement of the occipital bone [24]. In larger infants venous infarction from prolonged brain compression in long labours was previously frequently described [25]. It is possible that such a process may at least contribute to cerebral ischaemia in ELBW infants. If this were so the mode of delivery would be relevant. In infants below 1500 g a number of reports suggest that caesarian section has a protective effect for brain lesions such as periventricular haemorrhage. No reports specifically refer to infants under 1000 g in this respect, and any advantage might be masked by small numbers and the high mortality relating to gestational age. The data relating to infants under 1500 g, however, is uncontrolled and when other factors have been taken into account using multivariate analysis, no advantage for any particular mode of delivery is seen [26].

Apart from direct trauma, malformations, infections, and the effects of toxins such as aminoglycosides and bilirubin, lesions of the very preterm brain may be considered under three main groupings:

(1) Germinal matrix and intraventricular haemorrhage.
(2) Periventricular leucomalacia.
(3) Parenchymal haemorrhage and infarction.

These categories are not mutually exclusive and are likely to coexist and to be related by the causative mechanisms already discussed.

Germinal layer and intraventricular haemorrhage

Although the reported incidence of periventricular haemorrhage varies greatly, it is probably about 60–70% in ELBW infants. There is a strong association in most studies with birth asphyxia and hyaline membrane disease as already mentioned, and with factors seen with these two conditions such as hypercapnia, acidosis and pneumothorax. The haemorrhage begins in the great majority of cases in the germinal matrix, although a small proportion originate in the choroid plexus. It appears to be capillary in origin, is often multifocal, and may be confined to the germinal layer or extend to rupture into and even fill the ventricular system [27]. It has been proposed that the anatomy of the germinal matrix makes it vulnerable in that it is a primitive vascular rete, an irregular network of thin and poorly supported vessels. There is a relatively avascular central area in the germinal matrix which could make it more liable to infarction, and the arterial supply in this region is a boundary zone [6]. In the beagle puppy the germinal layer is a low flow area [28], although in the human infant injection studies show that at least in the superficial and deep layers of the germinal matrix there are plentiful small blood vessels. The association of germinal layer haemorrhage with an extended capillary bleeding time in the first six hours of life suggests that a platelet/capillary function disorder may be of importance [29]. The prostaglandins, and in particular prostacyclin, has an important influence in this area and the high levels of prostacyclin metabolites reported prior to haemorrhage may be relevant [13]. On the other hand the evidence for a role of major coagulation defects in germinal matrix haemorrhage is lacking [29]. Early studies reporting such associations were probably observing coagulation disorders occurring as the result of major haemorrhage rather than being the cause of it.

Recently a number of controlled therapeutic interventions aimed at reducing the incidence of periventricular haemorrhage have shed some light on its aetiology. The use of infusions of 10 ml/kg fresh frozen plasma soon after birth was associated with a substantial reduction in the rate of haemorrhage [30]. Although the rationale of the therapy was the correction of coagulation disorders, no significant alteration in coagulation status was achieved. The authors suggested that a correction of hypovolaemia at an early stage may have been the mode of action instead. The demonstration that fluctuating systemic blood pressure and consequently blood flow velocity in the anterior cerebral arteries was associated with an increase in haemorrhage, led another group to use pancuronium during mechanical ventilation to abolish the fluctuations. A significant reduction in the incidence of haemorrhage occurred implying that the fluctuations were causal [18]. A number of drugs have been used prophylactically with variable success. Both vitamin E and ethamsylate have shown significant reduction in haemorrhage in controlled trials [31,32]. They probably both act in a similar fashion by altering capillary leakage, vitamin E through its antioxidant effect protecting against the damage from superoxides generated after periods of ischaemia, and ethamsylate through an effect on prostacyclin release.

Most haemorrhages occur soon after birth, although a few are seen at post-mortem examination in stillborn infants. Using ultrasound scanning as many as 30% of haemorrhages are seen at the time of the first examination within an hour or two of birth. This particularly applies to the ELBW infant. Most bleeds will have occurred by 72 h and only a few thereafter. Extension of the original lesion may occur over a more extended period, however. The reason that haemorrhage is largely confined to the period immediately after birth may be due to the dilated and relatively unreactive cerebral vasculature at this time [19], or possibly to the timing of changes in vascular permeability. Prostacyclin metabolite levels are high immediately after birth but fall to low levels within 2–3 days even in sick infants [13].

Post-haemorrhagic hydrocephalus is commonly seen in ELBW infants following periventricular haemorrhage and relates to the extent of the lesion, being uncommon with germinal matrix haemorrhage alone but almost invariable when both ventricles are entirely filled with blood clot [33]. Some degree of ventricular enlargement almost always occurs after haemorrhage, but is transient and is resolving by 3–4 weeks of age [23]. This probably relates to a temporary abnormality in cerebrospinal fluid production and absorption induced by fibrin deposition. The majority of infants with post-haemorrhagic hydrocephalus have some degree of parenchymal involvement and the outcome in these infants following surgical treatment appears to relate to the extent of cystic changes seen on ultrasound scans rather than to the extent of the hydrocephalus or on any specific mode of management. In ELBW infants the results are particularly poor [34].

Periventricular leucomalacia (PVL)

Perinatal pathologists have long recognized neuronal loss and gliosis in the periventricular regions of the brains of small infants dying following perinatal difficulties, and have speculated about their possible significance in the aetiology of neurological deficits in survivors [35]. Although the introduction of *in vivo* diagnostic ultrasound initially showed the high incidence of haemorrhage in the brains of ELBW infants, the appearances of PVL were soon appreciated and their prognostic value recognized [36]. The aetiology of PVL has always been assumed to be ischaemic, at least in recent years. The nature of the mechanisms for the ischaemia has been debated and may result from hypotension leading to poor perfusion of the boundary zone between the ventriculopetal and ventriculofugal arteries supplying the periventricular region, or to venous stasis within the white matter induced by thrombosis of veins from the deep system as they pass through the germinal matrix [37].

The clinical associations of PVL in ELBW infants are similar to those of periventricular haemorrhage, except that PVL has been described as appearing in some cases at a much later stage such as after a period of septicaemia or necrotizing enterocolitis, whilst periventricular haemorrhage is usually confined to the first few days of life. Some authors claim that PVL is confined to infants of more than 900 g birth weight, but these reports are a little dated and probably reflect the fact that no sick infants of less than this weight survived long enough to develop the lesion. PVL has been put forward as the pathological lesion which in survivors leads to spastic diplegia, although there is very little evidence for this. In recent studies PVL of more than a very minor extent has been associated with a poor clinical outcome, and these survivors have had severe degrees of cerebral palsy, mental retardation or cortical blindness [36]. Recognition of PVL *in vivo* has depended on ultrasound as the resolution of CT scanning has proved inadequate for all but the most extensive lesions. As experience with the technique increases a wider range of appearances is being recognized, from small 'flares' in the first few days of life which may or may not develop into the more obvious cystic lesions more readily recognized later on [38]. A problem with the interpretation of these ultrasound findings is the paucity of autopsy correlations, as many of the infants developing them survive. At a later stage magnetic resonance imaging clearly defines the extent of disruption of myelination of tracts produced by PVL in ELBW infants [39]. Magnetic resonance spectroscopy has also had a role in clarifying the prognosis of early PVL appearances, low energy states being associated with poorer outcome [40].

Parenchymal haemorrhage and infarction

The extent of parenchymal involvement, whether due to haemorrhage or infarction, appears to be the most important determinant of outcome in follow-up studies of survivors [41]. There is, however, some debate as to the actual pathological lesion responsible for the ultrasound scan appearance of 'parenchymal echo-density'. The resolution of this debate is not merely academic, as any strategy for the ultimate improvement of outcome in ELBW infants must take account of the causative factors for these lesions.

Parenchymal lesions have often been assumed to be merely extensions of smaller periventricular haemorrhages. Certainly in many infants regular ultrasound scans show this to be the case, at least temporally. Direct extension of the haemorrhage, however, seems unlikely as unlike cerebral haemorrhage in a hypertensive adult, the bleeding is not from an arterial source and under pressure.

Two mechanisms at least can be considered. Firstly, as has already been described, the drainage of the greater part of the white matter in the ELBW infant is via the deep venous system and there is poor anastomosis with the more superficial system. Even small degrees of haemorrhage into the germinal matrix may produce thrombosis in these vessels, with subsequent venous infarction of the white matter supplied by them [42]. Alternatively, the presence of thrombus in the germinal matrix or ventricle may release substances which are themselves vasoactive, producing local ischaemia. This has been demonstrated in *in vitro* preparations [43] and is known to occur near the site of subarachnoid haemorrhage in adults, with a subsequent extension of the area of neuronal damage [44]. In either case the initial germinal matrix haemorrhage is the initiating factor. Other workers have suggested that most, if not all, extensive parenchymal lesions seen are caused by initial ischaemia followed by haemorrhage into the infarcted zone [45]. Certainly some extensive lesions are seen without a previous smaller intraventricular thrombus, but this is not the general pattern and there is no other evidence to suggest that this is the usual sequence of events. Whichever scenario is accepted, each is preceded by hypoxic and/or hypotensive events, and the prevention of such destructive lesions must depend on the avoidance of these antecedents.

Toxic neuronal damage

In the mature and intact human brain the neurones are protected from the effect of toxic substances by the integrity and selective behaviour of the blood-brain barrier (BBB). While it is unlikely that the BBB is functionally immature even in the ELBW infant, it is certainly vulnerable to the insults associated with neonatal diseases which are more frequent in the ELBW. Toxins may take the form of natural substances such as bilirubin, or administered ones such as gentamicin. Damage to the basal ganglia from the entry of bilirubin (kernicterus) has long been recognized in term infants with rhesus iso-immunization. Although the emphasis in prevention was always on keeping bilirubin levels low, more recent work suggests that the loss of integrity of the BBB due to intercurrent illness was probably more important in its causation. This is in keeping with the pathological findings of yellow staining of the basal ganglia in very preterm infants who had never experienced high bilirubin levels [46].

The nature of the clinical presentation of such bilirubin-induced injury in the very preterm survivor is uncertain. Classical choreoathetosis is a rare phenomenon in such infants, and it has been suggested that other forms of cerebral palsy or the high incidence of nerve deafness in ELBW infants is due to bilirubin toxicity. The occurrence of abnormalities of cortical evoked potentials in association with hyperbilirubinaemia might be seen as supportive evidence, although these changes are reversible [47].

The case for neurotoxicity of drugs such as gentamicin is even less clear. Streptomycin certainly caused deafness in babies in the early days of its use, but is no longer used in infants. Gentamicin is frequently used, but any association between its use and subsequent neurological deficit such as deafness is confounded by the presence of other adverse factors such as acidosis or meningitis. Other possible toxic substances include amino acids infused as part of total intravenous nutrition, some of which may reach potentially toxic levels in sick infants.

Conclusion

ELBW infants are at greater risk than any other group of newborn infants for acquiring neurological injury. This may be due in part to cerebral immaturity, but mainly to problems from immaturity of other systems such as the lungs, and to the problems which caused preterm birth. Whether the lesions which occur are due initially to haemorrhage or ischaemia the underlying aetiology is similar and strategies for the prevention of such problems must be along the traditional lines of prevention of preterm birth, avoidance of birth asphyxia, and better management of acute respiratory failure.

II. CLINICAL EVALUATION

Lilly M. S. Dubowitz

With the improvement in perinatal and neonatal care there has been a dramatic increase in the survival of ELBW infants in the last decade. This great improvement, unfortunately, has not been paralleled with a reduction in the rate of neurodevelopmental handicap in the survivors. The management of these infants has posed hitherto unknown problems to the neonatologists in intensive care units. There are differences both in nutrition and environment for these infants who are reared 12–16 weeks outside the uterus during a very critical period of neural development compared to a fetus at that gestation. It is to be expected that these differences will affect neural maturation. However, whether this artificial environment will produce deviant or delayed maturation by not providing the natural balance of nutrients or possibly accelerate it by earlier stimulation has not yet been established. In order to appreciate what represents abnormal development much more must be known about the maturational process of ELBW infants who had an optimal perinatal period and it will be necessary to document any changes which occur following a complication.

The aim of this section is to describe:

(1) The tools which are available for the neurological evaluation of the ELBW infant.
(2) What is now known of the similarity or differences in neurological maturation of extremely premature infants outside the uterus compared to the fetus in utero.
(3) The neurological findings in some of the more commonly encountered pathological conditions in these infants.

Neurological assessment

Estimation of gestational age

The relevance of gestational age (GA) for neonatal or follow-up studies cannot be sufficiently stressed. Not only will perinatal pathology differ according to the maturity of the neonate but various aspects of the early neurological examination and of later growth and development can only be correctly evaluated if gestational age is taken into account. The findings will be very different in an infant weighing 900 g at 25 weeks from one with similar weight but a GA of 35 weeks or more. In women with regular periods gestational age can be estimated from the date of the last menstrual period, but this is often uncertain. Thus a number of indirect methods have been utilized to estimate gestational age.

Ultrasound estimation of fetal size when used before 16 weeks gestation, such as the fetal crown–rump measurement [48] and the biparietal diameter [49] are probably the most accurate guides for gestational age. After 16 weeks gestation the latter becomes increasingly inaccurate [50]. Since nervous system and skin maturation are relatively spared in intrauterine growth retardation, the development of these has been employed in various schemes to estimate gestational age [51–57]. The argument in favour of neurological criteria is that they are least affected by fetal growth retardation even if it is very severe, while the argument against their use is that they might be difficult to elicit in ill infants and can be influenced by neurological abnormality [59]. Physical characteristics can be easily observed, but they are influenced by fetal growth failure [60], particularly if severe. Many also change rapidly in the extrauterine environment especially with the use of radiant heaters. In the author's experience, the best estimate of gestational age can be obtained when a combination of neurological and physical criteria are used [60,61]. The error is least when many types of observations are added together. However, in infants below 28–29 weeks gestation little change can be noted in either neurological or physical characteristics with decreasing gestational age, thus there will be a tendency to overestimate maturity. The only suitable and reliable estimate of gestational age in ELBW babies is the measurement of nerve conduction velocity [62–65]. This is a relatively simple technique which can be taught to ancillary staff and will give a reliable estimate of gestational age if performed within the first three weeks of life [66].

Systematic neurological evaluation

Until fairly recently there have been no adequate tools for the assessment of the neonatal nervous system. The impetus for standardized neurological examination for the newborn and particularly for the preterm infant came originally from André-Thomas and Saint-Anne Dargassies and their associates in Paris [67–71]. They mapped out the maturation of active and passive tone and primitive reflexes and developed an examination based mainly on these items. The more recent schemes included the assessment of hearing and vision as well [72]. The other main contribution came from Prechtl [73] in Holland who developed an examination geared for the full term infant. He particularly stressed the importance of age-specific techniques for any neonatal neurological examination and the impact the behavioural states have on nervous system functioning. He also suggested the use of the optimality concept to achieve objective scoring [74].

In the last two decades, interest has also developed in the behaviour of newborn babies. Brazelton [75] introduced a neurobehavioural scale to evaluate this. Although the examination has been frequently used as a neurological evaluation it is not suitable for that purpose as it is much more global and thus a less specific way of assessing neurological integrity [58].

The above examinations are not suitable for early or frequent monitoring of ELBW infants who often require life-support equipment or oxygen therapy. None has been developed for the ill infant as they require considerable expertise and are time consuming. In addition, some have only been standardized for full term infants [73,75]. Thus preterm infants can only be assessed when they have reached 40 weeks post-menstrual age (PMA). The validity of applying standards evolved for full term infants to preterm infants who might have spent as much as 10–16 weeks in an extrauterine, rather than an intrauterine, environment can also be questioned, particularly if the optimality scores developed for full term infants are applied to preterm infants at 40 weeks PMA [76].

A neurological examination suitable for ELBW infants must have as many items as possible which can be applied at birth, even to infants on ventilators, and must be suitable for longitudinal assessment. Good inter-observer correlation should be possible even when the examination is performed by relatively inexperienced staff, and it should take no longer than 10–15 min. By having a proforma with well defined instructions of how to elicit the requested items and aiding the recording with diagrams this can be achieved (Figure 19.1). The examination should include the assessment of behavioural states, tone and motility, some of the primitive reflexes and aspects of behaviour such as hearing, vision and consolability [77].

Items to be evaluated

BEHAVIOURAL STATE

The definition of behavioural states is important as they represent a centrally coordinated neural activity, which expresses itself in a variety of ways [78]. Thus the cause of the lower $P\text{O}_2$ in state 2 is not only due to the cardiorespiratory changes but also to different control of respiratory muscle activity and possibly to different reactivity to changes in arterial $P\text{O}_2$ and $P\text{CO}_2$. Behavioural state should be recorded for all items elicited. In infants above 36 weeks PMA this can be achieved easily by observing eye movements and alertness. At this age these show good correlation with other physiological variables such as electroencephalogram (EEG) pattern, respiratory rate and heart rate. In the younger preterm infants the well defined coordinated states do not exist but there are cycles of EEG activity, motility, regular and irregular breathing with or without eye movements. These may alternate independently or overlap. To what extent these rudimentary state cycles are responsible for the variability of heart rate, respiration, blood pressure and muscle tone in the extremely premature infant is not known. It is important to realize, however, that the cyclical variations in the cardiorespiratory status might be more a sign of good health than disease even in the most immature infant [58]. Examining infants halfway between feeds and following a set sequence through the examination will achieve comparable state for the same items.

ASSESSMENT OF TONE AND POSTURE

Observation of the infant in supine and prone positions (Figure 19.2), in sitting and ventral suspension, will give a good assessment of the tone of the muscles controlling the head and trunk, and also of the limbs. Further evaluation can be made by recording resistance to passive movement, but the objective recording of this requires familiarity of the norms for various gestational ages. Other methods used are the measurement of the power of recoil when the limbs are stretched or the angle of resistance either during passive movement or when traction is applied to the limbs (Figure 19.3*a* and *b*).

In infants who have been examined repeatedly longitudinally or at various gestational ages, it can be shown that with increasing maturity there is an increase in muscle tone [79,80]. In a normal infant this follows a predetermined pattern. Tone can be documented in the lower limbs before the upper limbs, and in the neck flexor muscles before the neck extensors. Limb tone can be assessed at birth even on infants on ventilators; some flexor tone in the lower limbs is found even at 25 weeks PMA, but is rarely observed in the upper limbs in well appropriate for gestational age (AGA) infants before 30 weeks gestation [79]. Increase in flexor tone in the arms is, however, common in all hyperexcitable infants; thus, it can be frequently observed in

NAME **D.O.B./TIME** **WEIGHT** **E.D.D. L.N.M.P.** **E.D.D. U/snd.**

HOSP. **NO.** **DATE OF EXAM** **HEIGHT**

RACE **SEX** **AGE** **HEAD CIRC.** **GESTATIONAL ASSESSMENT** **SCORE** **WEEKS**

STATES
1. Deep sleep, no movement, regular breathing.
2. Light sleep, eyes shut, some movement.
3. Dozing, eyes openign and closing.
4. Awake, eyes open, minimal movement.
5. Wide awake, vigorous movement.
6. Crying.

						STATE	COMMENT	ASYMMETRY
HABITUATION (⩽ state 3)								
LIGHT Repetitive flashlight stimuli (10) with 5 sec. gap. Shutdown = 2 consecutive negative responses	No response	A. Blink response to first stimulus only. B. Tonic blink response. C. Variable response.	A. Shutdown of movement but blink perists 2-5 stimuli. B. Complete shutdown 2-5 stimuli.	A. Shutdown of movement but blink perists 6-10 stimuli. B. Complete shutdown 6-10 stimuli.	A. Equal response to 10 stimuli. B. Infant comes to fully alert state. C. Startles + major responses throughout.			
RATTLE Respetitive stimuli (10) with 5 sec. gap.	No response	A. Slight movement to first stimulus. B. Variable response.	Startle or movement 2-5 stimuli, then shutdown	Startle or movement 6-10 stimuli, then shutdown	A. B. Grading as above C.			
MOVEMENT & TONE	Undress infant							
POSTURE ★ (At rest – predominant)			(hips abducted)	(hips adducted)	Abnormal postures: A. Oposthotonus. B. Unusual leg extension. C. Asymm. tonic neck reflex.			
ARM RECOIL Infant supine. Take both hands, extend parallel to the body; old approx. 2 sec. and release	No flexion within 5 sec. R L	Partial flexion at elbow > 100° within 4-5 sec. R L	Arms flex at elbow to < 100° within 2-3 sec. R L	Sudden jerky flexion at elbow immediately after release to < 60° R L	Difficult to extend; arm snaps back forcefully			
ARM TRACTION Infant supine; head midline; grasp wrist, slowly pull arm to vertical. Angle of arm scored and resistance noted at moment infant is initially lifted off and watched until shoulder off mattress. Do other arm.	Arm remains fully extended R L	Weak flexion maintain only momentarily R L	Arm flexed at elbow to 140° and maintained 5 sec. R L	Arm flex at approx. 100° and maintained R L	Strong flexion of arm < 100° and maintained R L			
LEG RECOIL First flex hips for 5 secs, then extend both legs of infant by traction on ankles; hold down on the bed for 2 secs. and release.	No flexion within 5 sec. R L	Incomplete flexion of hips within 5 sec. R L	Complete flexion within 5 sec. R L	Instantaneous complete flexion R L	Legs cannot be extended; snap back forcefully			
LEG TRACTION Infant supine. Grasp leg near ankle and slowly pull toward vertical until buttocks 1-2" off. Note resistance at knee and score angle. Do other leg.	No flexion R L	Partial flexion, rapidly lost R L	Knee flexion 140-160° and maintained R L	Knee flexion 100-140° and maintained R L	Strong resistance; flexion < 100° R L			
POPLITEAL ANGLE Infant supine. Approximate knee and thigh to abdomen; extend leg by gentle pressure with index finger behind ankle.	180-160° R L	150-140° R L	130-120° R L	110-90° R L	< 90° R L			
HEAD CONTROL (post. neck m.) Grasp infant by shoulder and raise to sitting position; allow head to fall forward; wait 30 sec.	No attempt to raise head	Unsuccessful attempt to raise head upright	Head raised smoothly to upright in 30 sec. but not maintained.	Head raised smoothly to upright in 30 sec. and maintained.	Head cannot be flexed forward.			
HEAD CONTROL (ant. neck m.) Allow head to fall backward as you hold shoulders; wait 30 secs.	Grading as above	Grading as above	Grading as above	Grading as above				
HEAD LAG ★ Pull infant toward sitting posture by traction on both wrists. Also note arm flexion.								
VENTRAL SUSPENSION ★ Hold infant in ventral suspension; observe curvature of back, flexion of limbs and relation of head to trunk.								
HEAD RAISING IN PRONE POSITON Infant in prone position with head in midline.	No response	Rolls head to one side	Weak effort to raise head and turns raised head to one side.	Infant lifts head, nose and chin off.	Strong prolonged head lifting.			
ARM RELEASE IN PRONE POSITION Head in midline. Infant in prone position; arms extended alongside body with palms up.	No effort	Some effort and wriggling.	Flexion effort but neither wrist brought to nipple level	One or both wrist brought at least to nipple level without excessive body movement.	Strong body movement with both wrists brought to face, or 'press-ups'.			
SPONTANEOUS BODY MOVEMENT During examination (supine). If no spont. movement try to induce by cutaneous stimulation.	None or minimal Induced	A. Sluggish. B. Random, incoordinated. C.	Smooth movements alternating with random, stretching, athetoid or jerky.	Smooth alernating movements of arms and legs with medium speed and intensity	Mainly: A. Jerky movement. B. Athetoid movement. C. Other abnormal movement.			
TREMORS Fast (> 6/sec.) Mark: or Slow (< 6/sec.)	No tremor	Tremors only in state 5-6.	Tremors only in sleep or after Moro and startles	Some tremors in state 4	Tremulousness in all states		1 2	
STARTLES	No startles	Startles to sudden noise. Moro, bank on table only.	Occasional spontaneous startle.	2-5 spontaneous startles.	6+ spontaneous startles.			
ABNORMAL MOVEMENT OR POSTURE	No abnormal movement	A. Hands clenched but open intermittently. B. Hands do not open with Moro.	A. Some mouthing movement. B. Intermittent adducted thumb.	A. Persistently adducted thumb. B. Hands clenched all the time.	A. Continuous mouthing movement. B. Abnormal toe posture. C. Abnormal finger posture. D. Convulsive movement.			

						STATE	COMMENT	ASYMMETRY
REFLEXES								
TENDON REFLEXES Biceps jerk. Knee jerk. Ankle jerk.	Absent		Present	Exaggerated	Clonus			
PALMAR GRASP Head in midline. Put index finger from ulnar side into hand and gently press palmar surface. Never touch dorsal side of hand.	Absent R L	Short, weak flexion R L	Medium strength and sustained flexion for several sec. R L	Strong flexion; contraction spreads to forearm R L	Very strong grasp. Infant easily lifts off couch. R L			
PLANTAR GRASP Press the thumb against the ball of the infants foot.	No response R L	Partial plantar flexion of toes. R L	Toes curl around examiners finger. R L					
ROOTING Infant supine, head midline. Touch each corner of the mouth in turn (stroke laterally).	No response	A. Partial weak head turn but no mouth opening. B. Mouth opening, no head turn.	Mouth opening on stimulated side with partial head turning.	Full head turning, with or without mouth opening.	Mouth opening with very jerky head turning.			
SUCKING Infant supine; place index finger (pad towards palate) in infant's mouth; judge power of sucking movement after 5 sec.	No attempt	Weak sucking movement: A. Regular. B. Irregular.	Strong sucking movement; poor stripping: A. Regular. B. Irregular.	Strong regular sucking movement with continuing sequence of 5 movements. Good stripping.	Clenching but no regular sucking.			
WALKING (state 4, 5) Hold infant upright, feet touching bed, neck held straight with fingers.	Absent		Some effort but not continuous with both legs.	At least 2 steps with both legs.	A. Stork posture; no movement. B. Automatic walking.			
PLACING Lift infant in an upright position and allow dorsum of foot to touch protruding edge of a flat surface.	No response R L	Dorsiflexion of ankle only R L	Full placing response with flexion fo hip and knee and placing sole of foot on surface. R L					
MORO One hand supports infant's head in midline, the other the back. Raise infant to 45° and when infant is relaxed let his head fall through 10°. Note if jerky. Repeat 3 times.	No response, or opening of hands only.	Full abduction at the shoulder and extension of the arm.	Full abduction but only delayed or partial adduction	Partial abduction at shoulder and extension of arms followed by smooth adduction. A. Abd > Add B. Abd = Add C. Abd < Add	A. No abduction or adduction; extension only. B. Marked adduction only.	J S		
NEUROBEHAVIOURAL ITEMS								
EYE APPEARANCES	Sunset sign Nerve palsy.	Transient nystagmus. Strabismus. Some roving eye movement.	Does not open eyes.	Normal conjugate eye movement.	A. Persistant nystagmus. B. Frequent roving movement C. Frequent rapid blinks.			
AUDITORY ORIENTATION (state 3, 4) To rattle. (Note presence of startle.)	A. No reaction. B. Auditory startle but no true orientation.	Brightens and stills; may turn toward stimuli with eyes closed.	Alerting and shiftign of eyes; head may or may not turn to source	Alerting; prolonged head turns to stimulus; search with eyes.	Turning and alerting to stimulus each time on both sides		S	
VISUAL ORIENTATION (State 4) To red woollen ball	Does not focus or follow stimulus	Stills; focuses on stimulus; may follow 30° jerkily; does not find stimulus again spontaneously	Follows 30-60° horizontally; may lose stimulus but finds it again. Brief vertical glance.	Follows with eyes and head horizontally and to some extend vertically, with frowning.	Sustained fixation; follows vertically, horizontally, and in circle.			
ALERTNESS/ RESPONSIVENESS Do **not** score appearance but responsiveness to visual stimulation.	Inattentive; rarely or never response to direct stimulation	When alert, periods rather brief; rather variable response to orientation	When alert, alertness moderately sustained; may use stimulus to come to alert state	Sustained alertness; orientation frequent, reliable to visual stimuli.	Continuous alertness, which does not seem to tire, to visual stimuli.			
DEFENSIVE REACTION A cloth or hand is placed over the infant's face to partially occlude the nasal airway.	No response	A. General quitening. B. Non-specific activity and long latency.	Rooting; lateral neck turning; possily neck stretching.	Swipes with arm.	Swipes with arm with rather violent body movement.			
PEAK OF EXCITEMENT	Low level arousal to all stimuli; never > state 3.	Infant reaches state 4-5 briefly but predominantly in lower states.	Infant predominantly state 4 or 5; may reach state 6 after stimulation but returns spontaneously to lower state.	Infant reaches state 6 but can be consoled relatively easily.	A. Mainly state 6. Difficult to console, if at all. B. Mainly state 4-5 but if reaches state 6 cannot be consoled.			
IRRITABILITY (states 3, 4, 5) Aversive stimuli: Uncover Ventral susp. Undress Moro Pull to sit Walking reflex Prone	No irritable crying to any of the stimuli	Cries to 1-2 stimuli	Cries to 3-4 stimuli	Cries to 5-6 stimuli	Cries to all stimuli			
CONSOLABILITY (state 6)	Never above state 5 during examination, therefore not needed	Consoling not needed. Consoles spontaneously	Consoled by talking, hand on belly or wrapping up.	Consoled by picking up and holding, may need finger in mouth.	Not consolable.			
CRY	No cry at all	Only whimpering cry	Cries to stimuli but normal pitch	Lusty cry to offensive stimuli; normal pitch	High pitched cry, often continuous			

NOTES ★ If asymmetrical or atypical, draw in on nearest figure. Record any abnormal signs (e.g. facial palsy, contractures, etc.). Draw if possible.

CHECK LIST OF ABNORMAL SIGNS

Head and trunk control	Orientation & alertness
Limb tone	Irritability
Motility	Consolability
Reflexes	Deviant sign

Modified from *The Neurological Assessment of the Preterm and Full-term Newborn Infant*, by Lilly and Victor Dubowitz

Record tape after feed

EXAMINER:

Figure 19.1 Neurological form for examination

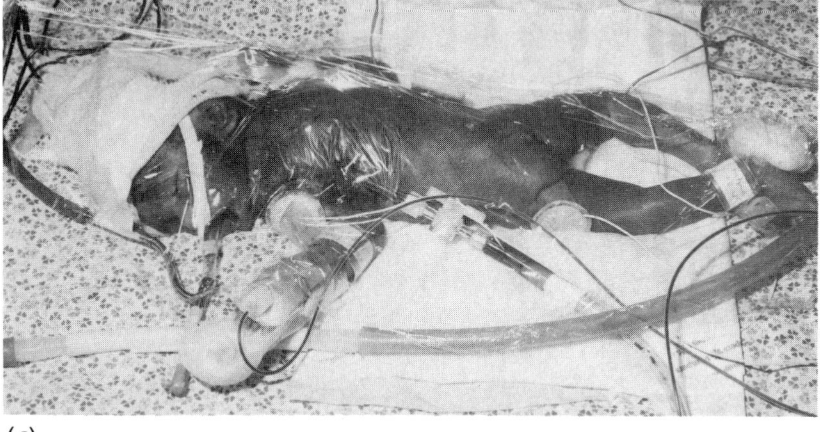

(*a*)

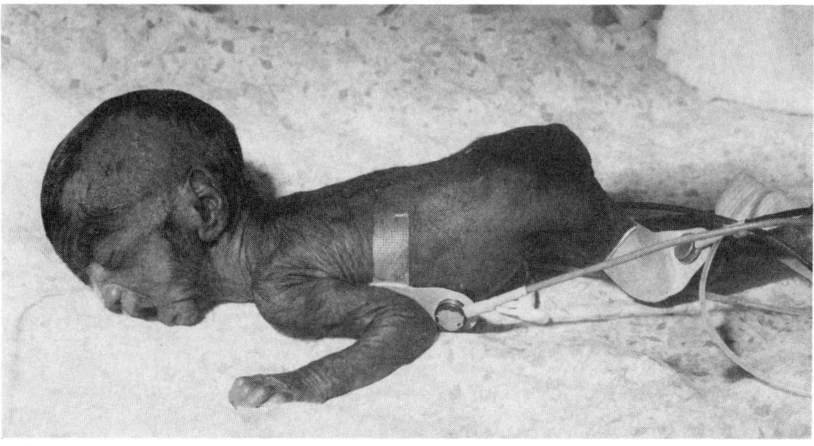

(*b*)

Figure 19.2 (*a*) Infant born at 26 weeks GA. BW 860 g. Aged 6 days. (*b*) Infant born at 28 weeks GA. BW 750 g. Aged 8 days. Note elevated hip in infant (*b*) who is SGA and well, indicating better tone

small for gestational age (SGA) infants under 1000 g, even before 29 weeks PMA. Longitudinal documentation allows the comparison in the pattern of development inside and outside the uterus in well and ill infants (Figure 19.4).

ASSESSMENT OF MOVEMENT

The quality, quantity and symmetry of spontaneous movements can be easily observed even in the smallest and most ill infants. Both quantity and quality can be noted to change with increasing maturity. The movements of the very immature infants often consist of slow assymetrical twisting and stretching movements of the trunk and limbs, which is often termed athetoid. This may be accompanied by rapid repetitive wide amplitude movements of the limbs resembling myoclonus. With increasing maturity there is a gradual change to smooth alternating movements with

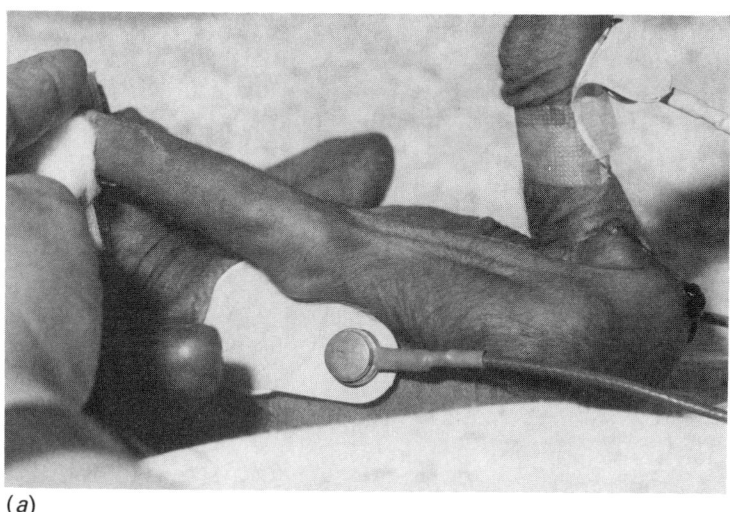

(*a*)

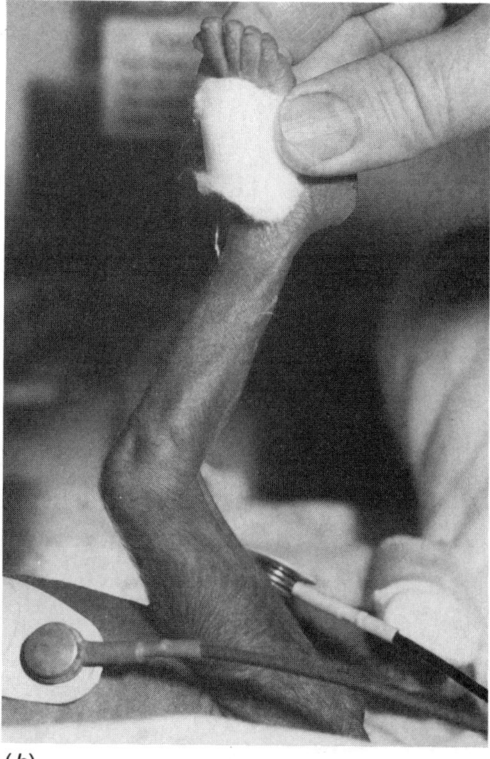

(*b*)

Figure 19.3 Assessment of limb tone by measuring angle of variance between leg and thigh: (*a*) to passive movement (180°); (*b*) to traction (160°)

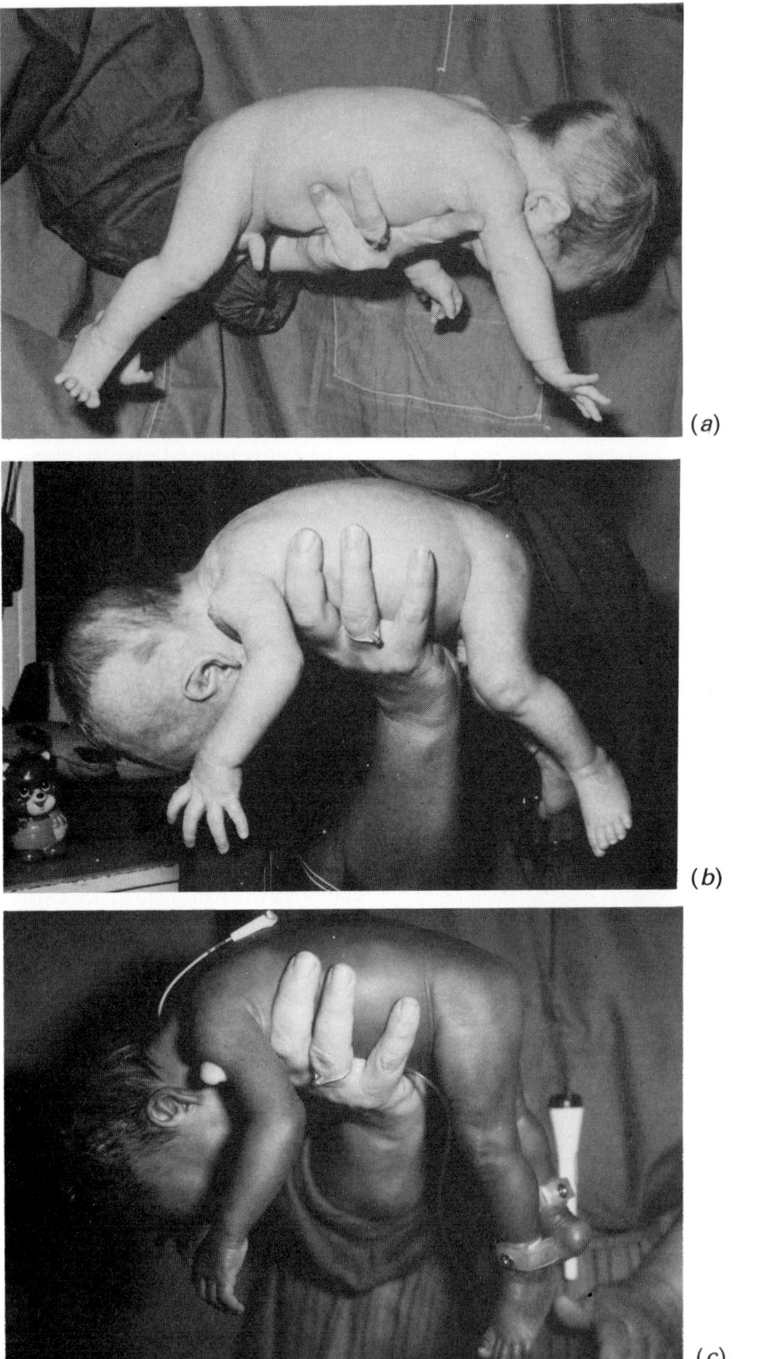

Figure 19.4 Ventral suspension at 40 weeks PMA. (*a*) Normal infant born at 29 weeks GA. BW 1100 g. (*b*) Normal infant born at 26 weeks GA. BW 780 g. (*c*) Infant with large PVH born at 28 weeks GA. BW 850 g. Note poorer head control in infant born at 26 weeks and even poorer in infant with PVH

medium speed and intensity. The quantity of motor activity changes little from approximately 28–35 weeks PMA, but decreases rapidly thereafter [81].

Abnormality of motor function may also be manifested by inappropriate quality and quantity of movement for the infant's maturity or by asymmetries. The norms for these are poorly defined for ELBW infants, thus the differentiation of abnormal movement and even convulsions can be difficult. The normal myoclonic movements can be interpreted as convulsions, while twitches representing seizures may be overlooked.

NEONATAL 'REFLEXES'

A number of transitory 'reflexes' which are unique to the neonate have been described. Many of them are already present at a very early gestation and show a distinctive developmental profile. In spite of the extensive literature on their description and development, little is known about the mechanisms which produce them. They tend to show certain common features in relation to neurological insults, similar to those in heavier infants. Absent and high threshold responses will be found in apathetic non-alert infants. Newborns who are hyperexcitable because of biochemical or central nervous system disturbances will have a low threshold or inappropriately mature responses for their PMA. These will therefore be common in otherwise well SGA infants at birth. Cortical injuries have no apparent effect on most of these reflexes. There are two notable exceptions. Poor plantar and placing reactions may be observed on the contralateral side of a large parenchymal haemorrhage. The probable mechanism is reduced afferent input so that the response is not elicited. In ELBW infants assymetry of the plantar grasp is commonly the earliest sign of a future hemiplegia.

SUCKING AND FEEDING

Feeding requires the coordinated action of sucking, swallowing and breathing. Adequate coordination already exists for this at 28 weeks gestation; but at this stage the sucking is neither powerful enough nor is there sufficient synchrony with swallowing to allow adequate feeding. With increasing maturity, sucking becomes more coordinated and a characteristic feeding posture develops [82].

ASSESSMENT OF VISUAL FUNCTION AND ALERTNESS

This function can and should be tested as part of the routine neurological assessment. A red woollen ball is an excellent stimulus which can be presented at a distance of 15–20 cm. Starting at the midline the ball is moved laterally in either direction, then vertically and finally in an arc (Figure 19.5). The infant's ability to focus and track this object is assessed [83]. From 29–30 weeks PMA, infants are able to focus and track briefly horizontally and vertically. The function is more consistent in SGA infants. With increasing maturity they can track the ball more smoothly and in an arc.

The integrity of the visual pathway can also be assessed by visually evoked potentials (VEP). VEP to flash stimulation can be consistently recorded from 27 weeks PMA [84] and again a maturational profile can be demonstrated. While studies of VEP maturation are of interest, their relevance to clinical diagnoses in the early neonatal period is doubtful.

Altertness should not be assessed from the infant's appearance but from his ability

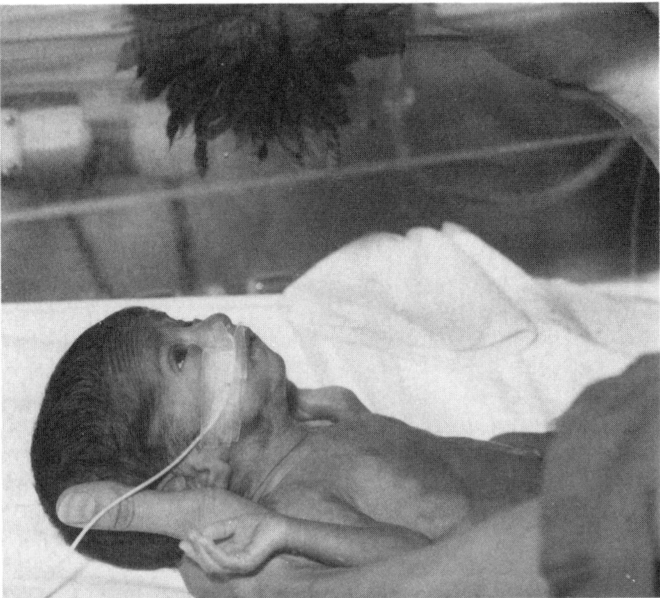

Figure 19.5 Visual tracking of a red woollen ball in an infant born at 29 weeks GA. BW 940 g. Assessed at two weeks of age. Note infant is able to track vertically

to respond to visual stimulation. In some ELBW infants treated with theophylline, staring eyes with retracted lids may give the appearance of alertness, yet they may have very poor responsiveness to stimuli.

ASSESSMENT OF HEARING

This should be part of a routine neurological examination. It can be tested either with a rattle producing a broad band of frequencies [77], an auditory cradle [85], or with auditory brainstem response (ABR) [86]. The former has the advantage that it is cheap, can be performed during the routine examination of the infant, and can be used with even the smallest infant from the moment of birth. Compared to the cradle, it has the disadvantage that a higher number of infants will fail the test even when the presence of good auditory evoked responses can be demonstrated at a 60 dB level. At present the cradle has not been evaluated for testing infants under 1500 g. Its advantage is that it is fully automated, thus is also free of any possible observer bias.

Our routine is to test infants with a rattle weekly from birth. The head is elevated about 20° and supported in the midline by the examiner's hand, leaving it free to rotate (Figure 19.6). The stimulus is presented on each side in turn with the hand and rattle out of sight. Infants in incubators and on ventilators can also be tested. Those who fail this test on repeated occasions are tested with an ABR before discharge or at 36 weeks PMA. At present, the ABR is the most reliable method for testing hearing in very small infants. The type of loss can be established and it can also test the hearing threshold [87].

The response to the rattle can be persistently elicited in neurologically normal infants from 27–28 weeks PMA. Assymetrical responses correspond with assymetri-

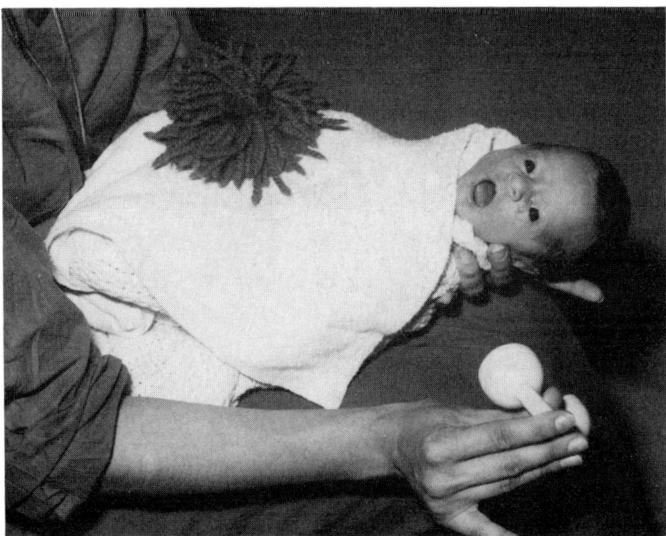

Figure 19.6 Assessment of hearing with a rattle. Infant assessed at 36 weeks PMA. GA 28 weeks. BW 950 g. Note that the baby becomes alert and the head turns to the side of the rattle

cal ABRs. Regular assessment of hearing in the neonatal period has been able to demonstrate that infants with periventricular haemorrhage (PVH) tend to have a poor auditory response at the time of the bleed; this tends to recover quickly and permanent hearing loss does not follow unless there is another complication. Jaundice, on the other hand, even at relatively low levels when it is persistent and associated with acidosis may cause permanent damage [88].

The incidence of mild hearing loss in ELBW infants in the early weeks of postnatal life is very common, even in the absence of PVH and jaundice. Most recover completely, often before their discharge from the unit. Although ABRs can be performed early they are time consuming; in view of the common but transient hearing loss, we recommend that ABRs should be performed later – at 36 weeks PMA. An exception to this is a persistent hearing loss in an otherwise well infant with marked growth retardation. This should raise the suspicion of cytomegalovirus infection, and in these babies the hearing loss should be confirmed with an ABR. In our experience hearing loss recovering by 36 weeks has no permanent effect but there is a higher incidence of neurodevelopmental abnormalities, including language delay, in infants where it persists beyond 40 weeks PMA, even if it recovers later.

Neurological profile of well infants and those with specific neurological insults

Neurological development in ELBW babies

Developmental profiles

Early reports claimed that neurological development is similar inside and outside the uterus [69]. More recently differences in the pattern of development have been noted and their variation with postnatal age [76,79,80,89,90]. The reports have not shown consistent findings. They probably reflect not only differences in the population studied and the criteria used for assessment, but also differences in the environment of these infants, such as nutrition, position of nursing and exposure to stimulation. These factors also interact in the same nursery, and norms are thus difficult to establish. We found that, in infants born between 28 and 35 weeks gestation, at 40 weeks PMA there is increasingly better head control with increasing postnatal age. The difference may be the result of placing very preterm infants in a prone position, thus promoting head control, however even well infants below 28 weeks gestation have much poorer development of head control. In this case it is possible that their nutritional state was less satisfactory, affecting both neuronal and muscle maturation.

There are also a number of other neurological functions which show definite acceleration in development in the extrauterine environment. Thus in well infants the development of sucking and sucking posture relates more to postnatal age than PMA [82]. The same may be observed for visual tracking responses [77]. Thus a visual performance in a preterm infant at 40 weeks PMA which is similar to that of the full term infant during the first few days of life, represents delayed development and is observed in infants who have suffered a neurological insult, particulary PVH/IVH [91]. This delay does not appear to be a marker for later abnormality in neurological or visual development. Similar delay in development may be observed in the maturation of VEP under these circumstances; again this does not seem to have a prognostic significance [92]. However, absent or deviant VEPs do seem to be associated with future abnormalities [93].

We have found that repeated neurological examination can also document deviant patterns in the development outside the uterus compared to that within, both in well and ill infants. By correlating these with early cranial ultrasound and electrophysiological findings, and also with later neuro-developmental outcome, one might identify those differences which are normal for ELBW babies and need no intervention, from those which are abnormal and need attention.

Marked arm and leg extension in ventral suspension is normal in preterm infants born at less than 35 weeks gestational age when they reach 40 weeks PMA [79] (Figure 19.4*a*). A similar posture in a full term infant would suggest later spasticity. Flexor tone in the arm equal to that in the legs is normal in full term infants, but in the preterm infant at 40 weeks PMA it is usually associated with later shoulder retraction and this will need attention. Although in the absence of other neurological abnormality this rectifies itself, it interferes with early bimanual manipulation [94] and produces a rather frustrated infant (Figure 19.7*a* and *b*).

High frequency, low amplitude tremors and startles were commonly noted in apparently well premature infants reaching 40 weeks PMA, particularly in those with extreme prematurity, by Piper *et al.* [76]. In our experience they are frequently associated with other abnormal signs or cranial ultrasound abnormalities and thus should not be regarded as normal.

When abnormal signs are present their significance is generally quite different from those in a full term infant. Thus hypotonia and weak responses are common in infants with prolonged illness such as bronchopulmonary dysplasia (BPD) [76], even in the absence of a neurological insult. In these infants they represent a delay in maturation rather than loss of function and thus they carry a more favourable prognosis than in a full term infant. Deviant patterns of development and the persistence of deviant signs appear to be prognostically much more significant.

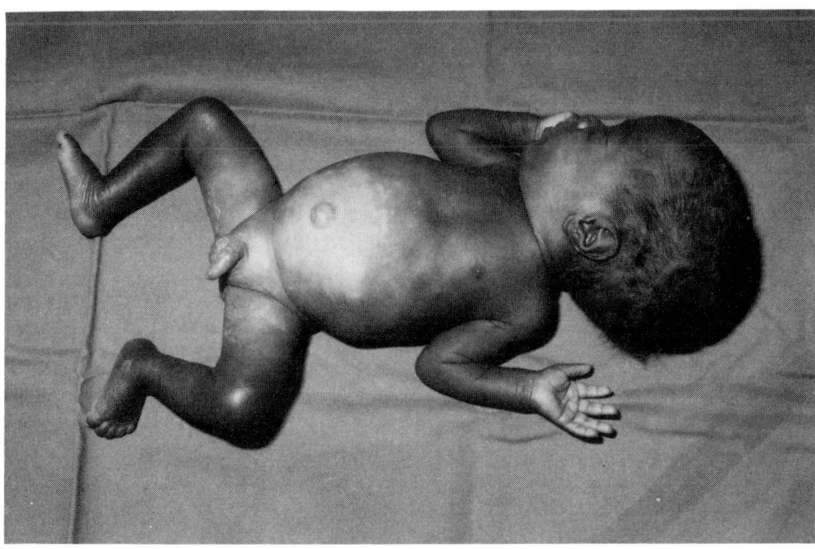

(a)

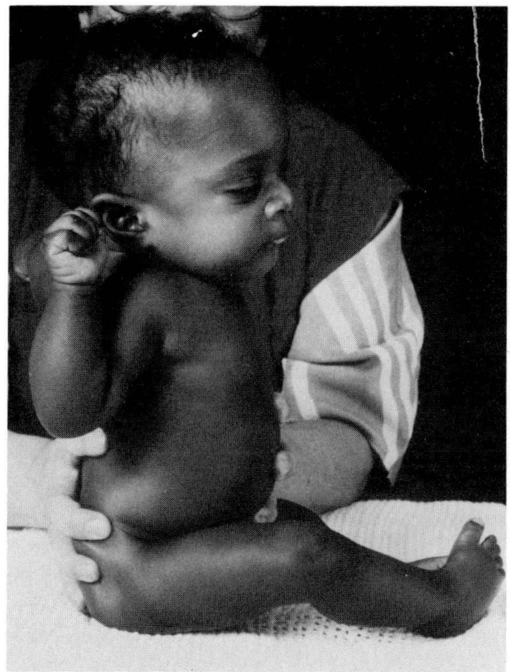

(b)

Figure 19.7 Marked arm flexor tone at 40 weeks PMA. (*a*) Compared with normal for premature infants at this age. (*b*) This is often associated with shoulder retraction in infancy

Neurological profiles of specific insults

Repeated neurological examinations also allow the documentation of the signs associated with some specific insults.

Periventricular and intraventricular haemorrhage

This is by far the commonest neurological insult seen in ELBW infants. Although many of these lesions have been 'clinically silent' [95], careful examination reveals abnormal neurological signs in nearly all cases.

Volpe [96] described two characteristic syndromes associated with the larger intraventricular haemorrhages. The first was the characteristic deterioration which occurs in the infants that usually do not survive. They passed from stupor to coma, developed apnoea, generalized tonic seizures, fixed pupils and flaccid quadriplegia. With the advent of cranial ultrasonography it has been possible to study the evolution of these haemorrhages. It has been noted that while the above findings do accompany some of the larger bleeds, they can also be noted in their absence. The second syndrome he described was the saltatory syndrome, which consisted of alteration of levels of consciousness, change in the quality and quantity of movement. Deterioration and improvement occurred for many hours.

By closely correlating ultrasound findings with repeated clinical examinations, we were able to identify most haemorrhages clinically [97] and map out the signs related to their evolution [98]. Preceding the haemorrhage or at the time of onset, hypertonicity is more marked in the arms and excessive motility with tremors and startles may be noted. Tendon reflexes are brisk, the Moro response is abnormal, and visual and auditory orientation is absent. The infant is usually irritable. Stage 2 occurs after the haemorrhage has occurred. Tone and motility are decreased but the popliteal angle is relatively tight. There is poor reactivity and visual orientation is absent. Stage 3 is the phase of recovery. Limb tone becomes normal first, including the popliteal angle, and motility improves next. First auditory then visual orientation recovers, and head and trunk control are the last to become normal. During this phase, roving eye movements are often noted. Also at this stage, a number of deviant signs become apparent in infants who later show an abnormal outcome. These include persistent assymetry of tone, spontaneously up-going toes (Figure 19.8*a* and *b*), adducted thumbs (Figure 19.9) and primitive reflexes.

It is interesting that the severity of the signs in the early stages do not necessarily correlate either with the size of the lesion or with later outcome. There is, however, a good correlation between the speed of recovery and later outcome, and the number of deviant signs as opposed to delayed maturation are also good markers [99]. Posthaemorrhagic ventricular dilatation produces practically no abnormal signs even when there is considerable increase in the head size provided intracranial pressure is not markedly elevated. The only abnormal sign related to the hydrocephalus is poor head control, the severity of which correlates with head size. The hydrocephalus only rarely produces deterioration in either visual or auditory evoked potential. They may even become normal when there is progressive ventricular dilatation. With rising pressure the infant often becomes irritable and tremulous; increased arm flexor tone and neck extensor hypertonia may also be noted. Auditory and visually evoked potentials may remain remarkably normal during the neonatal period despite considerably elevated intracranial pressure. If the potentials are abnormal, they may not revert to normal after ventricular drainage. Thus, in contrast to older infants,

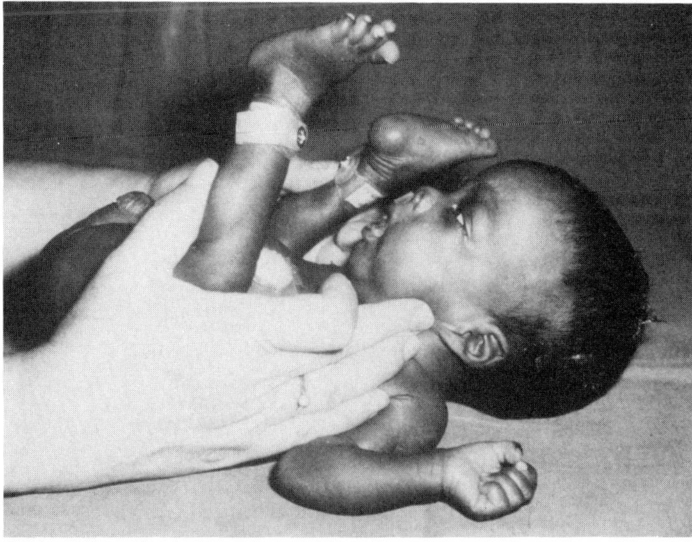

(a)

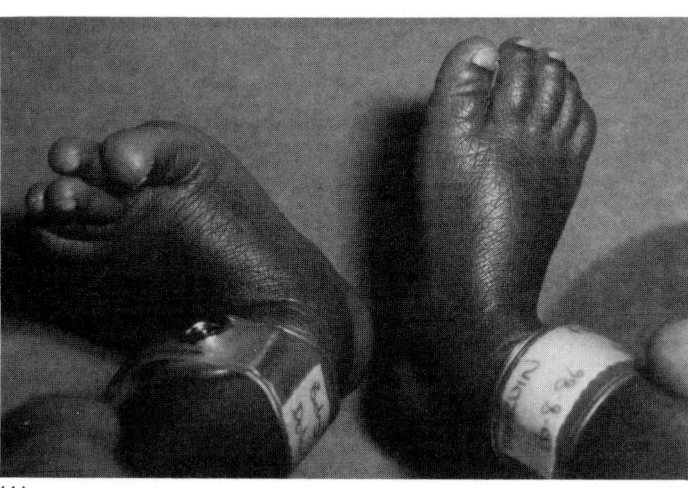

(b)

Figure 19.8 Infant born at 28 weeks GA. BW 880 g. Large PVH on the right on day 2. Examined 36 weeks PMA. Note (*a*) assymetric popliteal angle tighter on the left and (*b*) spontaneously up-going toe on the left

they are of little use in monitoring the effect of ventricular dilatation in this population.

Cystic periventricular leucomalacia (PVL)

Generalized severe ischaemia in the absence of a significant PVH does not seem to produce cystic leucomalacia in the very immature infant. Thus, in these babies the

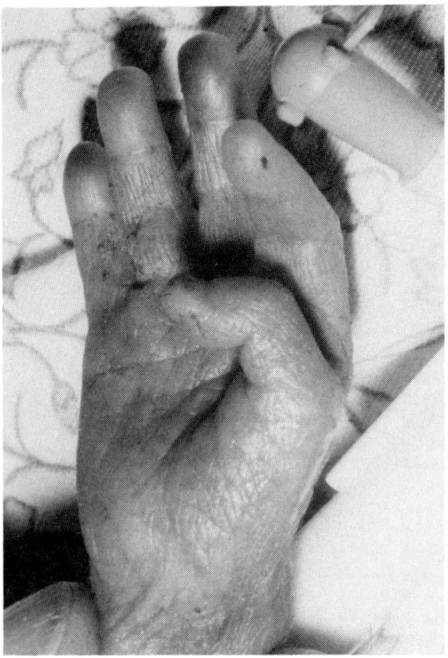

Figure 19.9 Adducted thumb in neurologically abnormal preterm infant not associated with fisting which would be common in the more mature infant

lesions are not usually seen at the time of birth or soon after. However, if they suffer a severe collapse, repeated prolonged bradycardia or, particulary, necrotizing enterocolitis, the lesion may develop even at several weeks of age [100]. This is in marked contrast to PVH which rarely develops after the first week of life. The early signs of the lesion are hypotonia and lethargy which may be masked by the illness which actually produces the lesions. Auditory and visual responses tend to be appropriate.

The infants then improve and for a period in fact may appear normal; however, between six and ten weeks after the insult a characteristic picture emerges. They gradually become more irritable and although they can be pacified with feeding, very little else is of use. Abnormal tone pattern with an increase in flexor tone in the arms and extensor tone in the legs and marked neck extensor hypertonia may be observed (Figure 19.10). This abnormal tone pattern is much less marked in infants with BPD. Movement may be abnormal or stereotyped. Tongue protrusion is often present giving the appearance of hypothyroidism. Fisting and adducted thumbs are usually rare at this stage, but abnormal finger and toe posture are common. This includes flexion of the index finger with other fingers extended and spontaneously up-going toes in a supine infant lying quietly (Figure 19.11). The placing reaction is poor. The Moro response is abnormal, consisting of extension at the elbow only without any abduction or adduction of the arms. At this stage visual and auditory functions are normal [101]. In the neonatal period there is no difference in the clinical signs between the infants with periventricular and subcortical leucomalacia, but the EEG and VEPs are always abnormal in the latter while they are usually normal at this stage in the former.

If these infants are evaluated only at the time of discharge, the abnormal

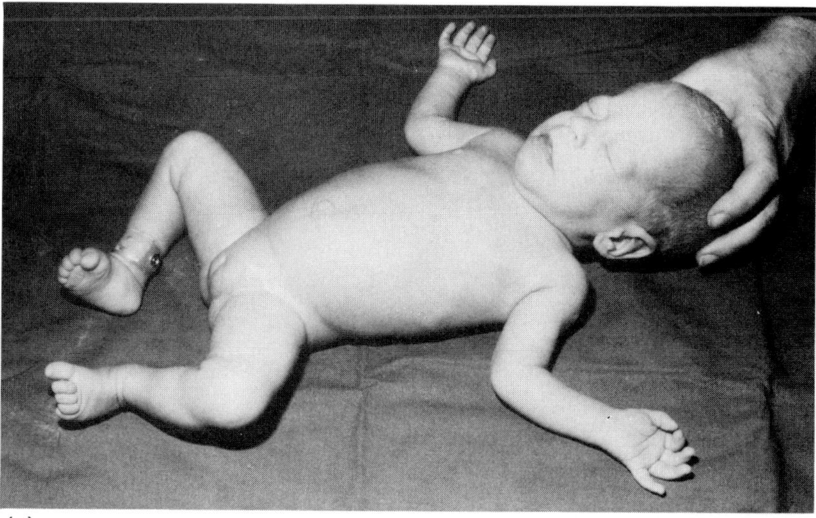

(*a*)

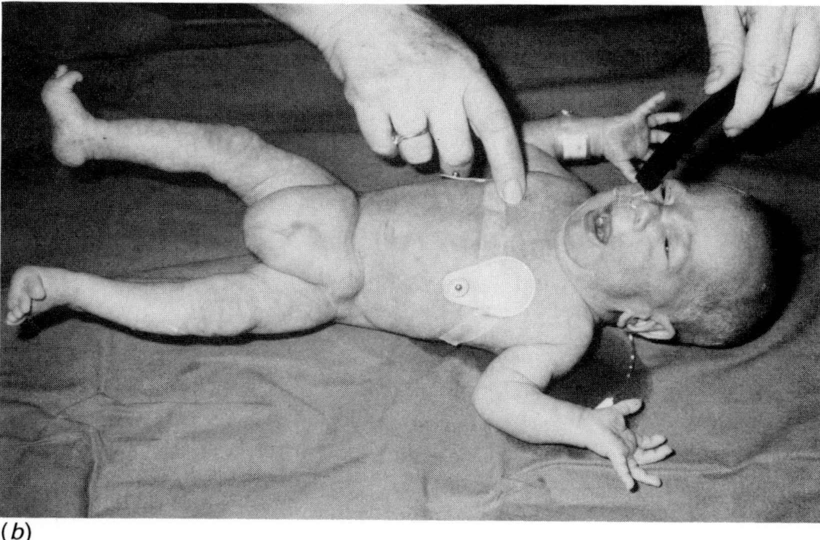

(*b*)

Figure 19.10 Twins born at 28 weeks Ga. Twin (*a*) BW 950 g. Small PVH day 2. Twin (*b*) BW 720 g. Periventricular cystic leucomalacia. Note normal supine posture appropriate for age (40 weeks PMA) in twin (*a*), extended posture with flexed arms and up-going toes in twin (*b*)

neurological signs may be minimal and thus easily missed. At 40 weeks PMA the cysts are often no longer visible while the clinical signs are prominent. At this stage there is clinically no difference in visual function between the infants who maintain their vision and those who are later cortically blind, but there is a marked difference in the appearance of the VEPs. This condition illustrates not only the importance of repeated evaluations but also the value of an integrated approach.

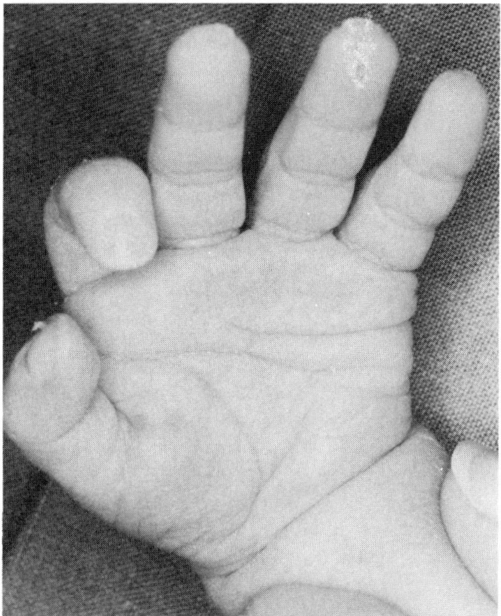

Figure 19.11 Abnormal finger posture consisting of flexion in index finger and thumb with other fingers extended. This sign is frequently noted in infants with PVL even when quiet. It may be seen in normal infants when crying

Conclusion

The neurological evaluation of ELBW infants is not only feasible but essential. It provides a means of studying the effect of the environment – both stimulation and deprivation – on the maturing nervous system. Manipulation of this environment might show us to what extent this neurological development can be altered through the plasticity of the nervous system in normal and abnormal infants. Regular assessments will also allow earlier recognition of disability. By instituting treatment early, the impact of these could be reduced. Finally, a knowledge of the normal for the infants reared outside the uterus can also help the paediatrician to reassure parents about some of their anxieties and thus promote better parent and infant relationships.

III. THE NORMAL ELECTROENCEPHALOGRAM

Janet Eyre

The period from 24 weeks gestation to term is a critical time for maturation and organization of the cerebral cortex; those born very prematurely are at greatest risk of a disturbance in this process. It has been known for many years that there are striking changes in the electroencephalogram (EEG) of the preterm infant with increasing post-conceptional age. These changes are a reflection of the progressive maturation of the central nervous system. Repeated recording of the EEG can provide a simple and non-invasive means to monitor cerebrocortical maturation but only if the ontogenesis of the EEG is well understood.

The pattern of the EEG in a healthy baby is dependent upon the baby's gestational age and so is related only indirectly to birth weight. In this section, therefore, the EEG of babies of less than 32 weeks gestational age will be discussed because 1000 g is the third centile for the birth weight of girls at 32 weeks of gestation [102].

Development of the cerebral cortex

The ontogenesis of the human central nervous system begins during embryogenesis. In these first 30 days of life the neural plate and groove are formed to be followed by the development of the primitive neural tube [103]. In the second month of life the rostral end of the neural tube (the prosencephalon) differentiates into the diencephalon, from which the thalami and the hypothalamus are formed, and the telencephalon, which gives rise to the basal ganglia, the lateral ventricles and the cerebral hemispheres [103,104]. It is during this period of ventral induction that neural proliferation and migration begins. The neurones are derived from cells lying in the subependymal region and migrate from there to their ultimate position. The cerebral cortex is derived therefore from cells arising in the periventricular region, with the earliest cells forming the deepest layer of the cortex (layer six) and the later neurones passing through these cells to form the more superficial layers [105,106]. The peak period for neural proliferation is 2–4 months of gestation and for neural migration is 3–5 months. It is not completely clear when neuronal proliferation ceases in the cerebral cortex; however, by the end of the sixth month mitotic figures are no longer observed and the cortex presumably has acquired its full complement of nerve cells [107].

The differentiation and the organization of the cerebral cortex occurs between 24 and 40 weeks of gestational age. At 24 weeks a rapid multiplication of glial cells commences. This is accompanied by the differentiation, alignment and orientation of cortical neurones into identifiable layers. In addition there is the elaboration of neuronal dendritic processes, the formation of synapses between cortical neurones and the establishment of thalamocortical connections [108–110]. The arborization of dendrites is perhaps the most critical factor in the development of the central nervous system since dendrites provide the major part of the membrane surface area for the integration of both excitatory and inhibitory synaptic activity.

It is assumed from animal studies and from detailed recordings in adults that the EEG recorded from scalp electrodes represents the summation of excitatory and inhibitory post-synaptic potentials generated in the superficial cortical neurones. The rhythmicity and the rate of firing of the neurones, however, is influenced by subcortical centres, primarily in the thalamus [111]. It is not surprising therefore to find that there are striking changes in the EEG over this period of rapid differentiation and maturation of the cortical neurones. The changes in the pattern of the EEG in the preterm newborn with increasing gestational age reflect the differentiation of cortical neurones and the development of dendrites and dendritic spines. The appearance of cyclical changes in the pattern of the EEG with sleep and wakefulness, and the synchronization of these rhythms with changes in the pattern of other physiological parameters are thought to correspond with the development of thalamocortical connections. A knowledge of the age-related changes in the EEG and repeated recordings in individual babies will allow the process of cortical maturation to be monitored during this critical period of development.

Maturation of the EEG from 24 to 32 weeks gestational age

The systematic study of the EEG of newly born babies began with the pioneering descriptions of Gibbs and Gibbs in 1950 [112]. The description by Askerinsky and his colleagues [113,114] of the cyclical organization of sleep by the use of polygraphic studies aroused interest in studies of the EEG in the newborn and in the premature infant in relationship to sleep and wakefulness. The healthy full-term infant has since been shown to have well developed and easily recognizable sleep-wake cycles [115]. These states can be identified by the EEG, the polygraphic and the behavioural criteria defined by Prechtl [116], and by Anders and colleagues [117] (Figures 19.12, 19.13 and 19.14). Unlike the term baby, the very preterm baby does not have clearly defined sleep states. This is because there are no consistent temporal relationships between the eye movements, body motility, the pattern of respiration, the variability of the heart rate and the EEG which together define sleep states.

The first signs of behavioural state organization do begin, however, well before 24 weeks of gestational age with the emergence of two distinct patterns of EEG (Figure 19.15). The first pattern, comprising clusters of bursts of high voltage slow wave activity interpersed between periods of suppressed EEG activity, is called *tracé alternant* or burst suppression pattern, and is characteristic of the EEG during quiet sleep in the term baby (Figure 19.14). The second, a continuous EEG of mixed frequencies with a predominance of slow wave activity, is the precursor of the EEG patterns later associated with wakefulness and active sleep in more mature babies (Figure 19.12).

It is often stated that the EEG of the very preterm baby comprises almost entirely the second, discontinuous, pattern with little or no continuous activity [119]. This

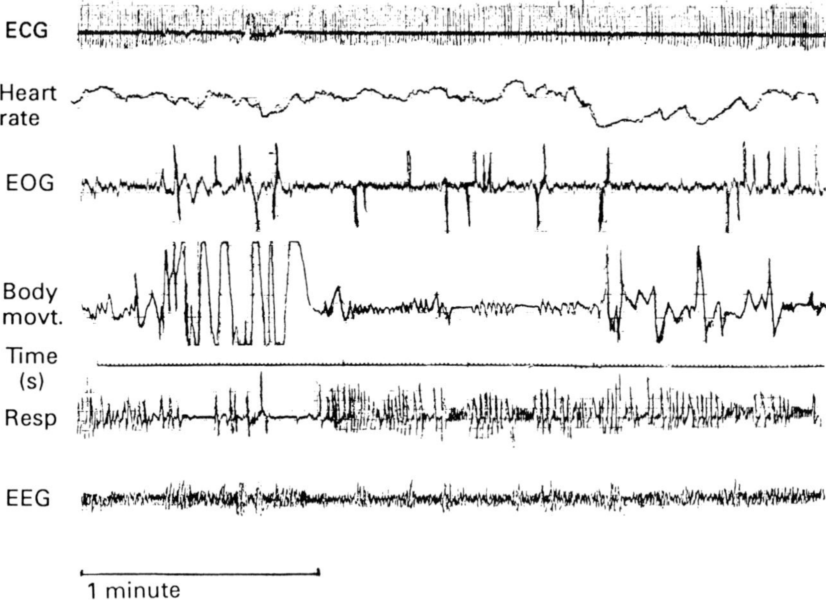

Figure 19.12 A polygraphic record during active sleep or wakefulness in a term baby. It shows an irregular heart rate, frequent eye movements, body movements, an irregular respiration rate and a fast, mixed voltage EEG

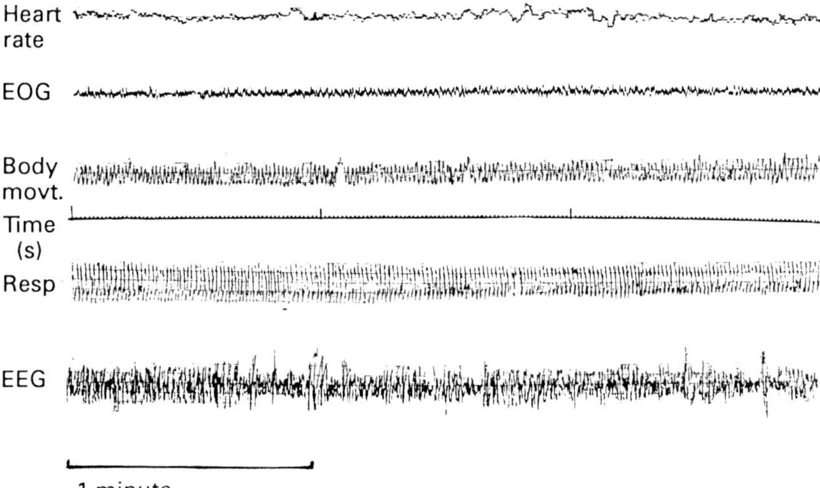

Figure 19.13 A polygraphic record during quiet sleep in a term baby. It shows a regular heart rate, an absence of eye movements, no body movements, a regular respiration rate and a slow high voltage EEG

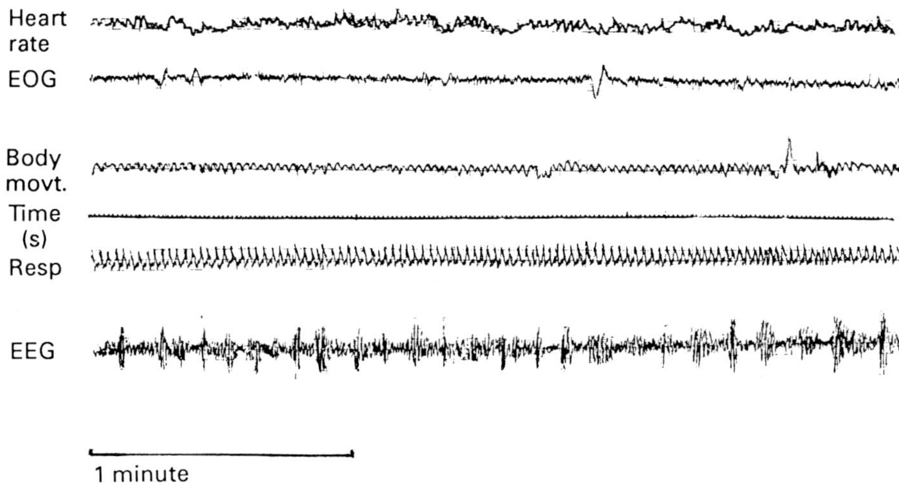

Figure 19.14 A polygraphic record during quiet sleep in a term baby. It shows a regular heart rate, an absence of eye movements, no body movements, a regular respiration rate and a discontinuous, *tracé alternant* pattern of the EEG

conclusion, however, has been based either on the findings of early studies of the EEG when such preterm babies were previable and the subjects were very ill and subsequently died, or from recordings made from sleeping infants. Continuous electrical activity has in fact been recorded in the pons of human fetuses from as early as 10 weeks. A second, intermittent pattern of EEG was recorded from 17 weeks gestational age in the rostral part of the brainstem and from the hippocampus [120]. Thus the two distinct patterns of the EEG can be recorded from fetuses well before 24 weeks gestational age.

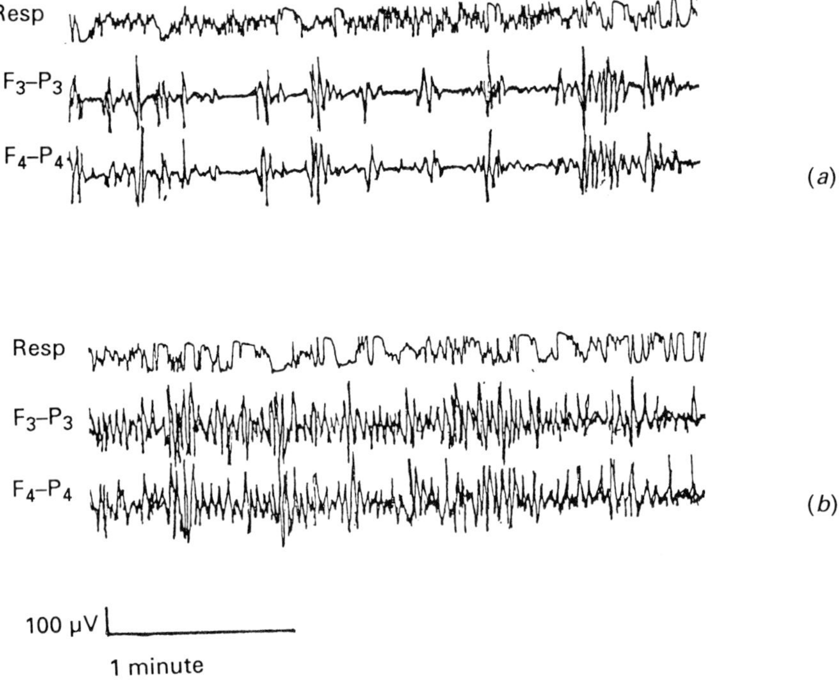

Figure 19.15 EEG recorded from a 24-week gestation healthy preterm infant showing the two patterns of the EEG; (*a*) a discontinuous *tracé alternant* pattern and (*b*) a continuous EEG

Recently it has become possible to make continuous recordings of the EEG over many days [121] in healthy preterm babies. These studies have demonstrated that although the EEG of babies born as prematurely as 24 weeks gestational age is predominantly discontinuous, there are periods of continuous activity particularly during wakefulness [122]. The duration of individual epochs of continuous activity and the percentage of the total EEG which is continuous increase progressively as the child matures and there is a reciprocal reduction in the duration of the discontinuous activity so that the EEG changes rapidly from being predominantly discontinuous at 24 weeks to predominantly continuous by 28 weeks (Table 19.1).

While the two basic patterns of EEG exist in very preterm babies there is little synchronization of the EEG with the other parameters which together define sleep states in the older baby. Thus eye movements, body movements, irregularity of the respiratory pattern and spontaneous fluctuations of the skin resistance can and do occur independently and with either pattern of the EEG. It is not until 32 weeks of gestation that organization of these parameters into recognizable sleep states begins; from then until 40 weeks post-conceptional age the interrelations between different elements become more clearly defined and organized into the two sleep states termed active and quiet sleep. The two sleep states appear to mature independently and studies by Dreyfus-Brisac [123] show that active sleep is seen in its typical form by 35 weeks and quiet sleep by 37 weeks gestational age.

The measurement of the relative durations of continuous and discontinuous EEG activity in any individual baby requires continuous recording of the EEG for at least 24 h and this may not be practical for the clinical assessment of very preterm babies.

Table 19.1 The duration of continuous and *tracé alternant* (discontinuous) EEG activity in relation to gestational age

Gestation (weeks)	*Total CA/24 h* (h)		*Duration of epochs of CA* (min)		*Duration of epochs of TA* (min)	
	Median	*Range*	*Median*	*Range*	*Mean*	*± 1s.d.*
26	10.5	8.9–11.5	13	10–36	21	1.5
28	16.7	8.3–16.9	17	12–36	19	1.1
30	18.5	18.1–20.0	25	15–38	15	0.9
32	19.4	18.0–21.2	38	25–52	12	0.75

CA = continuous activity; TA = *tracé alternant*.
Table adapted from Eyre, Nanei and Wilkinson [122]

There are, however, changes in the background activity of the EEG which are age dependent and which also reflect the increasing maturity of the cerebral cortex. Two variables, the progressive changes in the *tracé alternant* pattern and the incidence of delta brush, can easily be quantified from short recordings of the EEG and these provide useful indices of cortical maturity.

Changes in the background activity of the discontinuous EEG with increasing gestational age

There are progressive changes in the discontinuous or *tracé alternant* pattern of the EEG with increasing gestational age (Figure 19.16). Perhaps the most striking change is a progressive reduction in the duration of the individual periods of suppression between the bursts of the high voltage slow waves [122,124]. The mean durations of these intervals in relation to gestational age can be calculated and are tabulated in Table 19.2. In addition to the longer mean duration of suppression between bursts, a much greater variability of this duration about the mean is found in very preterm babies, and this too decreases markedly with increasing maturity.

In contrast to the duration of suppression, the duration of each burst of high voltage slow waves does not change with increasing gestation and remains between 2 and 5 s [122,124]. The amplitude of the high voltage slow wave activity during bursts does, however, change with gestational age; it is significantly greater in very preterm babies in comparison to more mature babies (Table 19.2). The mean voltage does not change, however, until 31 weeks gestation and, from then until term there is a progressive decrease from a mean of 440 μV at 31 weeks to 130 μV at 42 weeks. The variability of the maximum voltage is much greater in very preterm babies and this variability decreases significantly over the same period.

To summarize these data: with increasing maturity the duration of the suppressed intervals becomes shorter, the difference between the amplitude of the activity in the suppressed periods and the bursts becomes less marked and the minute to variability of the pattern becomes less pronounced. The overall tendency is for the *discontinuous* pattern to become essentially more *continuous* in nature with increasing gestational age; in fact this discontinuous pattern of EEG is no longer seen in the EEG of a normal child from three months after term.

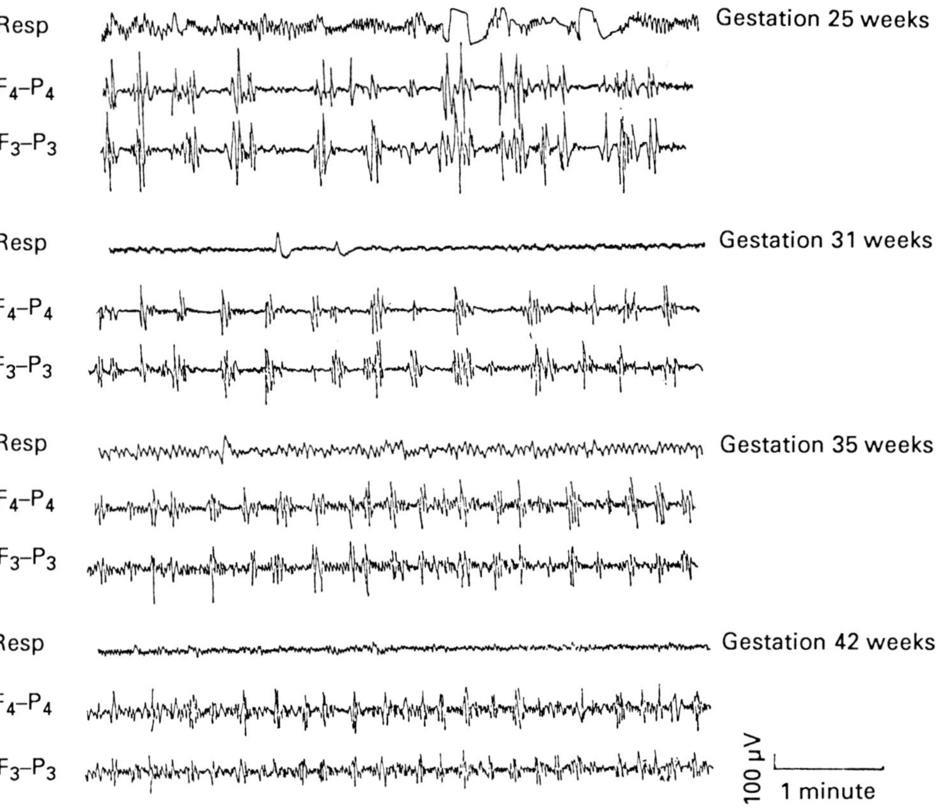

Figure 19.16 Discontinuous or *tracé alternant* EEG recorded from healthy preterm babies illustrating the progressive changes with increasing maturity

Table 19.2 The characteristics of the *tracé alternant* in relation to gestational age

Gestation	*Interval of suppression* (s)		*Duration of bursts* (s)		*Maximum voltage in bursts* (μV)	
(weeks)	*Mean*	± 1*s.d.*	*Mean*	± 1*s.d.*	*Mean*	± 1*s.d.*
26	26	7.3	3.3	0.7	420	75
28	24	6.5	2.9	0.5	432	80
30	16	4.1	3.0	0.4	435	70
32	13	3.1	2.5	0.6	300	65

Table adapted from Eyre, Nanei and Wilkinson [122]

Delta brush

Delta brush is the name given to high frequency spindle-like activity which is superimposed on slow wave delta activity (Figure 19.17). While the origin of this activity is unknown, this pattern of activity is recognized to be one of the characteristic signatures of the EEG of very preterm babies [125,126]. The presence and the frequency of the occurrence of the delta brush is highly dependent upon gestational age and so it provides a useful index of the degree of cortical maturity. Delta brush is

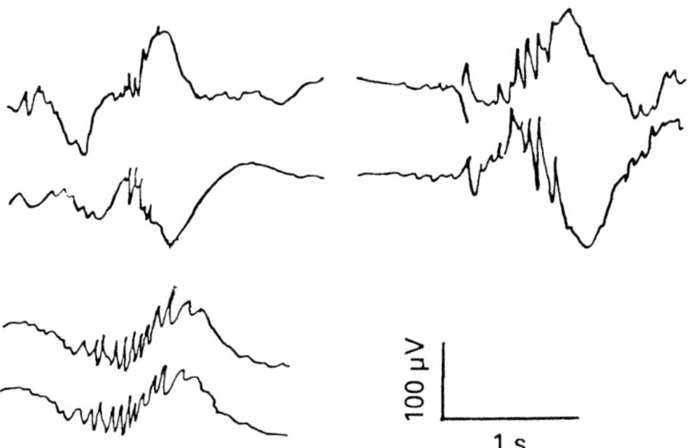

Figure 19.17 Delta brush recorded from a 31-week gestation baby

seen only very infrequently, less than once in 5 min of EEG recording in babies of 27 or less weeks gestation [124]; from 27–31 weeks the frequency of its occurrence increases rapidly so that by 31 weeks it occurs as often as 30–50 times in a 5 min period of EEG recording [126]. The incidence of delta brush then becomes progressively smaller and it is rarely seen in the EEG of a baby of greater than 36 weeks gestation (1–2 delta brushes in 5 min).

The data presented concerning the pattern of the normal EEG in relation to gestational age clearly show that there are progressive changes which are a reflection of increasing cerebral maturity. There is a wide normal range at any given gestational age and so it is not possible to assess an individual baby's cortical maturity from one single EEG recording. A longitudinal study of the EEG will, however, allow the measurement electrophysiologically of the increasing maturity of the cerebral cortex in an individual baby [126].

The significance of abnormality in the EEG of very preterm babies

The premature infant's brain is very vulnerable to a variety of stresses and insults. This is reflected in the high incidence of EEG abnormalities recorded from these infants in a neonatal intensive care nursery. It is beyond the scope of this review to discuss in detail every type of EEG abnormality associated with neurological illness or complications in the premature infant. This would not in any case be helpful because the abnormalities are non-specific and only rarely, if ever, can an aetiological diagnosis be assigned to a particular EEG pattern. Instead evidence is presented to support the proposal that abnormalities in the EEG provide a means to assess acutely the severity of a brain injury even in these very preterm infants.

The value of the EEG in the prediction of the long-term neurological outcome of neonates who have sustained a variety of brain injuries has been assessed many times [125,127–129]. Although a statistical relationship between the EEG findings and the long-term outcome has been established in these studies, the EEG findings proved unreliable in correctly predicting the outcome for at least 25% of babies [125]. This unreliability has made the EEG an unsatisfactory method to assess the prognosis of individual babies in the clinical situation. The majority of the studies, however, used

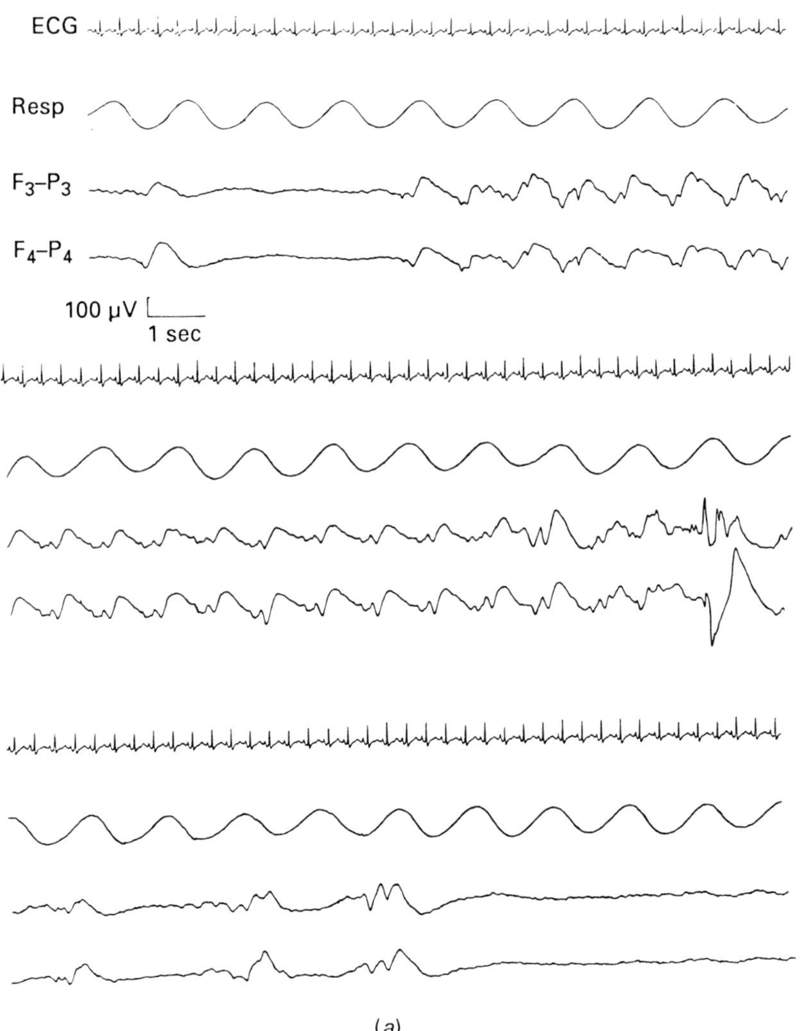

Figure 19.18 (*a*) Electroencephalographic seizure activity recorded in a 26-week gestation infant showing rhythmical sharp and slow wave activity; (*b*) Electroencephalographic seizure activity recorded in a 24-week gestation infant showing a burst of rhythmical activity of a single frequency

intermittent and short recordings of the EEG. This made it impossible to determine in which babies the EEG abnormality was only present transiently and in which there was a much longer period of EEG abnormality. It is likely that transient abnormalities have less prognostic significance than similar abnormalities which persist for long periods. The use of intermittent EEG recordings is likely to introduce an error which interferes significantly with the prediction of outcome in individual babies.

We have recently completed a study to determine if data obtained prospectively from the continuous recording of the EEG during the period of acute illness and the intensive care could be predictive of the eventual outcome in babies of all gestational ages, including very preterm babies [122]. In this study the EEG of babies who

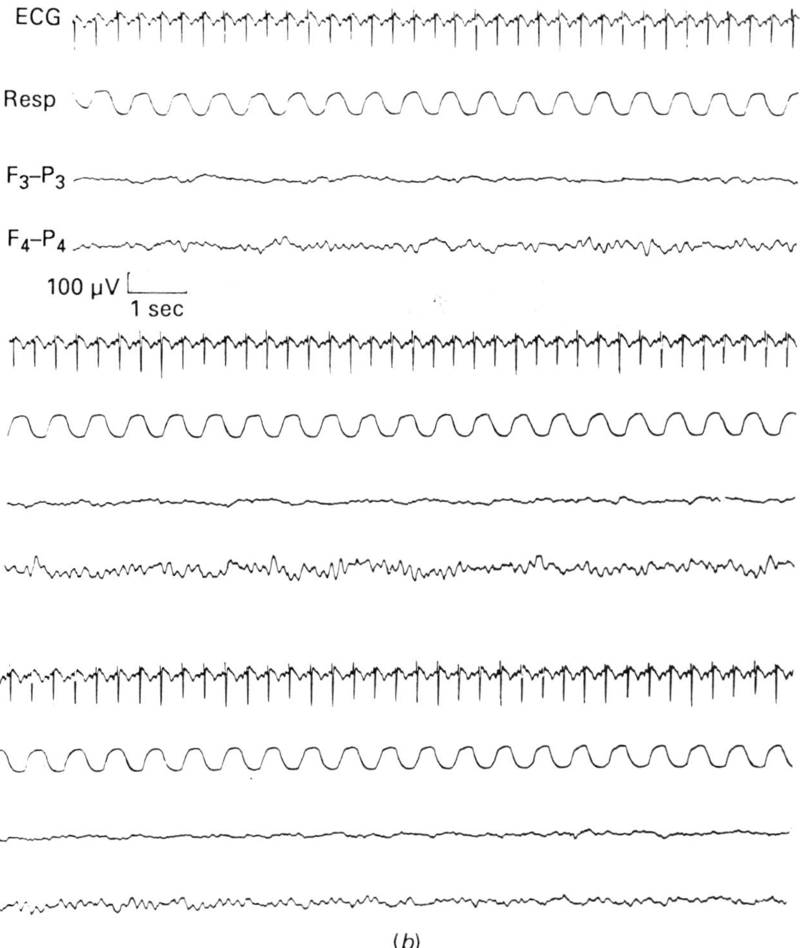

(b)

required ventilation from within 5 h after birth was recorded continuously while they received intensive care; 35 of these babies were less than 32 weeks in gestation (range 25–31 weeks) and their data are presented below. The EEG was analysed for the presence and the total duration of electroencephalographic seizure activity and for the degree and duration of abnormalities in the background activity. The results of the EEG analyses were then correlated with the findings of an independent assessment of neuro-developmental outcome at 18 months.

Seizures

Seizures in the newborn, particularly in the very preterm infant, may be very difficult to recognize from clinical signs alone. Subclinical seizures have frequently been reported in the newborn [119]. When there are clinical signs accompanying electrographic seizure acivity, these are frequently atypical and subtle, e.g. eye movements, abnormal postures or apnoea. This makes diagnosis difficult. It has been proposed that seizures in the very preterm baby are much less common than in more mature babies because the preterm brain is too immature to sustain synchronized electrical activity. In addition, because of immature myelination, it has been proposed that the preterm baby rarely has generalized seizure activity.

In contrast to the clinical diagnosis, electrographic seizure activity in the newborn is easily recognized. There are two basic forms: the sudden onset of rhythmical sharp and slow waves (Figure 19.18*a*) or the paroxysmal appearance of rhythmic activity of a single frequency within the frequency range 5–13 Hz (Figure 19.18*b*). The spike and wave pattern typical of seizure activity in older children and adults is not seen in the newborn presumably because the immature myelination of pathways slows the conduction of spikes to scalp electrodes.

In the 35 babies of less than 32 weeks gestation seizure activity was recorded in 13 (37%). The seizures began between 2 and 63 h after birth with a median time of onset of 10 h. Ten of the 13 babies began to have seizure activity within 24 h after birth. The seizures persisted for between one and five days; however in 11 of the 13 babies (85%) the seizures were present for less than 72 h. The total duration of seizure activity for each baby was greatest on the first day after seizure onset and decreased markedly over the subsequent days.

These results suggest that seizures represent an acute reaction to a perinatal insult. Discriminant analysis identified five perinatal factors strongly predictive of seizure onset:

(1) The degree and duration of abnormal background EEG activity.
(2) The Apgar scores at 1 and 5 min.
(3) The maximum percentage of oxygen required.
(4) The total number of pneumothoraces.
(5) The lowest blood pH measured.

These data suggest that ischaemic hypoxic encephalopathy was the commonest cause of seizures during the period of intensive care of these very preterm babies. In total 755 separate episodes of seizure activity were recorded in these 13 babies; 36% of the seizures had a focal onset and remained confined to one hemisphere, 63% were primarily or became secondarily generalized. No significant differences could be found between these very preterm babies and the more mature babies in the study when the incidence, the predictive factors, the duration and the time course of seizure activity were considered.

A detailed assessment was made of the babies by an independent observer at 18 months. Nine had died, nine of the survivors had neuro-developmental abnormalities and 17 were normal. Both the occurrence and the duration of electrographic seizures were strongly related to outcome (Table 19.3). Seizures during the acute period of illness predicted death or abnormal survival with a sensitivity of 85%, a specificity of 94%, a positive predictive value of 0.92 and a negative predictive value of 72%.

Table 19.3 The incidence and duration of seizures in relation to outcome

Outcome	*No. of patients with no seizures*	*No. of patients with seizures*	*Mean total duration of seizure activity* (h)
Died	1	8	3.70
Abnormal	5	4	1.31
Normal	16	1	0.49

Table 19.4 The duration of normal and abnormal EEG in relation to outcome at 18 months

Outcome	*Mean percentage of the EEG*			
	Normal	*Mildly abnormal*	*Moderately abnormal*	*Severely abnormal*
Normal	82	13	6	0
Abnormal	45	17	16	17
Died	0	3	34	67

The background EEG was classified into normal, mildly, moderately and severely abnormal activity and the total duration of each was measured during the recording period. These durations were then subsequently related to the neuro-developmental outcome (Table 19.4). The strong relationship between the degree and duration of abnormality in the EEG and the neuro-developmental outcome makes the quantitative analysis of an EEG recorded continuously during the period of acute illness useful for the assessment of the severity of the brain injury sustained.

Conclusion

The recording of the EEG in newborn babies is relatively simple and non-invasive. The interpretation of the EEG is not, however, simple and requires considerable experience. The rapid development of the cortex in babies less than 32 weeks in gestation results in dramatic changes in the pattern of the EEG with increasing gestational age. Longitudinal studies of the EEG in individual babies therefore will allow the process of cortical maturation and development to be followed electrophysiologically. In ill babies, acute abnormalities in the EEG are not usually diagnostic of the aetiology of the brain injury; the severity of the abnormality and its duration, however, are useful in the acute assessment of the severity of the injury sustained.

IV. CRANIAL ULTRASONOGRAPHY

Richard W. I. Cooke

Real time ultrasound scanning of the cranium of newborn infants was introduced less than a decade ago but has rapidly become accepted as the best technique for visualizing the brain in this age group. This is especially true when one considers the infant under 1000 g, because of their general fragility and their small size relative to the resolving power of equipment such as CT scanners. The details of the techniques used to obtain suitable images of the brain with ultrasound in the newborn have been widely described [130–132], and mention here will only be of points especially relevant to the ELBW infant.

Technique

Although with a little skill information may be obtained on brain scan with almost any type of ultrasound imaging device, a real time sector scanner with 5 and 7.5 MHz transducers is required to produce the most useful images in the tiniest infant. Most sector scanners are mechanical devices although an increasing number of phased array devices are being produced. The latter have the advantage of a steadier image and no moving parts, but often have fewer lines per sector and therefore a poorer lateral resolution. The linear resolution is higher with higher frequency transducers, although the actual resolution achieved will depend on a number of image processing factors and in practice the difference in resolution between a 5 MHz and 7.5 MHz transducer may not be as great as theoretically expected.

The use of a sector format is essential in ELBW infants if more than the midline structures of the brain are to be seen. The transfontanelle approach produces the clearest images, and since most ELBW infants have a relatively large anterior fontanelle this is usually no problem. By nature of the way in which the sector image is presented, structures very close to the transducer may be hidden in bright echoes from the scalp. The surface of the brain beneath the fontanelle may be more easily seen if a spacer device is used to provide an offset of 2–3 cm. This at its simplest is a water-filled rubber glove, but commercially available slabs of jelly are more convenient to use although a great deal more expensive. Small superficial collections of blood are only visible by such means.

Images are best recorded on a digital image recorder using silver coated plastic film. 'Polaroid' prints and videofilm are less convenient and more expensive. For both clinical and research purposes it is best to record each examination in descriptive terms as well as by a representative series of photographs. At the minimum, mid-coronal and right and left parasaggital 'cuts' should be recorded.

The purpose of scanning

Ultrasound scanning in ELBW infants can provide clinical diagnostic, management, and prognostic information. Diagnostic information includes gestational age assessment, congenital malformations of the brain, periventricular and superficial cerebral haemorrhage, cerebral infarction, periventricular leucomalacia, hydrocephaly and ventriculitis. Evidence of haemorrhage or hydrocephalus may be an adequate explanation for convulsions or clinical deterioration at the bedside. The management of hydrocephaly is aided by having daily measurements of the ventricular size as a guide to the effectiveness of treatment, and the presence of extensive bilateral brain destruction may, together with clinical neurological data, enable the discontinuation of intensive therapy in some cases. Long-term follow-up from a number of centres now enables a reasonably accurate prognosis to be given with regard to neurological and cognitive development in ELBW survivors [133–135].

Ultrasound diagnosis

When using cranial ultrasound in the very preterm infant, it is important to be aware of the differences which exist in anatomy between such infants and more mature ones. In the very preterm infant the brain itself is much less reflective of sound and appears consequently less detailed and darker. Structures such as the choroid plexus in comparison appear relatively more reflective and brighter, and may be confused with blood clot in the lateral ventricles. The lateral ventricles are larger relative to their size in term infants and are clearly seen, although the posterior horns of the lateral ventricles do not develop until after about 30 weeks of gestation. The immature brain itself is rather smaller than the skull and so the subarachnoid space is relatively larger and easily seen around the brain (Figure 19.19). Blood clot from subarachnoid haemorrhage not normally visible in older infants can be seen especially if it is in the lateral sulcus or the interhemispheric fissure (Figure 19.20*a* and *b*). Tangential views of the brain in a parasagittal direction used to show the surface of the parietal and temporal lobes appear almost featureless in infants of under 27 weeks of gestation, except for the lateral sulcus. Gyral development may be used as a guide to gestational age (Figure 19.21*a* and *b*).

Several cerebral malformations are relatively easy to diagnose using ultrasound. In many cases the diagnosis may be made clinically. The presence and extent of hydrocephaly in conjunction with meningomyelocoele is easily assessed. Holoprosencephaly is not uncommon in ELBW infants and not always immediately clinically apparent. The ultrasound appearances are, however, very striking (Figure 19.22). Although porencephaly is regularly recognized as a consequence of postnatal cerebral insults, it is also seen in otherwise fit ELBW infants. Figure 19.23 shows the brain of an 800 g girl with extensive cystic development in the parietal and temporal lobes on one side and in the temporal lobe on the other. This was associated with the spontaneous abortion of the twin sibling at 16 weeks of the pregnancy. There were no external or neurological signs in this otherwise apparently well infant.

Perinatal infections may give rise to characteristic ultrasound appearances. Intrauterine viral infections such as cytomegalovirus may produce hydrocephaly, but also periventricular calcification which may be obvious on ultrasound before it can be seen on X-ray (Figure 19.24). Infants with hydrocephaly from malformation or as the

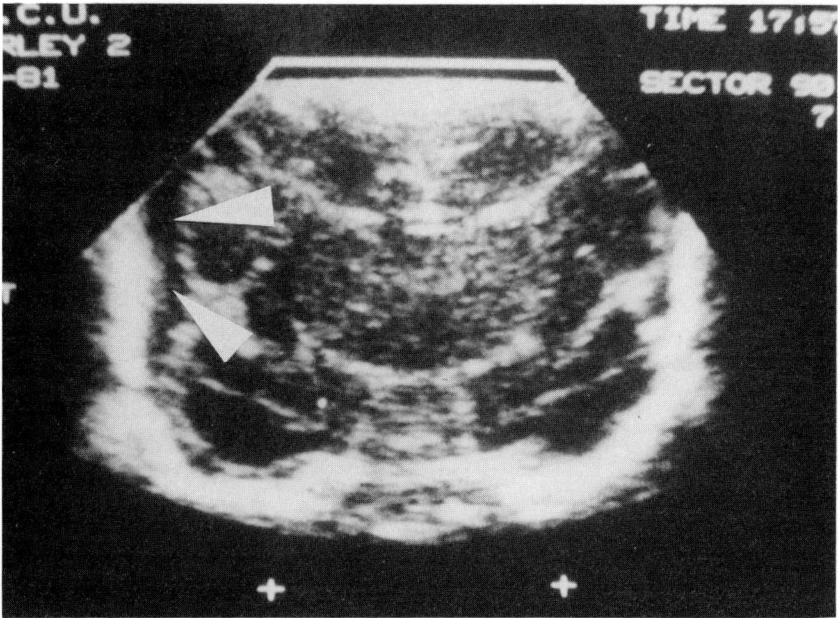

Figure 19.19 Coronal scan of brain of 26-week infant showing wide subarachnoid space

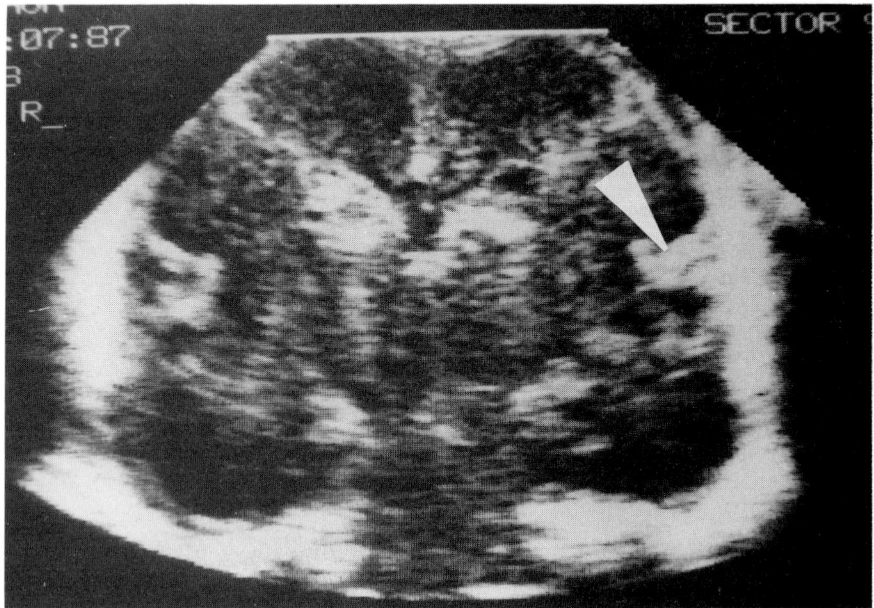

(*a*)

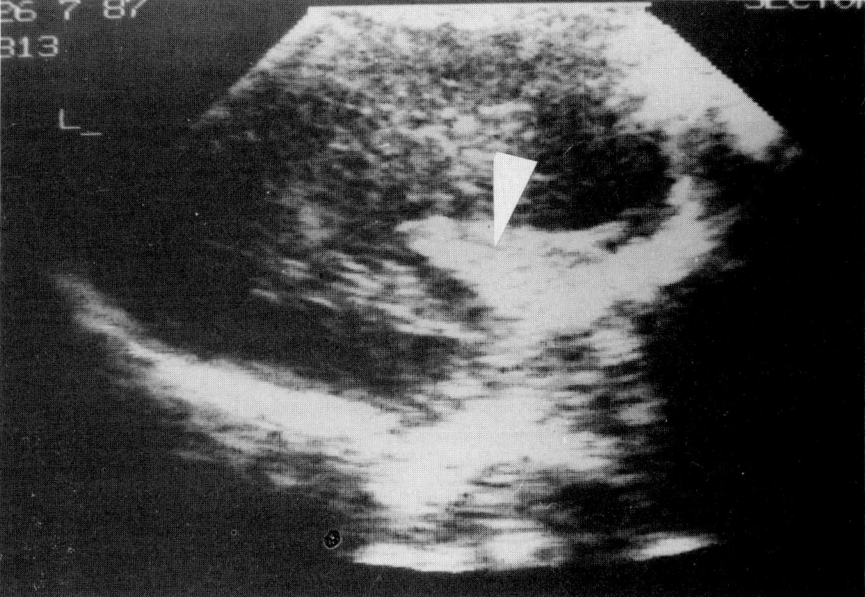

(*b*)

Figure 19.20 (*a*) Coronal and (*b*) tangential parasagittal scans of brain of 25-week infant showing blood clot in lateral sulcus

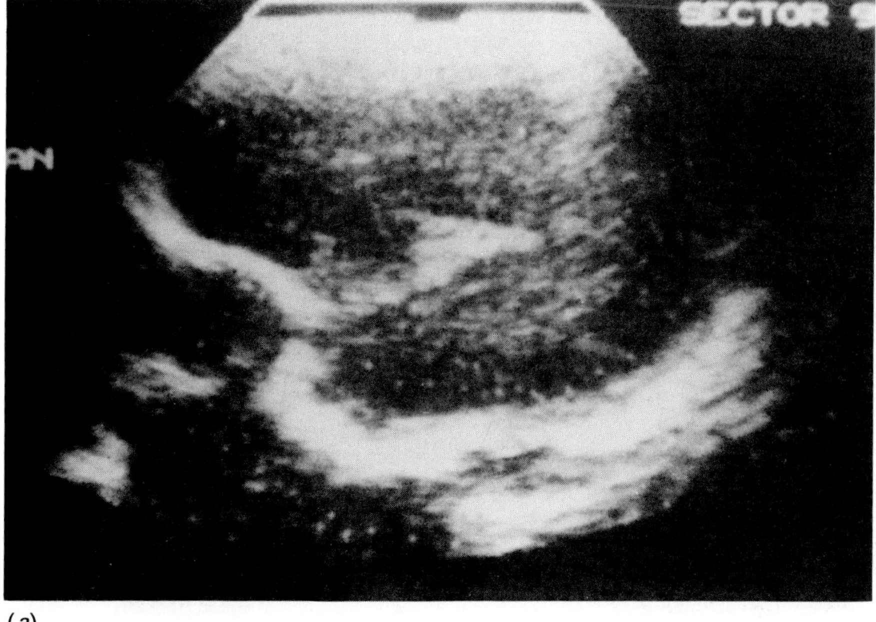

(*a*)

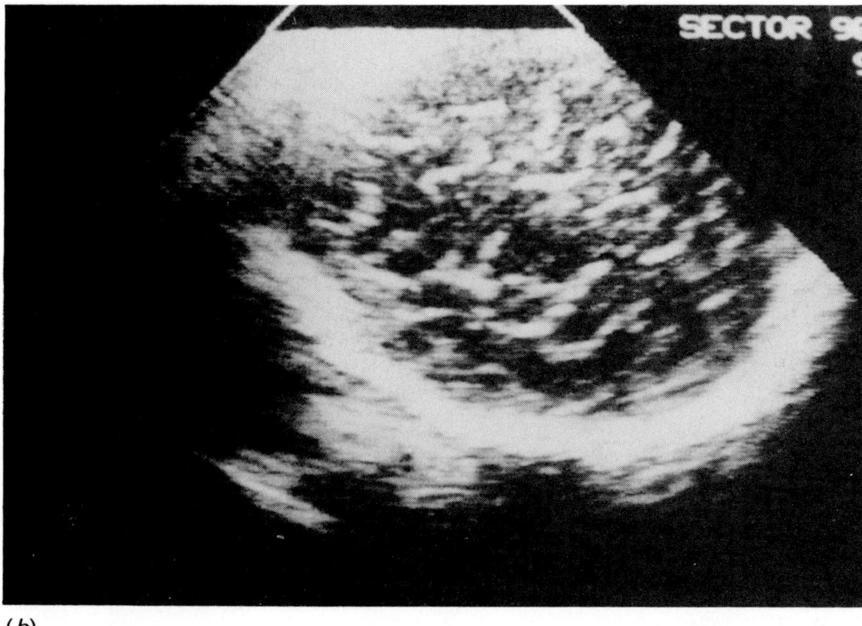

(*b*)

Figure 19.21 Tangential parasagittal scans of the parietal and temporal lobes of (*a*) a 26-week and (*b*) a term infant

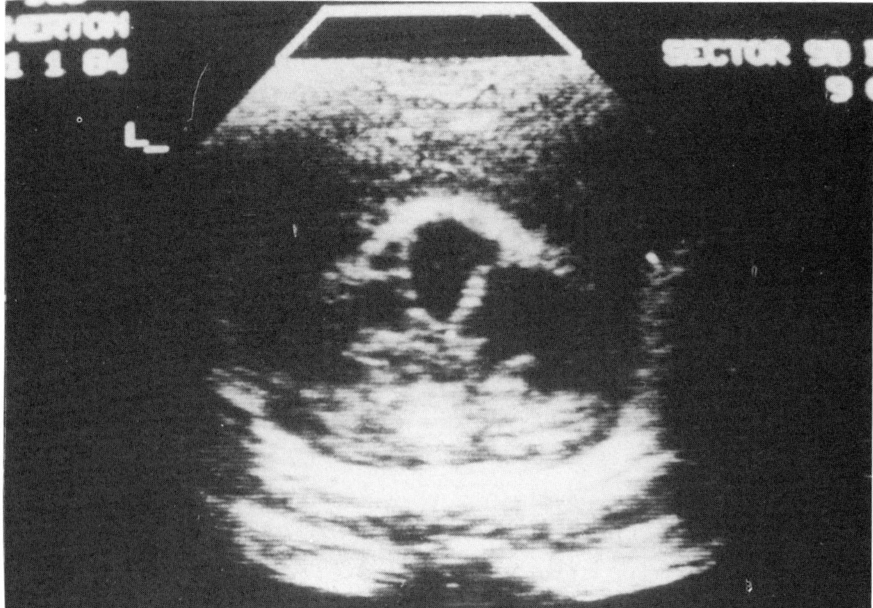

Figure 19.22 Coronal scan of brain of preterm infant with holoprosencephaly. Note the central single ventricle

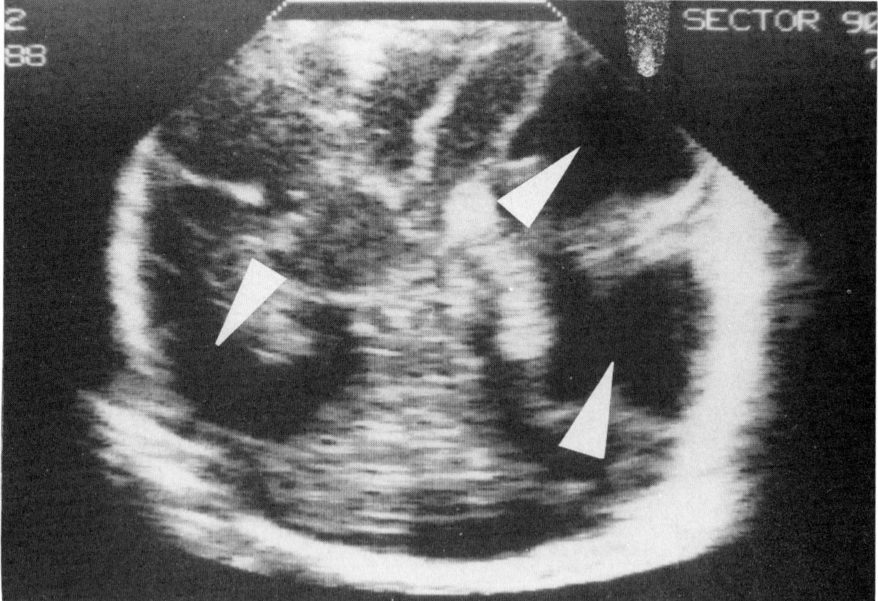

Figure 19.23 Coronal scan of brain of 27-week infant at 1 h of age. Note atrophy of parietal and temporal lobes

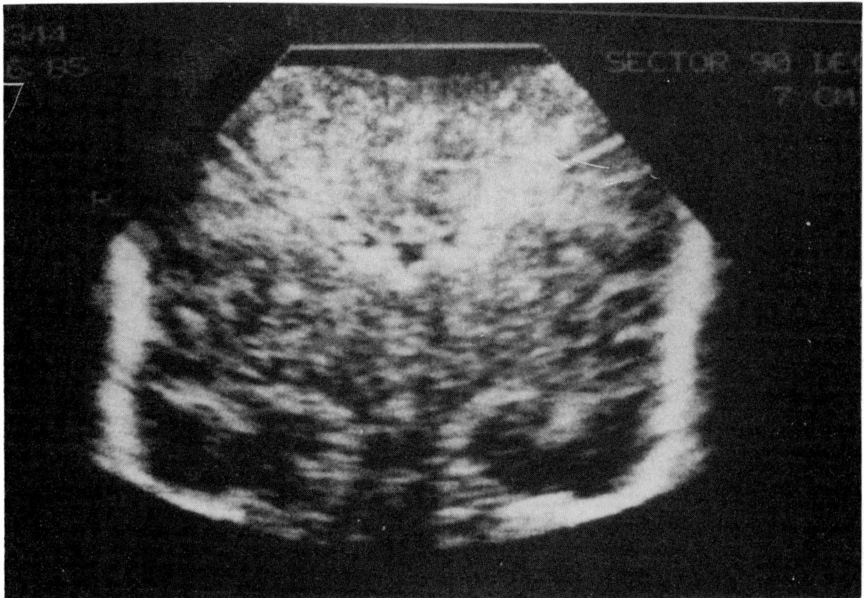

Figure 19.24 Coronal scan of brain of 1000 g infant with congenital cytomegalovirus infection. Note periventricular echoes from cerebral calcification

result of intraventricular haemorrhage may develop ventriculitis. In the early stages a bright periventricular halo may be seen, and later either intraventricular strands of fibrin crossing the ventricles (Figure 19.25), or debris resembling snowflakes when the infant's head is moved.

The various appearances of periventricular haemorrhage in preterm infants are well described and do not differ substantially in the ELBW infant. More recently interest has focused on periventricular leucomalacia which is very common in these infants, and in particular its early ultrasound appearances. Small flare-like echoes are frequently seen extending from the lateral angles of the lateral ventricles on the first few days of life (Figure 19.26). Many of these fade early and appear to be of little consequence. Their aetiology is uncertain. In some cases these 'flares' are brighter and persist for a week or more, frequently resulting in localized cyst formation at 2–3 weeks of age (Figure 19.27). These are the appearances of early periventricular leucomalacia. The areas most often affected as seen on a parasagittal scan are frontal and occipital. Cyst formation may be minimal and the cysts fill in after a month or two, or they may be much more extensive and even extend well into the cerebral subcortical areas (Figure 19.28*a* and *b*). When such major lesions are seen, and especially when they occur bilaterally, cortical blindness, spastic quadriplegia and severe developmental delay are usually seen. Gross ventricular enlargement is easily seen on ultrasound and may reflect hydrocephaly with a raised intraventricular pressure, or simply local periventricular atrophy usually with a normal pressure. In the case of hydrocephaly the ventricular enlargement is smooth and balloon-like, but is irregular and 'craggy' in the case of atrophy (Figure 19.29*a* and *b*). Both states may coexist, however. Further evidence of periventricular cerebral atrophy may often be seen in the form of small periventricular cysts. These may not be evident when the hydrocephaly is rapidly progressive, but appear after it has been treated by drainage

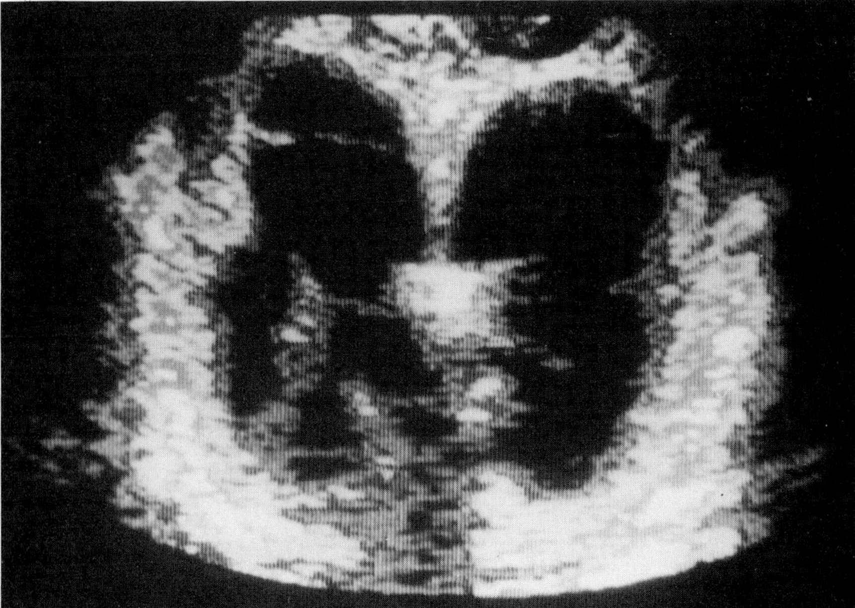

Figure 19.25 Coronal scan of brain of 880 g infant with ventriculitis showing strands of fibrin in lateral ventricles

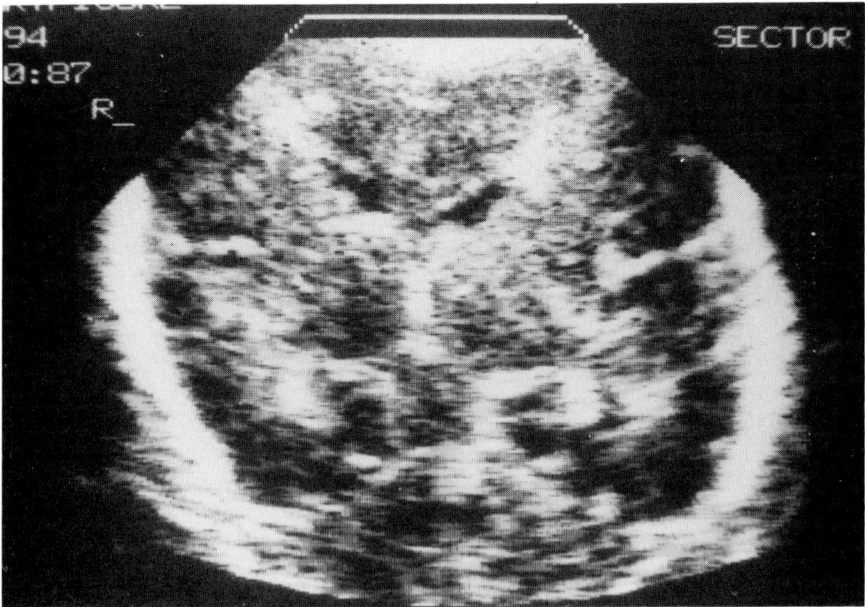

Figure 19.26 Coronal scan of brain showing 'flares' at upper angles of the lateral ventricles

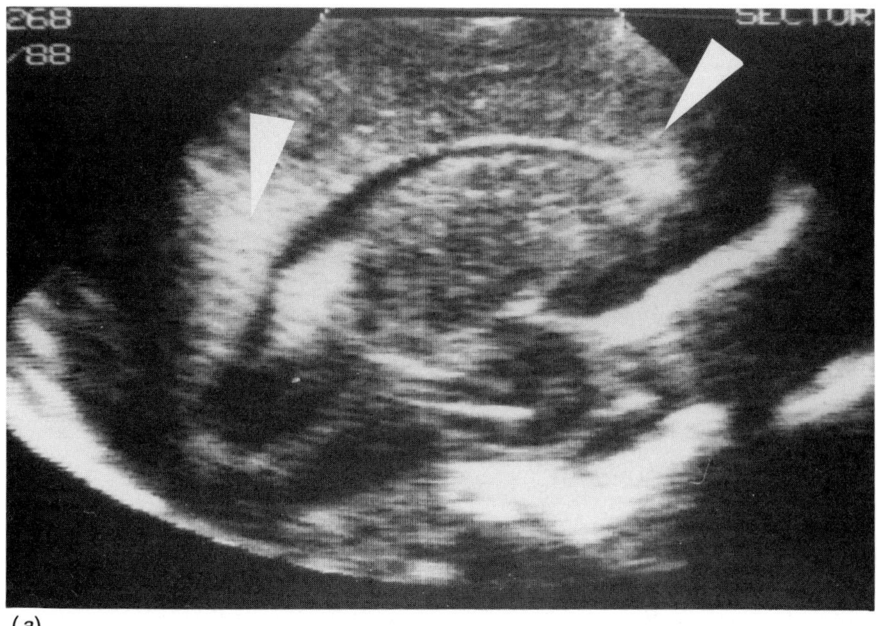

(*a*)

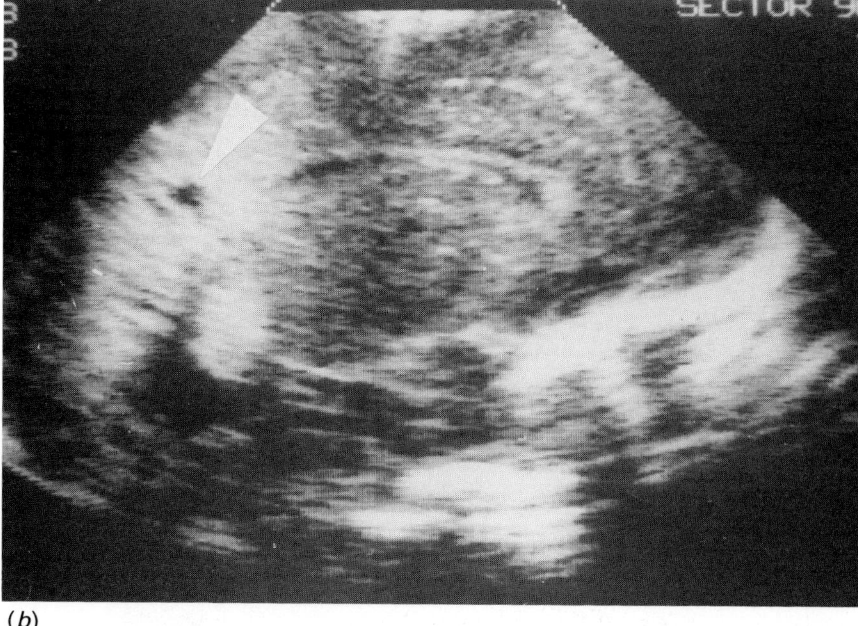

(*b*)

Figure 19.27 Parasagittal scans of brain of 27-week infant showing (*a*) two areas of increased echo (flare) at day 3 and (*b*) an area of cystic degeneration three weeks later in the occipital area at the site of the early flare

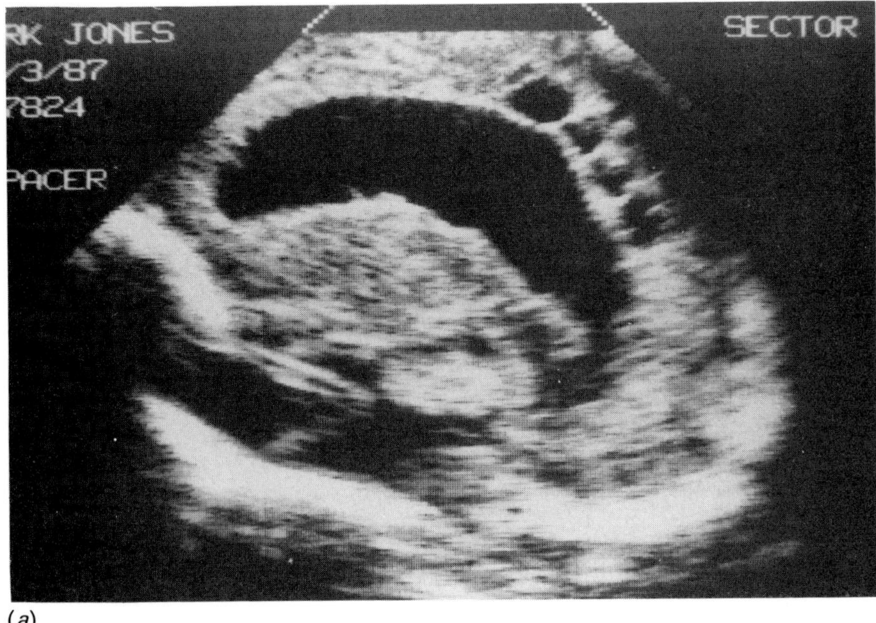

(*a*)

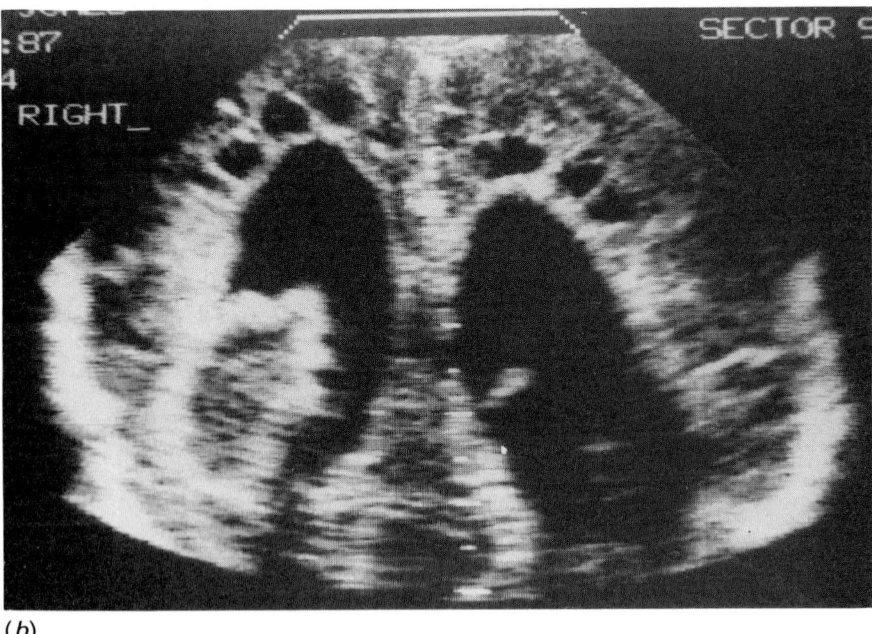

(*b*)

Figure 19.28 (*a*) Parasagittal and (*b*) coronal scans showing extensive periventricular cystic leucomalacia

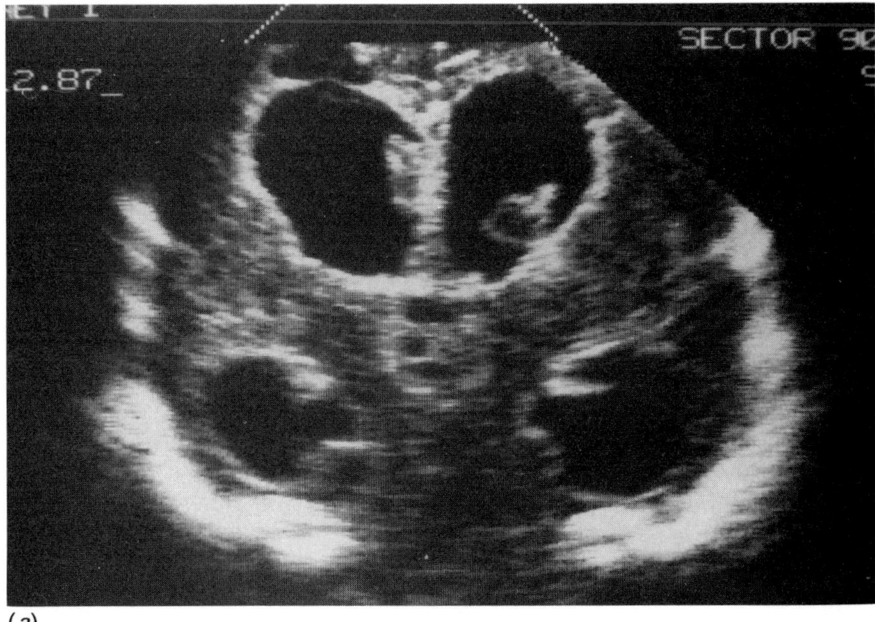

(*a*)

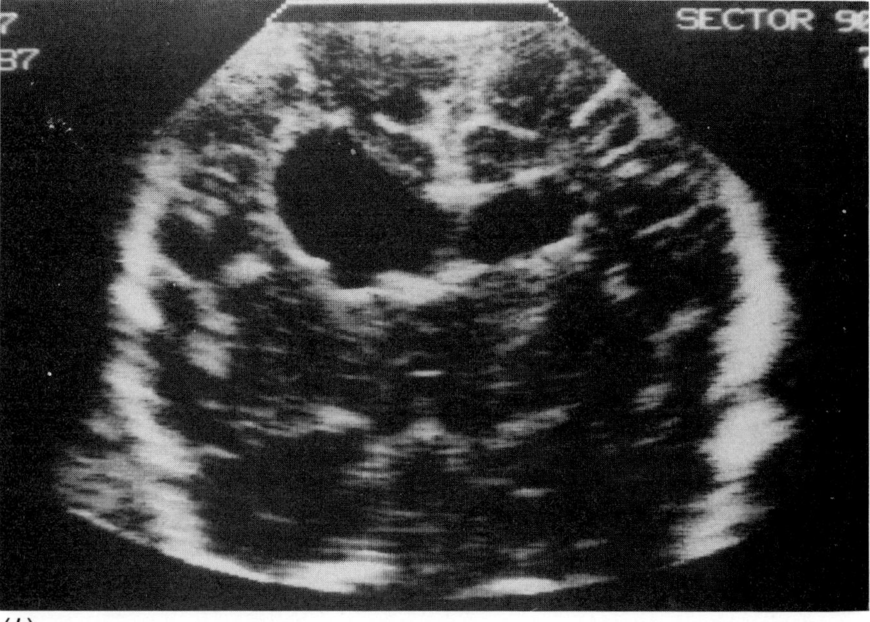

(*b*)

Figure 19.29 Coronal scans showing ventricular enlargement due to (*a*) post-haemorrhagic hydrocephalus and (*b*) periventricular atrophy

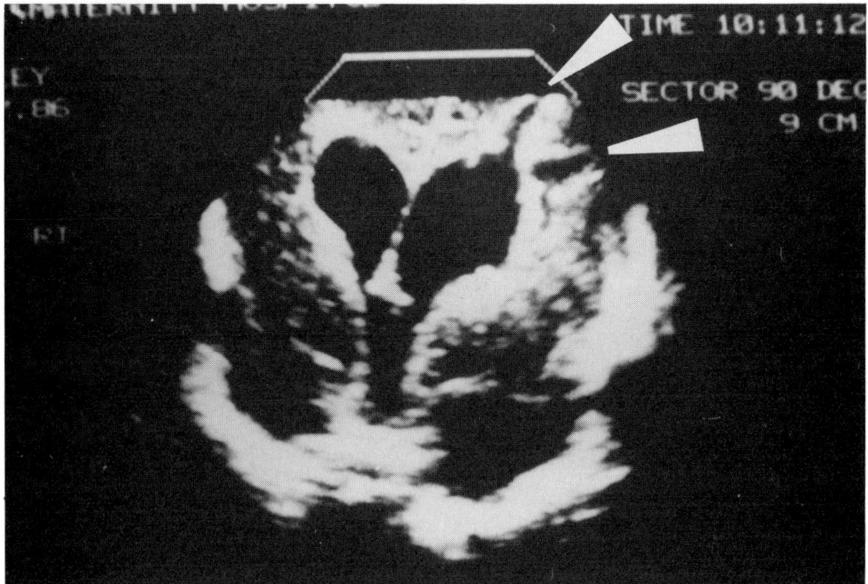

(*a*)

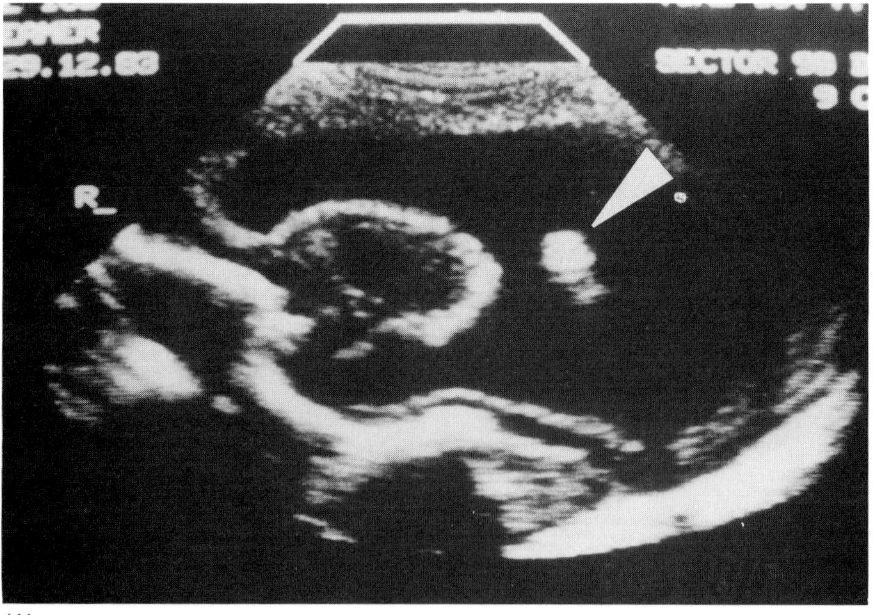

(*b*)

Figure 19.30 (*a*) Coronal scan showing needle tracks following repeated ventricular taps to relieve hydrocephaly. (*b*) Parasagittal scan showing catheter following insertion of ventriculoperitoneal shunt

or shunting. Ultrasound may be useful in the monitoring of such procedures, showing their effectiveness or otherwise, and some of the complications that may result (Figure 19.30*a* and *b*).

Perhaps the greatest value of cerebral ultrasound is in neurological prognosis. In the acute stage of neonatal management, ultrasound apearances usually only confirm the clinical diagnosis of extensive brain injury and allow cessation of intensive care to be considered. In infants without parenchymal lesions on ultrasound most follow-up studies show the risk of major developmental problems to be less than 5%, allowing the clinician to be confident in reassuring parents of good outcome in the majority of infants at discharge. Details of outcome relating to specific lesions seen on ultrasound have only been published for infants of under 1500 g or 32 weeks gestation [133–135], although these are not likely to be much different in infants of under 1000 g. The main difference is that the mortality of ELBW infants with major lesions is much higher, and so proportionately fewer disabled survivors with these lesions are seen in ELBW infants. Haemorrhages into the cerebral ventricles which do not involve the parenchyma are regarded as relatively benign by most workers, although intraventricular haemorrhage may be associated with localized secondary parenchymal extension in many cases which is associated with poorer outcome.

Parenchymal unilateral cystic lesions are followed by major disabilities in over 60% of cases, mostly spastic hemiplegias. Bilateral cystic lesions are almost invariably followed by major disabilities and these may be multiple and severe. The results from neonatal cerebral ultrasound are proving valuable as a method of assessing the probable long-term effects of new procedures in neonatal care as well as a method for identifying high risk groups for follow-up purposes. Future developments are likely to include more precise delineation of minor lesions, allowing prognoses to be more accurate.

V. TREATMENT OF NEUROLOGICAL DISORDERS

Andrew Whitelaw

Whereas resuscitation and mechanical ventilation are the main problems in the immediate treatment of a small baby, the prevention and treatment of disorders of the brain will determine whether the child is severely disabled or not. New techniques, especially ultrasound, have allowed cerebral lesions to be identified early. They have also shown that some disorders, particularly periventricular haemorrhage, can disappear without trace. Other lesions, such as periventricular leucomalacia generally have a worse prognosis but are often more difficult to identify. In the next few years it will be important to apply ourselves to the prevention of serious neurological disability and to find out which type of management will improve prognosis.

Treatment of convulsions

After even one brief convulsion it is important to investigate and treat possible causes such as hypoglycaemia, hypocalcaemia, hyponatraemia and meningitis. Repeated convulsions, a convulsion lasting longer than 3 min, or a fit destabilizing blood pressure or respiration merit anticonvulsant therapy.

It can be argued that fits which do not impair oxygenation or perfusion are not intrinsically damaging and that anticonvulsant drugs may do more harm than good. Perhaps the strongest evidence that repeated seizures are likely to be harmful to the developing brain comes from a study by Wasterlain and Plum [136]. They administered 150 V shocks daily across the head of newborn rats. Compared to control littermates, animals subjected to seizures between days 2 and 11 had a 14% reduction in brain weight and a 15% reduction in brain cell number. Rats having convulsions between days 9 and 18 subsequently had an 8% reduction in brain weight but no reduction in cell number. Animals who had convulsions after 18 days showed no change in brain weight or cell number. None of the brains showed any histological evidence of necrosis. The authors concluded that the brain still undergoing mitosis is more vulnerable to repeated seizures than the brain which is post-mitotic. Considerable cell division takes place in the human brain after 28 weeks gestation particularly in the cerebellum, brainstem and glial tissue. Other investigators have demonstrated that seizures are associated with a fall in brain glucose, high energy phosphates, DNA, RNA, protein and cholesterol and a rise in intracellular lactate [137,138].

We have observed that tonic and clonic seizures are often associated with a drop in $P\text{O}_2$, and a rise in arterial pressure and intracranial pressure. Thus it has been our practice to treat definite clinical seizures if they have lasted over 3 min or have been recurrent.

Phenobarbitone

The drug of first choice is phenobarbitone. Different doses are quoted in the literature. Volpe [139] suggests 10 mg/kg intravenously, repeated after 20 min if necessary. He suggests that maintenance at 3–4 mg/kg/day should be started. O'Donohoe [140] starts with 15 mg/kg/day followed by maintenance therapy. In older textbooks dosage regimens beginning with 5 mg/kg/day, 8 mg/kg/day and 10 mg/kg/day have been suggested. Lockman *et al.* [141] studied the relationship between phenobarbitone loading dose, gestational age, blood level and seizure control in 39 neonates. Figure 19.31 shows that all twelve neonates who achieved seizure control had blood levels of phenobarbitone exceeding 16.9 mg/l. The 26 infants who continued to have seizures had blood levels between 4 and 25 mg/l. A mean dose of 16.2 mg/kg was required to give a therapeutic blood level over 16.9 mg/l. No toxic effects were recognized with blood levels up to 25.8 mg/l. The mean dose:peak plasma concentration was 0.81 ± 0.19 for intravenous injection. Absorption was found to be more variable from intramuscular injection; for babies under 1000 g the intravenous route should be used as there is very little muscle into which to inject.

Pippenger and Rosen [142] found that loading doses of 5 mg/kg did not produce therapeutic levels at all and doses of 10 mg/kg produced levels above 10 mg/l after 1–2 days. In our own study at Hammersmith Hospital [143] a single loading dose of 20 mg/kg gave mean phenobarbitone levels of 20.8 mg/l at 24 h, 19.2 mg/l at 48 h and 18.1 mg/l at 72 h.

Are maintenance doses of phenobarbitone required?

Painter *et al.* [144] found that maintenance doses of 5 mg/kg/day following a loading dose of 20 mg/kg resulted in accumulation of the drug with mean plasma concentration reaching 40 mg/l after one week. As the renal and hepatic elimination of virtually all drugs is slower in babies under 1000 g birth weight than in larger neonates,

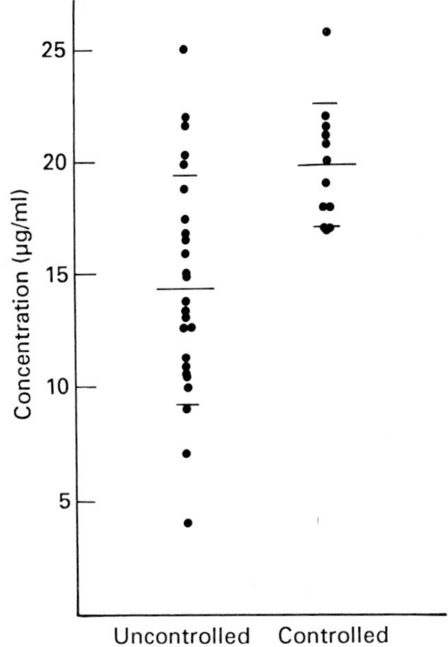

Figure 19.31 Phenobarbitone concentrations in controlled versus uncontrolled neontal seizures

accumulation is likely to be even more of a problem. The Hammersmith phenobarbitone trial was confined to babies below 1500 g birth weight and therapeutic plasma levels were maintained for several days without maintenance [143].

Our approach is to give a loading dose of 20 mg/kg. If this achieves seizure control no maintenance therapy is given. Often neonates have convulsions in response to an acute insult which is transient and has gone by the time the loading dose is eliminated. If seizures which were initially controlled with phenobarbitone recur after a few days, then maintenance phenobarbitone should be started at 4 mg/kg/day. Monitoring of plasma levels is essential, with the aim of a concentration of 17–25 mg/l. Because the Hammersmith trial was double blind it was possible to look for adverse effects. Babies under 1500 g who had received 20 mg/kg phenobarbitone were significantly more likely to develop respiratory failure and require ventilation after the injection than were controls who received only placebo. Because of this, great care must be taken with the administration of phenobarbitone to non-ventilated infants below 1000 g as respiratory depression may occur. As respiratory depression may result from convulsions or from treatment, it is important to monitor arterial blood gases. Heart rate and blood pressure should also be monitored and hypotension or hypovolaemia promptly corrected.

Paraldehyde

If convulsions continue despite 20 mg/kg phenobarbitone, paraldehyde should be given. Because of the relative absence of muscle, paraldehyde is given intravenously or rectally. Paraldehyde dissolves rubber and some types of plastic (e.g. polyvinyl) including three-way taps, but does not dissolve Teflon cannulae or polypropylene or polyethylene syringes and connecting tubes [145]. A solution of 5% paraldehyde in 5% dextrose has been used for many years at 1–3 ml/kg/h [146]. A bolus of 1 ml of 5%

paraldehyde can be given to initiate treatment. We have found paraldehyde to be well tolerated even by infants under 1000 g, with no evidence of respiratory depression at these doses. Elimination is partly through the lungs. The plasma half life of paraldehyde is considerably shorter (10.2 h in term infants) than that of phenobarbitone or phenytoin, but is probably longer in infants under 1000 g who have lung disease. Paraldehyde can be administered rectally by mixing 0.3 ml/kg with an equal volume of mineral oil and injecting it through a Teflon, polypropylene or polyethylene tube passed a few centimetres into the rectum. This can be repeated every 4 h but should be avoided if there is any clinical suspicion of necrotizing enterocolitis.

Phenytoin

Concern has been expressed about adverse effects of long-term phenytoin therapy on cerebellar development. However, short-term use is still advocated [139]. We use phenytoin as third choice for neonatal seizures. Painter *et al.* [144] showed that a loading dose of 15–20 mg/kg intravenously produced a mean plasma concentration of 14.5 mg/l. The intravenous loading dose must be given slowly (1 mg/kg/min) as phenytoin can affect cardiac rhythm. They found that oral administration of phenytoin did not give adequate blood levels in newborns. Intramuscular administration was also ineffective. If maintenance dosage is necessary after a few days, 5 mg/kg/day is a reasonable starting dose although monitoring of plasma levels is also necessary as accumulation can occur at this dose.

Diazepam

Diazepam is not recommended for initial treatment of neonatal convulsions for a number of reasons:

(1) Diazepam has an extremely unpredictable duration of action and its therapeutic dose is very varied (0.1–0.5 mg/kg)

(2) Intravenous diazepam in addition contains sodium benzoate and this may increase the risk of kernicterus by uncoupling bilirubin from albumin. Diazemuls, a new formulation of diazepam in an oil–water emulsion, may not carry this risk

(3) Respiratory depression is a well-documented side effect of diazepam

(4) Lastly, diazepam is unsuitable for maintenance. A second drug is often needed because of the variability of duration of action.

Thus diazepam should only be used if seizures do not stop after 20 mg/kg of phenobarbitone, 0.1 mg/kg paraldehyde and 20 mg/kg of phenytoin have been given.

We have no experience with very high doses of barbiturates such as are used to induce a brain-protecting coma. However, high doses of thiopentone have been reported to reduce arterial blood pressure in neonates [147]. In our view this would be a particularly undesirable effect because of the crucial importance of maintaining cerebral perfusion.

Treatment of periventricular haemorrhage (PVH)

The aetiology, prevention and diagnosis of PVH have been dealt with elsewhere. This section deals with the management of:

(1) The acute consequences of loss of blood.

(2) Post-haemorrhagic ventricular dilatation.

Blood loss

Large amounts of blood (half the circulating blood volume) may be lost in a massive PVH. Clinical observation of perfusion (capillary filling time should not exceed 3 s), blood pressure monitoring and regular acid-base and haematocrit measurements are the best guides to loss of blood in babies weighing less than 1000 g. Arterial catheter insertion is justified in any baby weighing less than 1000 g if there is any respiratory problem. This facilitates serial arterial blood gas sampling and the use of a blood pressure transducer for continuous arterial pressure measurement.

What is the minimum safe blood pressure for cerebral perfusion?

Using mean arterial pressure because it is less subject to damping than systolic or diastolic pressure and because mean pressure is used in the calculation of cerebral perfusion pressure, infants below 1000 g who develop normally and have no cerebral lesions on ultrasound scan have been reported to maintain their mean arterial pressure above 30 mmHg [148].

In some neonatal intensive care units an umbilical venous catheter is inserted into the inferior vena cava or right atrium of ill infants weighing less than 1000 g. It is argued that a secure route can thus be established for fluids and drugs, that the risks of sepsis are much reduced if the catheter is inserted soon after birth rather than after the umbilical cord has become colonized, and that the peripheral veins of such tiny infants should be preserved for future infusions. We do not do this on a routine basis but, in selected cases, such a catheter provides a route for central venous pressure (CVP) measurement. There are no published guidelines on CVP in babies below 1000 g, but we have used a range of 2–8 mmHg.

Large PVH may give rise to consumption of clotting factors and thrombocytopenia as well as anaemia. Thus our immediate management plan is:

(1) Transfuse 10 ml/kg of plasma protein fraction or 4% albumin to raise arterial pressure above 30 mmHg, improve perfusion and elevate pH.
(2) Use whole blood or packed red cells if the haematocrit is below 0.36 or haemoglobin below 12 g/dl.
(3) Use fresh frozen plasma if there is evidence of a coagulation abnormality.
(4) Transfuse 10 ml/kg of platelet-rich plasma if the platelet count is less than 20 000 μl.

If there is no improvement after 10 ml/kg over 10–20 min, the transfusion should be repeated. If there is a CVP line in place and mean arterial pressure remains below 30 mmHg, colloid should be given until the CVP reaches 5 mmHg. If clinical examination suggests that the baby is still hypovolaemic after 20 ml/kg (pallor, poor capillary filling, collapsed veins), a third infusion of 10 ml/kg should be given with dopamine at 5 μg/kg/min by continuous intravenous infusion. Dopamine increases cardiac output and improves renal perfusion but is no substitute for replacing circulating volume. The rate of infusion can be increased to 10 or 15 μg/kg/min.

Post-haemorrhagic ventricular dilatation (PHVD)

ELBW infants who develop large intraventricular haemorrhage are at risk of developing progressive ventricular dilatation. This may result from particles of blood clot obstructing the interventricular foramina, aqueduct of Silvius, basal cisternae or the arachnoid villi. Gliosis and arachnoiditis may occur to add to the obstruction [149]. Infants who develop PHVD generally have a worse neuro-developmental prognosis than babies who have had only intraventricular haemorrhage [141]. Reviewing the available reports of survivors with persistent or progressive ventricular dilatation gives an overall cerebral palsy rate of approximately 60% and a 36% rate of severe developmental delay [150–158]. These can only be approximate figures because of differences in definitions of PHVD, different methods of assessment and variations in age and completeness of follow-up. Allan, Dransfield and Tito [151] concluded that neuro-developmental outcome is related more to the degree of original hypoxic ischaemic parenchymal damage than to the hydrocephalus.

Our criteria of PHVD are (a) intraventricular haemorrhage diagnosed with ultrasound and (b) progressive increase in both ventricular widths reaching 4 mm over the 97th centile of Levine [159] (Figure 19.32). This means for most babies weighing less than 1000 g that each ventricular width must reach 15 mm; this is measured in the transfontanelle coronal view just posterior to the interventricular foramina, taking the distance from the midline to the most lateral border of the ventricle. In cases of cerebral atrophy the ventricles usually dilate, but this process should be distinguishable from CSF-driven dilatation by the following features:

(1) In CSF-driven PHVD the ventricles are usually rounded (ballooned), but in cerebral atrophy the ventricles have an irregular outline.
(2) In PHVD ventricular enlargement can be rapid with considerable growth within 24 h, whereas cerebral atrophy is much slower in enlarging the ventricles.

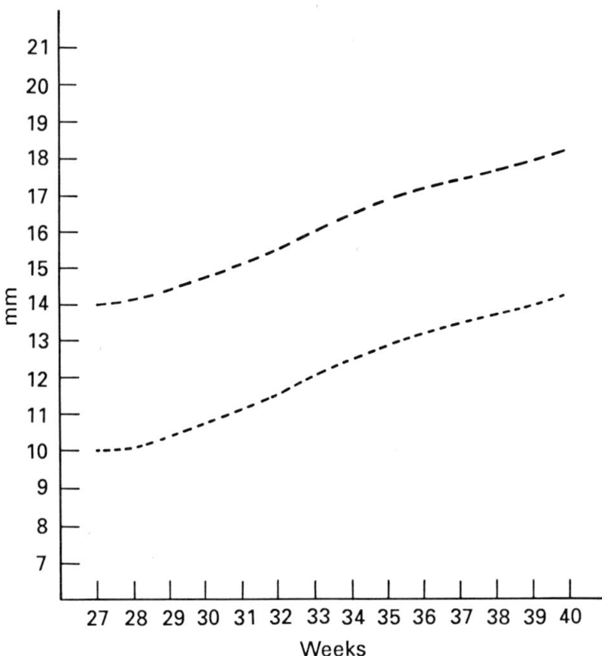

Figure 19.32 The lower line shows the 97th centile for ventricular width [159]. The upper line shows our criteria for post-haemorragic ventricular dilatation (4mm over the 97th centile)

(3) Head circumference does not usually increase much in the early stages of PHVD, but with progressive ventricular enlargement head growth does eventually accelerate. In cerebral atrophy head growth is not accelerated. It may be subnormal or nonnal in rate.
(4) In pure cerebral atrophy intracranial pressure is not raised.

We have established a normal range for intracranial pressure in newborn infants. By measuring the pressure at lumbar puncture under standardized conditions in normal newborns, mean CSF pressure was found to be 2.8 ± 1.4 mmHg. This applies to babies under 1000 g [160]. We studied a series of 16 infants with PHVD; Figure 19.33 shows the CSF pressure measurements. During ventricular expansion CSF pressure mean was 8.8 ± 4.6 mmHg. It is noteworthy that in some of the babies under 1000 g ventricular enlargement can occur at very modest pressures because the immature brain and soft skull are highly compliant [161].

It can be hypothesized that infants with PHVD have such an adverse outcome because of additional later damage resulting from a period of raised CSF pressure with periventricular oedema, distortion of developing pathways and possibly decreased cerebral perfusion. Is ventricular dilatation with a pressure of 7 or 8 mmHg directly harmful to the brain? Simultaneous blood pressure measurements in our babies did not suggest that cerebral perfusion would be seriously impaired.

Treatment of PHVD

The immediate aims of treatment are to control intracranial pressure and excessive head enlargement. Approximately 50% of the babies reaching 4 mm over the 97th centile for ventricular width will regress spontaneously without any treatment. What

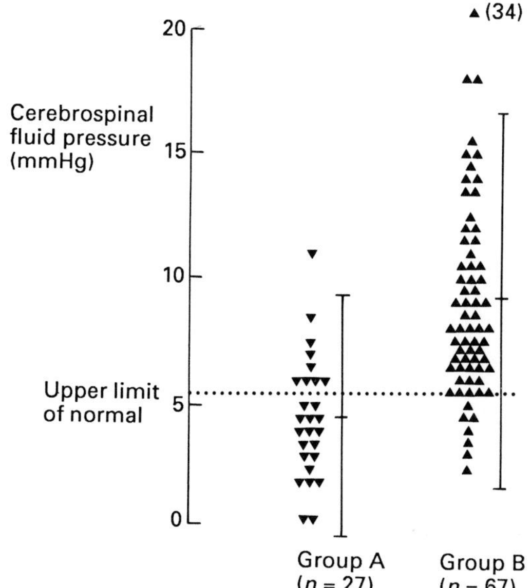

Figure 19.33 CSF pressure in infants with post-haemorrhagic ventricular dilatation. Group A, static or contracting; Group B, active ventricular expansion

level of intracranial pressure should be considered undesirable? We have considered that 12 mmHg is excessive. This is four times the normal mean and 100% over the upper limit of normal. This pressure is not necessarily associated with specific signs but we have often noted irritability and a tense fontanelle in these cases. A fontanelle pressure sensor such as that developed by Dr Martin Wright (available from SLE, 15 Campbell Road, Croydon, Surrey CR0 2SQ) can help as a screening test for intracranial hypertension when it is applied to the fontanelle with collodion.

One approach to treatment of PHVD has been to carry out repeated lumbar punctures. Kreusser *et al.* [162] showed that removal of 10–20 ml CSF by lumbar puncture could temporarily control ventricular enlargement. Mantovani *et al.* [163] and Anwar *et al.* [164] carried out randomized trials of serial lumbar puncture in babies with large intraventricular haemorrhage. Both studies concluded that these measures did not prevent eventual progression to hydrocephalus requiring insertion of a shunt system. Other authors have suggested that early drainage of CSF by lumbar puncture might improve neuro-developmental outcome by reducing pressure, oedema and distortion. On the other hand, the extra handling of vulnerable tiny infants, with the additional risk of trauma and infection, might be harmful. The issue is currently being tested by a multicentre trial.

Another approach to PHVD is to reduce CSF formation with drugs. Isosorbide has been used by Lorber [165]. However, his study did not involve babies under 1000 g and there was a high incidence of adverse effects such as vomiting with this osmotic agent.

Acetazolamide, a carbonic anhydrase inhibitor, has been used by a number of investigators. The most encouraging report was by Shinnar *et al.* [166]. They described a selected uncontrolled group of infants with hydrocephalus some of whom were below 1000 g, in whom acetazolamide 100 mg/kg/day was combined with frusemide 1–3 mg/kg/day. The authors concluded that they avoided shunt insertion in over 50% of the patients who would otherwise have been certain candidates for surgery. We have not had any success with acetazolamide in avoiding surgery. Furthermore, considerable doses of buffering agents such as sodium bicarbonate or potassium bicarbonate are needed to control the metabolic acidosis. In infants under 1000 g with any respiratory or renal problem such metabolic stress could be undesirable.

Shunt surgery

For control of persistent intracranial hypertension and excessive head growth, a ventriculoperitoneal (V-P) shunt system is the most widely used treatment. Under general anaesthesia a small burr hole is made in the parietal bone above and behind the right ear. A ventricular catheter is passed with its tip lying in the anterior horn. The ventricular catheter is brought out to a subcutaneous Rickham reservoir. This in turn connects to a one-way valve which may be a Spitz-Holter, Pudenz, Hakim or any small low pressure valve. Distal to the valve is connected a catheter which runs subcutaneously to the peritoneal cavity; 25–30 cm of tubing can be placed within the peritoneal cavity and this allows for growth. Such a shunt may last for 3–4 years before needing replacement. In contrast, a ventriculo-atrial shunt requires repeated lengthening as the child grows and infection in this site results in septicaemia, with additional risks of emboli and glomerulonephritis. Because the ventricular pressure may be only 5–7 mmHg, the valve must be very compliant to allow flow at such low pressures. If a V-P shunt does not drain well, it may help to lay the infant on an incline of 30 ° to create a differential hydrostatic pressure between the ventricles and the peritoneal cavity.

V-P shunting will usually be delayed until the CSF has cleared of visible blood and the CSF protein has fallen to below 1.5–2.0 g/l. This is done because it is thought that the shunt would block more readily in the presence of a high CSF protein. The CSF must be free of infection before shunt insertion. Despite the simple principles of the V-P shunt, most centres have experienced a high rate of complications in infants shunted after intraventricular haemorrhage compared to other causes of hydrocephalus. This may be because these infants tend to be smaller, with cardiorespiratory problems, blood and protein in the CSF and more prone to infection. Cooke reported very good results from Liverpool [167]. In a series of 54 VLBW infants with shunts for PHVD, only 38% needed revision within 12 months; 12% required three or more revisions. Significantly only 27% of the 54 were neuro-developmentally normal.

TIMING OF SHUNT SURGERY

In infants weighing less than 1000 g it is desirable to postpone shunt surgery for as long as possible. Such infants may withstand surgery and general anaesthesia poorly because of chronic lung disease and patent ductus arteriosus. Furthermore the surgeon usually finds it easier to operate on a larger patient. The initially blood-stained CSF and high protein level also contraindicate early surgery. Thus non-surgical management is appropriate. The head circumference and ventricular widths should ideally be measured daily to monitor progress. If the fontanelle is tense, or the baby is excessively irritable, a fontanelle sensor can be used with collodion adhesion. If the fontanelle pressure reads over 10 mmHg or the fontanelle is tense and bulging, then a direct CSF pressure measurement via lumbar puncture should be carried out. If the pressure is over 12 mmHg fluid should be allowed to drain to a maximum of 2% of body weight. When there is minimal flow of CSF from the lumbar route on two occasions, non-communication should be assumed and CSF pressure measured by ventricular tap. In asymmetrical ventricular dilatation it is better to insert the needle into the larger ventricle and thus traverse the shorter depth of cerebral tissue.

Lumbar puncture or ventricular tap should be repeated as often as required to maintain intracranial pressure below 12 mmHg. Excessive head growth is arbitrarily defined as an increase of 3 cm over two weeks or less *or* crossing from below the 50th centile to 2 cm over the 90th centile on the Gairdner chart [168]. If repeated taps have been necessary for four weeks, V-P shunting can be considered. If the baby's cardiorespiratory state is still poor or the CSF protein greater than 2 g/l, non-surgical management should continue until these contraindications to surgery improve.

References

1. Cooke, R. W. I., Lucas, A., Pryse–Davies, J. and Yudkin, P. L. N. (1977) Head circumference as an index of brain-weight in the fetus and newborn infant. *Early Hum. Dev.*, **1**, 145–149
2. Van den Bergh, R. (1967) The periventricular intracerebral blood supply. In *Research on the Cerebral Circulation* (3rd International Salzburg Conference), (eds J. S. Meyer, M. Lechner and O. Eickhorn), C. C. Thomas, Springfield, Illinois, pp. 52–63
3. Dorovini–Zis, K. and Dolman, C. L. (1977) Gestational development of the brain. *Arch. Pathol. Lab. Med.*, **101**, 192–195
4. Duckett, S. (1971) The establishment of internal vascularisation in the human telencephalon. *Acta Anat.*, **80**, 107–113

5. Keir, E. L. (1974) Fetal cerebral arteries; a phylogenetic and ontogenetic study. In *Radiology of the Skull and Brain*, Vol. 2, Book 1 (eds T. H. Newton and D. G. Potts), C. V. Mosby, St. Louis, pp. 1089–1130
6. Pape, K. E. and Wigglesworth, J. S. (1979) Blood supply to the developing brain. In *Haemorrhage, Ischaemia and the Perinatal Brain, Clin. Dev. Med.*, **69/70**, pp. 16–17, SIMS, Heinemann, London
7. Dobbing, J. and Sands, J. (1970) Timing of neuroblast multiplication in developing human brain. *Nature*, **226**, 639–640
8. Pape, K. E. and Wigglesworth, J. S. (1979) Blood supply to the developing brain. In *Haemorrhage, Ischaemia and the Perinatal Brain, Clin. Dev. Med.*, **69/70**, pp. 26–27, SIMS, Heinemann, London
9. Hauw, J. J., Berger, B. and Escourolle, R. (1975) Electron microscopic study of the developing capillaries of human brain. *Acta Neuropathol.*, **31**, 229–242
10. Gruner, J. E. (1970) The maturation of human cerebral cortex in electron microscopy study of post-mortem punctures in premature infants. *Biol. Neonate*, **16**, 243–255
11. Takashima, S. and Tanaka, K. (1978) Microangiography and vascular permeability of the subependymal matrix in the premature infant. *Can. J. Neurosci.*, **5**, 45–50
12. Grontoft, O. (1958) Intracerebral and meningeal haemorrhages in perinatally decreased infants; intracerebral haemorrhages: pathologic-anatomical and obstetrical study. *Acta Obstet. Gynecol. Scand.*, **3**, 308–334
13. Rennie, J. M., Doyle, J. and Cooke, R. W. I. (1987) Elevated levels of immunoreactive prostacyclin metabolite in babies who develop intraventricular haemorrhage. *Acta Paediatr. Scand.*, **76**, 19–23
14. Elund, A., Bomfim, W., Kaijser, L. *et al.* (1981) Pulmonary formation of prostacyclin in man *Prostaglandins*, **22**, 323–331
15. Ment, L. R., Duncan, C.C., Ehrenkranz, R. A. *et al.* (1984) Intraventricular haemorrhage in the preterm neonate: timing and cerebral blood flow changes. *J. Pediatr.*, **104**, 419–425
16. Volpe, J. J., Herscovitch, P., Perlman, J. M. and Raichle, M. E. (1983) Positron emission tomography in the newborn: extensive impairment of regional cerebral blood flow with intraventricular hemorrhage and hemorrhagic cerebral involvement. *Pediatrics*, **72**, 589–601
17. Perlman, J. M., McMenamin, J. B. and Volpe, J. J. (1983) Fluctuating cerebral blood flow velocity in respiratory distress syndrome. *N. Engl. J. Med.*, **309**, 204–209
18. Perlman, J. M., Goodman, S., Kreusser, K. L. and Volpe, J. J. (1985) Reduction in intraventricular hemorrhage by elimination of fluctuating cerebral bloodflow velocity in preterm infants with respiratory distress syndrome. *N. Engl. J. Med.*, **312**, 1353–1357
19. Drayton, M. R. and Skidmore, R. (1987) Vasoactivity of the major intracranial arteries in newborn infants. *Arch. Dis. Child.*, **62**, 236–240
20. Fujimura, M., Salisbury, D. M., Robinson, R. O. *et al.* (1979) Clinical events relating to intraventricular haemorrhage in the newborn. *Arch. Dis. Child.*, **54**, 409–414
21. Watkins, A., West, C. and Cooke, R. W. I. (1987) Blood pressure and cerebral injury in sick very low birthweight infants. *Arch. Dis. Child.*, **62**, 648–649
22. Weindling, A. M., Rochfort, M. J., Calvert, S. A., Fok, T-F. and Wilkinson, A. (1985) Development of cerebral palsy after ultrasonographic detection of periventricular cysts in the newborn. *Dev. Med. Child Neurol.*, **27**, 800–806
23. Cooke, R. W. I. (1981) Factors associated with periventricular haemorrhage in very low birthweight infants. *Arch. Dis. Child.*, **56**, 425–431
24. Wigglesworth, J. S. and Husemeyer, R. P. (1977) Intracranial birth trauma in vaginal breach delivery: the continued importance of injury to the occipital bone. *Br. J. Obstet. Gynaecol.*, **84**, 684–691
25. Schwartz, P. (1961) *Birth Injuries in the Newborn*, S. Karger, Basel
26. Clark, C. E., Clyman, R. I., Roth, R. S., Sniderman, S. H., Lane, B. and Ballard, R. A. (1981) Risk factor analysis of intraventricular hemorrhage in low-birth-weight infants. *J. Pediatr.*, **99**, 625–628
27. Hambleton, G. and Wigglesworth, J. S. (1976) Origin of intraventricular haemorrhage in the preterm infant. *Arch. Dis. Child.*, **51**, 651–659
28. Pasternak, J. F., Groothuis, D. R., Fischer, J. M. and Fischer, D. P. (1982) Regional cerebral blood flow in the newborn beagle pup: the germinal matrix is a 'low-flow' structure. *Pediatr. Res.*, **16**, 499–503
29. Setzer, E. S., Webb, L. B., Wassenaar, J. W., Reeder, J. D., Mehta, P. S. and Eitzman, D. V. (1982)

Platelet dysfunction and coagulopathy in intraventricular hemorrhage in the premature infant. *J. Pediatr.*, **100**, 599–605

30. Beverley, D. W., Pitts–Tucker, T. J., Congdon, P. J. Arthur, R. J. and Tate, G. (1985) Prevention of intraventricular haemorrhage by fresh frozen plasma. *Arch. Dis. Child.*, **60**, 710–713
31. Sinha, S., Davies, J., Toner, N., Bogle, S. and Chiswick, M. (1987) Vitamin E supplementation reduces frequency of periventricular haemorrhage in very preterm babies. *Lancet*, **i**, 466–470
32. Benson, J. W. T., Drayton, M. R., Hayward, C. *et al.* (1986) Multicentre trial of ethamsylate for prevention of periventricular haemorrhage in very low birthweight infants. *Lancet*, **ii**, 1297–1299
33. Hill, A. and Volpe, J. J. (1981) Normal pressure hydrocephalus in the newborn. *Pediatrics*, **68**, 623–629
34. Cooke, R. W. I. (1987) Determinants of major handicap in post-haemorrhagic hydrocephalus. *Arch. Dis. Child.*, **62**, 504–506
35. Banker, B. Q. and Larroche, J. C. (1962); Periventricular leukomalacia in infancy. *Arch. Neurol.*, **7**, 386–410
36. de Vries, L. S., Dubowitz, L. M. S., Dubowitz, V. *et al.* (1985) Predictive value of cranial ultrasound in the newborn baby: a reappraisal. *Lancet*, **ii**, 137–140
37. Armstrong, D. and Norman, M. G. (1974) Periventricular leucomalacia in neonates: complications and sequelae. *Arch. Dis. Child.*, **49**, 367–375
38. Sinha, S., Davies, J. M., Sims, D. G. and Chiswick, M. L. (1985) Relation between periventricular haemorrhage and ischaemic brain lesions diagnosed by ultrasound in preterm infants. *Lancet*, **ii**, 1154–1155
39. Dubowitz, L. M. S., Bydder, G. M. and Mushin, J. (1985) Developmental sequence of periventricular leucomalacia. Correlation of ultrasound, clinical, and nuclear magnetic resonance functions. *Arch. Dis. Child.*, **60**, 349–355
40. Hamilton, P. A., Hope, P. L., Cady, E. B., Delpy, D. T., Wyatt, J. S. and Reynolds, E. O. R. (1986) Impaired energy metabolism in brains of newborn infants with increased cerebral echodensities. *Lancet*, **i**, 1242–1246
41. Stewart, A. L., Thorburn, R. J., Hope, P. L., Goldsmith, M., Lipscomb, A. P. and Reynolds, E. O. R. (1983) Ultrasound appearance of the brain in very preterm infants and neurodevelopmental outcome at 18 months of age. *Arch. Dis. Child.*, **58**, 589–604
42. Gould, S. J., Howard, S., Hope, P. L. and Reynolds, E. O. R. (1987) Periventricular intraparenchymal cerebral haemorrhage in preterm infants: the role of venous infarction. *J. Pathol.*, **151**, 197–202
43. Edvinsson, L., Lou, H. C. and Tvede, K. (1986) On the pathogenesis of regional cerebral ischaemia in intracranial hemorrhage: a causal influence of potassium? *Pediatr. Res.*, **20**, 478–480
44. Fisher, C. M., Roberson, G. H. and Ojemann, R. G. (1972) Cerebral vasospasm with ruptured saccular aneurysm – the clinical manifestations. *Neurosurgery*, **1**, 245–248
45. Rushton, D. I., Preston, P. R. and Durbin, G. M. (1985) Structure and evolution of echodense lesions in the neonatal brain. A combined ultrasound and necropsy study. *Arch. Dis. Child.*, **60**, 798–808
46. Levine, R. L., Fredericks, W. R. and Rapoport, S. I. (1982) Entry of bilirubin into the brain due to opening of the blood-brain barrier. *Pediatrics*, **69**, 255–259
47. Wennberg, R. P., Ahlfors, C. E., Bickers, R. G., McMurty, C. A. and Shetter, J. L. (1982) Abnormal auditory brain stem response in a newborn infant with hyperbilirubinaemia: improvement with exchange transfusion. *J. Pediatr.*, **100**, 624–626
48. Robinson, H. P. and Fleming, J. E. E. (1975) A critical evaluation of sonar crown–rump length measurements. *Br. J. Obstet. Gynaecol.*, **82**, 702–710
49. Campbell, S. (1969) The prediction of fetal maturity by ultrasonic measurement of the biparietal diameter. *J. Obstet. Gynaecol.*, **76**, 603–609
50. Dubowitz, L. M. S. and Goldberg, G. (1976) Assessment of gestational age in various stages of pregnancy in infants differing in size and ethnic origin. *Br. J. Obstet. Gynaecol.*, **83**, 255–259
51. Brett, E. (1963) The estimation of foetal maturity by the neurological examination of the neonate. In *Gestational Age, Size and Maturity* (eds M. Dawkins and B. MacGregor), *Clin. Dev. Med.*, **19**, SSMEIU/Heinemann, London
52. Robinson, R. J. (1966) Assessment of gestational age by neurological examination. *Arch. Dis. Child.*, **41**, 437–447

53. Mitchell, R. G and Farr, V. (1965) The meaning of maturity and the assessment of maturity at birth. In *Gestational Age, Size and Maturity* (eds M. Dawkins and B. MacGregor), *Clin. Dev. Med.*, **19**, 83–99, SSMEIU/Heinemann, London
54. Farr, V., Mitchell, R. G., Nelligan, G. A. and Parkins, J. M. (1966) The definition of some external characteristics used in the assessment of gestational age in newborn infants. *Dev. Med. Child Neurol.*, **8**, 657
55. Usher, R., McLean, F. and Scott, K. E. (1966) Clinical significance of gestational age and an objective method for its assessment. *Pediatr. Clin. North Am.*, **13**, 835–848
56. Amiel-Tison, C. (1968) Neurological evaluation of the maturity of newborn infants. *Arch. Dis. Child.*, **43**, 89–93
57. Hittner, H. M., Hirsh, N. J. and Rudolph, A. J. (1977) The lens in the assessment of gestational age. *J. Pediatr.*, **91**, 455–460
58. Casear, P., Eggermont, E. and Volpe, P. J. (1986) Neurological problems in the newborn. In *Textbook of Neonatology* (ed N. R. C. Roberton), Churchill Livingstone, Edinburgh, pp. 527–537
59. Farr, V. and Mitchell, R. G. (1967) The effect of birthweight on maturity scoring. *Dev. Med. Child Neurol.*, **9**, 745
60. Dubowitz, L. M. S., Dubowitz, V. and Goldberg, C. (1970) Clinical assessment of gestational age in the newborn infant. *J. Pediatr.*, **77**, 1–10
61. Dubowitz, L. M. S. and Dubowitz, V. (1977) *Gestational Age of the Newborn: A Clinical Manual*, Addison-Wesley, California
62. Dubowitz, V., Whittaker, G. F., Brown, B. H. and Robinson, A. (1968) Nerve conduction velocity: an index of neurological maturity of the newborn infant. *Dev. Med. Child Neurol.*, **10**, 741–749
63. Schulte, F. J., Michaelis, R., Linke, I. and Nolter, R. (1968) Motor nerve conduction velocity in term, preterm and small for date infants. *Pediatrics*, **42**, 17–21
64. Moosa, A. and Dubowitz, V. (1971) Postnatal maturation of peripheral nerves in preterm and full term infants. *J. Pediatr.*, **79**, 915–922
65. Miller, G., Heckmatt, J. Z., Dubowitz, L. M. S. and Dubowitz, V. (1983) Use of nerve conduction velocity to determine gestational age in infants at risk and in very low birth weight infants. *J. Pediatr.*, **103**, 109–112
66. De Vries, L. S., Heckmatt, J. Z., Burrin, J. M., Dubowitz, L. M. S. and Dubowitz, V. (1986) Low serum thyroxine concentrations and neural maturation in preterm infants. *Arch. Dis. Child.*, **61**, 862–866
67. André Thomas and Saint-Anne Dargassies, S. (1952) *Etudes Neurologiques sur le Nouveau-né et la Jeune Nourisson*, Masson, Paris
68. André Thomas, Chesni, Y. and Saint-Anne Dargassies, S. (1960) The neurological examination of the infant. *Little Club Clinics in Developmental Medicine*, No. 1, National Spastics Society, London
69. Amiel-Tison, C. and Grenier, A. (1980) *Evaluation Neurologique du Nouveau-né et du Nourisson*, Masson, Paris
70. Amiel-Tison, C., Barrier, G., Shnider, S. M., Levinson, S. C. and Stefani, S. J. (1982) A new neurologic and adaptive scoring system for evaluating obstetric medications in full term newborn infants. *Anesthesiology*, **56**, 340–350
71. Saint-Anne Dargassies, S. (1966) Neurological maturation of the premature infant of 28 to 41 weeks gestational age. In *Human Development* (ed F. Falkner), Saunders, Philadelphia, pp. 302–325
72. Saint-Anne Dargassies, S. (1977) *Neurological Development in Full Term and Premature Neonates*, Elsevier/North Holland/Excerpta Medica, Amsterdam
73. Prechtl, H. F. R. (1977) *The Neurological Examination of the Full Term Newborn Infant*, 2nd edn, *Clin. Dev. Med.*, **63**, SIMP/Heinemann, London
74. Prechtl, H. F. R. (1980) The optimality concept. *Early Hum. Dev.*, **4**, 201–206
75. Brazelton, T. B. (1973) Neonatal behavioural assessment scale. *Clin. Dev. Med.*, **50**, SIMP/Heinemann, London
76. Piper, M. C., Kunos, I., Willis, D. M. and Mazer, B. (1975) Effect of gestational age on neurological functioning of the very low birthweight infant at 40 weeks. *Dev. Med. Child Neurol.*, **27**, 596–605
77. Dubowitz, L. and Dubowitz, V. (1981) The neurological assessment of the preterm and full term newborn infant. *Clin. Dev. Med.*, **79**, SIMP/Heinemann, London
78. Prechtl, H. F. R. and O'Brien, M. J. (1982) Behavioural states of the full term newborn: the

emergence of a concept. In *Psychobiology of the Human Newborn* (ed. P. Statton), Wiley, New York, pp. 53–73

79. Palmer, P. G., Dubowitz, L. M. S., Verghote, M. and Dubowitz, V. (1982) Neurological and neurobehavioural differences between preterm infants at term and full term newborn infants. *Neuropediatrics*, **13**, 183–189
80. Lacey, J. L., Henderson–Smart, D. J., Edwards, D. A. and Storey, B. (1985) The early development of head control in preterm infants. *Early Hum. Dev.*, **ii**, 199–212
81. Prechtl, H. F. R., Fargel, J. W., Weinmann, H. M. and Bakker, H. H. (1979) Postures, motility and respiration of low risk preterm infants. *Dev. Med. Child Neurol.*, **21**, 3–27
82. Casaer, P., Daniels, H., Devlieger, H., de Cock, P. and Eggermont, E. (1982) Feeding behaviour in preterm neonates. *Early Hum. Dev.*, **7**, 331–346
83. Dubowitz, L. M. S., Dubowitz, V., Morante, A. and Verghote, M. (1980) Visual function in the premature and full term newborn infant. *Dev. Med. Child Neurol.*, **22**, 465–475
84. Hrbek, A., Karlberg, P. and Olsson, T. (1973) Development of visual and somatosensory evoked responses in low birthweight infants. *Electroencephalogr. Clin. Neurophysiol.*, **34**, 225–232
85. Bhaitacharia, J., Beneh, M. J. and Tucker, S. M. (1984) Long term follow up of newborns tested with the auditory response cradle. *Arch. Dis. Child.*, **59**, 504–511
86. Stockard, J. E. and Stockard, J. J. (1981) Brainstem auditory evoked potentials in normal and otoneurologically impaired newborns and infants. In *Current Clinical Neurophysiology: Update on EEG and Evoked Potentials* (ed. C. E. Henry), Elsevier/North Holland, Amsterdam, pp. 9–71
87. Lary, S., Briassoulis, G., de Vries, L., Dubowitz, L. M. S. and Dubowitz, V. (1985) Hearing threshold in preterm and term infants by auditory brainstem response. *J. Pediatr.*, **107**, 593–599
88. De Vries, L. S., Lary, S. and Dubowitz, L. M. S. (1985) Relationship of serum bilirubin levels to ototoxicity and deafness in high risk low birthweight infants. *Pediatrics*, **76**, 415–417
89. Howard J., Parmelee, A. H., Kopp, C. B. and Littman, B. (1976) A neurological comparison of preterm and full term infants at term conceptual age. *J. Pediatr.*, **88**, 995–1002
90. Kutzberg, D., Vaughan, H. G., Dau, M. C., Grellong, B. A., Albin, S. and Rotkin, L. (1979) Neurobehavioural performances of low birthweight infants at 40 weeks conceptional age. Comparison with full term infants. *Dev Med. Child Neurol.*, **21**, 596–607
91. Morante, A., Dubowitz, L. M. S., Levene, M. and Dubowitz, V. (1982) The development of visual function in normal and neurologically abnormal preterm and full term infants. *Dev. Med. Child Neurol.*, **24**, 771–784
92. Placzek, M., Mushin, J. and Dubowitz, L. M. S. (1985) Maturation of the visual evoked response and its correlation with visual acuity in preterm infants. *Dev. Med. Child Neurol.*, **27**, 448–454
93. Kutzberg, D. and Vaughan, H. G. (1985) Electrophysiological assessment of auditory and visual function in the newborn. *Clin. Perinatol.*, **12**, 277–298
94. Touwen, B. C. L. and Hadders Algra, M. (1983) Hyperextension of the neck and trunk and shoulder retraction in infancy: a prognostic study. *Neuropediatrics*, **14**, 202
95. Papile, L., Burnstein, J., Burnstein, R. and Koffler, H. (1978) Incidence and evolution of subependymal and intraventricular haemorrhage: a study of infants with birthweight less than 1500 g. *J. Pediatr.*, **92**, 529–534
96. Volpe, J. J. (1978) Neonatal periventricular hemorrhage, past, present and future. *Pediatrics*, **92**, 693–696
97. Dubowitz, L. M. S., Levene, M. I., Morante, A., Palmer, P. and Dubowitz, V. (1981) Neurological signs in neonatal intraventricular hemorrhage: correlation with real-time ultrasound. *J. Pediatr.*, **99**, 127–133
98. Dubowitz, L. M. S. (1985) Neurological assessment of the full term and preterm newborn infant. In *The At-Risk Infant: Psycho/Social/Medical Aspects* (eds S. Harel and N. Y. Anastolsiow), Paul H. Brooks, Baltimore, pp. 185–196
99. Dubowitz, L. M. S., Dubowitz, V., Palmer, P. G., Miller, G., Fawer, C. L. and Levene, M. I. (1984) Correlation of neurological assessment in the preterm newborn infant with outcome at one year. *J. Pediatr.*, **105**, 452–456
100. De Vries, L. S., Regev, R. and Dubowitz, L. M. S. (1986) Late onset cystic leukomalacia. *Arch. Dis. Child.*, **61**, 298–299

101. De Vries, L. S., Dubowitz, L. M. S., Dubowitz, V. *et al.* (1985) Predictive value of cranial ultrasound in the newborn baby: a reappraisal. *Lancet*, **ii**, 137–140
102. Yudkin, P. L., Aboualfa, M., Eyre, J. A., Redman, C. W. G. and Wilkinson, A. R. (1987) Influence of elective delivery on birthweight and head circumference standards. *Arch. Dis. Child.*, **62**, 24–29
103. Lemire, R. J., Loeser, J. D., Leech, R. W. and Alvord, E. C. Jr (1975) *Normal and Abnormal Development of the Human Nervous System*, Harper and Row, Hagerstown, Maryland
104. Yakovlev, P. I. (1959) Pathoarchitectonic studies of cerebral malformations. I. Arrhinencephalies (holoprosencephalies). *J. Neuropathol. Exp. Neurol.*, **18**, 22–35
105. Sidman, R. L., Miale, I. L. and Feder, N. (1959) Cell proliferation and migration in the primitive ependymal zone: an autoradiographic study of histogenesis in the nervous system. *Exp. Neurol.*, **1**, 322–326
106. Berry, M., Rogers, A. W. and Eayrs, J. F. (1964) Pattern of cell migration during cortical histogenesis. *Nature*, **203**, 591–593
107. Sidman, R. L. and Rakic, P. (1973) Neuronal migration with special reference to developing human brain: a review. *Brain Res.*, **62**, 1–15
108. Gruner, J. E. (1970) The maturation of human cerebral cortex in electron microsopy study of post-mortem punctures in preterm infants. *Biol. Neonate*, **16**, 243–247
109. Marin-Padilla, M. (1970) Prenatal and early postnatal ontogenesis of the human cortex: a Golgi study. 1. The sequential development of the cortical layers. *Brain Res.*, **23**, 167–169
110. Molliver, M. E., Kostovic, I. and Van Der Loos, H. (1973) The development of synapses in cerebral cortex of the human fetus. *Brain Res.*, **50**, 403–407
111. Purpura, D. P. (1959) Nature of electrocortical potentials and synaptic organisations in the cerebral and cerebellar cortex. *Int. Rev. Neurobiol.*, **1**, 47–163
112. Gibbs, F. A. and Gibbs, E. L. (1950) *Atlas of Encephalography*, Addison-Wesley, Reading, Massachusetts
113. Askerinsky, K. E. and Kleitman, N. (1953) Regularly occurring periods of eye motility and concomitant phenomena during sleep. *Science*, **118**, 273–274
114. Askerinsky, K. E., Dement, W. and Klietman, N. (1957) Cyclical variations in EEG during sleep and their relation to eye movement, body motility, and dreaming. *Electroencephalogr. Clin. Neurophysiol.*, **9**, 680–690
115. Wolfe, P. H. (1959) State and neonatal activity. *Psychosom. Med.*, **21**, 110–118
116. Prechtl, H. F. R. (1968) States of the infant. *Clin. Dev. Med.*, **28**, 27–41
117. Anders, T. F., Emde, R. and Parmelee, A. H. (1971) *A Manual of Standardized Terminology, Techniques and Criteria for Scoring States of Sleep and Wakefulness in Newborn Infants*, UCLA Brain Information Service, BRI Publications Office, Los Angeles, California, NNDS Neurological Information Network
118. Dreyfus-Brisac, C. (1968) Sleep ontogenesis in early human prematures from 24 to 27 weeks of conceptional age. *Dev. Psychol.*, **1**, 162–169
119. Dreyfus-Brisac, C. (1979) Neonatal electroencephalography. In *Reviews in Perinatal Medicine*, Vol. 3, (eds E. M. Scarpelli and E. V. Cosmi), Raven Press, New York
120. Bergstrom, R. M. (1969) Electrical parameters of the brain during ontogeny. In *Brain and Early Behaviour* (ed. R. J. Robinson), Academic Press, London, pp. 15–36
121. Eyre, J. A., Oozeer, R. C. and Wilkinson, A. R. (1983) Diagnosis of neonatal seizure by continuous recording and rapid analysis of the electroencephalogram. *Arch. Dis. Child.*, **58**, 785–790
122. Eyre, J. A., Nanei, S. and Wilkinson, A. R. (1988) Quantification of changes of the normal neonatal electroencephalogram in relation to gestational age from continuous five day recordings. *Early Hum. Dev.*
123. Dreyfus-Brisac, C. (1970) Ontogenesis of sleep in human prematures after 32 weeks of conceptional age. *Dev. Psychol.*, **3**, 91–121
124. Anderson, C. M., Torres, F. and Faoro, A. (1985) The EEG of the early premature. *Electroencephalogr. Clin. Neurophysiol.*, **60**, 95–105
125. Watanabe, K. (1978) Neurophysiological approaches to the normal and abnormal development of CNS in early life. *Asian Med. J.*, **21**, 421–450
126. Lombroso, C. T. (1979) Quantified electrographic scales on 10 pre-term healthy newborns followed up to 40–43 weeks of conceptional age by serial polygraphic recording. *Electroencephalogr. Clin. Neurophysiol.*, **46**, 460–471

127. Monod, N. and Ducas, P. (1968) The prognostic value of the encephalogram in the first two years of life. In *Clinical Electroencephalography of Children* (eds P. Kellawat and Petersen), Grune and Stratton, New York, pp. 61–76
128. Rose, A. L. and Lombroso, C. T. (1970) Neonatal seizure states. A study of clinical, pathological and electroencephalographic features in 137 full term babies with a long term followup. *Pediatrics*, **45**, 404–442
129. Engel, R. C. H. (1975) *Abnormal Electroencephalograms in the Neonatal Period*, C. C. Thomas, Springfield, Illinois
130. Rumack, C. M. and Johnson, M. L. (1984) *Perinatal and Infant Brain Imaging*, Year Book Medical Publishers, Chicago.
131. Fischer, A. Q., Anderson, J. C., Shuman, R. M. and Stinson, W. (1985) *Pediatric Neurosonography. Clinical Tomography and Neuropathological Correlates*, Wiley, Chichester
132. Levine M. I., Williams, J. L. and Fawer, C–L. (1985) *Ultrasound of the Infant Brain*, Spastics International Medical Publications 92, Blackwell Scientific Publications, Oxford
133. Stewart, A. L., Thorburn, R. J., Hope, P. L., Goldsmith, M., Lipscombe, A. P. and Reynolds, E. O. R. (1983) Ultrasound appearances of the brain in very preterm infants and neurodevelopmental outcome at 18 months of age. *Arch. Dis. Child.*, **58**, 598–604
134. De Vries, L. S., Dubowitz, L. M. S., Dubowitz, V. *et al.* (1985) Predictive value of cranial ultrasound in the newborn baby; a reappraisal. *Lancet*, **ii**, 137–140
135. Cooke, R. W. I. (1987) Early and late cranial ultrasonographic appearances and outcome in very low birthweight infants. *Arch. Dis. Child.*, **62**, 931–937
136. Wasterlain, C. G. and Plum, F. (1973) Vulnerability of developing rat brain to electroconvulsive seizures. *Arch. Neurol.*, **29**, 38–45
137. King, L. J. *et al.* (1967) Effects of convulsants on energy reserves in the cerebral cortex. *J. Neurochem.*, **14**, 599–611
138. Plum, F., House, D. C. and Duffy, T. E. (1974) Metabolic effects of seizures. In *Brain Dysfunction in Metabolic Disorders* (ed. F. Plum), Raven Press, New York
139. Volpe, J. (1981) Neurological disorders. In *Neonatology* (ed. G. Avery), Lippincott, Philadelphia
140. O'Donohoe, N. V. (1979) *Epilepsies of Childhood*, Butterworths, London
141. Lockman, L. A., Kriel, R., Zaske, D., Thompson, T. and Virnig, N. (1979) Phenobarbital dosage for control of neonatal seizures. *Neurology*, **29**, 1445–1449
142. Pippenger, C. and Rosen, T. V. (1975) Phenobarbital plasma levels in neonates. *Clin. Perinatol.*, **2**, 111–115
143. Whitelaw, A., Placzek, M., Dubowitz, L., Lary, S. and Levene, M. (1983) Phenobarbitone for prevention of periventricular haemorrhage in very low birth weight infants. A randomised double blind trial. *Lancet*, **ii**, 1168–1170
144. Painter, M. J., Pippenger, C., MacDonald, H. and Pitlick, W. (1978) Phenobarbital and diphenylhydantoin levels in neonates with seizures. *J. Pediatr.*, **9**, 315–319
145. Johnson, C. E. and Vigoreaux, J. A. (1984) Compatibility of paraldehyde with plastic syringes and needle hubs. *Am. J. Hosp. Pharm.*, **41**, 306–308
146. Giacoia, G. P., Gessner, P. K., Zaleska, M. M. and Boutwell, W. C. (1984) Pharmacokinetics of paraldehyde disposition in the neonate. *J. Pediatr.*, **104**, 291–295
147. Eyre, J. A. and Wilkinson, A. R. (1986) Thiopentone-induced coma after severe birth asphyxia. *Arch. Dis. Child.*, **61**, 1084–1089
148. Miall-Allen, V. and Whitelaw, A. (1986) Neonates who develop large intraventricular haemorrhages have lower arterial pressure in the first 22 hours. Paper presented to the Neonatal Society, Marstrand, Sweden, May 1986
149. Larroche, J. C. (1972) Post-haemorrhagic hydrocephalus in infancy: anatomical study. *Biol. Neonate*, **20**, 287–299
150. Palmer, P., Dubowitz, L. M. S., Levene, M. I. and Dubowitz, V. (1982) Developmental and neurological progress of preterm infants with IVH and ventricular dilatation. *Arch. Dis. Child.*, **57**, 748–753
151. Allan, W. C., Dransfield, D. A. and Tito, A. M. (1984) Ventricular dilatation following periventricular-intraventricular hemorrhage: outcome at one year. *Pediatrics*, **73**, 158–162
152. Cooke, R. W. I. (1983) Early prognosis of low birth weight infants treated for progressive post-haemorrhagic hydrocephalus. *Arch. Dis. Child.*, **58**, 410–414

153. Lipscomb, A. P., Thorburn, R. J., Stewart, A. L., Reynolds, E. O. R. and Hope, P. L. (1983) Early treatment for rapidly progressive post-haemorrhagic hydrocephalus. *Lancet*, **i**, 1438–1439
154. Liechty, E. A., Gilmor, R. L., Bryson, C. Q. and Bull, M. J. (1983) Outcome of high-risk neonates with ventriculomegaly. *Dev. Med. Child Neurol.*, **25**, 162–168
155. Papille, L. A., Munswick-Bruno, G. and Schaefer, A. (1983) Relationship of cerebral intraventricular haemorrhage and early childhood neurologic handicaps. *J. Pediatr.*, **103**, 273–277
156. Chaplin, E. R., Goldstein, G. W., Myerberg, D. Z., Hunt, J. V. and Tooley, W. H. (1980) Post-hemorrhagic hydrocephalus in the preterm infant. *Pediatrics*, **65**, 901–909
157. Shankaran, S., Slovis, T. L., Bedard, M. P. and Poland, R. L. (1982) Sonographic classification of intracranial hemorrhage. A prognostic indicator of mortality, morbidity and short-term neurologic outcome. *J. Pediatr.*, **100**, 469–475
158. Williamson, W. D., Desmond, M. M., Wilson, G. S., Murphy, M. A., Rozelle, J. and Garcia-Prats, J. A. (1983) Survival of low-birth weight infants with neonatal intraventricular hemorrhage. *Am. J. Dis. Child.*, **137**, 1181–1184
159. Levene, M. I. (1981) Measurement of the growth of the lateral ventricles in preterm infants with real time ultrasound. *Arch. Dis. Child.*, **56**, 900–904
160. Kaiser, A. and Whitelaw, A. (1986) Normal cerebrospinal fluid pressure in the newborn. *Neuropediatrics*, **17**, 100–102
161. Kaiser, A. and Whitelaw, A. (1985) Cerebrospinal fluid pressure in infants with post-haemorrhagic ventricular dilatation. *Arch. Dis. Child.*, **60**, 920–924
162. Kreusser, K. L., Tarby, T. J., Kovnar, E., Taylor, D. A., Hill, A. and Volpe, J. (1985) Serial lumbar punctures for at least temporary amelioration of neonatal post-hemorrhagic hydrocephalus. *Pediatrics*, **75**, 715–723
163. Mantovani, J. F., Pasternak, J. F., Mathew, O. P. *et al.* (1980) Failure of daily lumbar punctures to prevent the development of hydrocephalus following intraventricular hemorrhage. *J. Pediatr.*, **97**, 278–281
164. Anwar, M., Kadam, S., Hiatt, I. M. and Hegyi, T. (1985) Serial lumbar punctures in prevention of post-hemorrhagic hydrocephalus in preterm infants. *J. Pediatr.*, **107**, 446–449
165. Lorber, J. (1975) Isosorbide in treatment of infantile hydrocephalus. *Arch. Dis. Child.*, **50**, 431–436
166. Shinnar, S., Gammon, K., Bergman, E. W., Epstein, M. and Freedom, J. M. (1985) Management of hydrocephalus in infancy: use of acetazolamide and furosemide to avoid cerebrospinal fluid shunts. *J. Pediatr.*, **107**, 31–36
167. Cooke, R. W. I. (1986) Ventriculoperitoneal shunt for post-haemorrhagic hydrocephalus in low birth weight infants. Paper presented to the British Paediatric Association, York, April 1986
168. Gairdner, D. and Pearson, J. (1971) A growth chart for premature and other infants. *Arch. Dis. Child.*, **46**, 783–787

Chapter 20

Iatrogenic disease

Jean W. Keeling and Elizabeth M. Bryan

The baby who weighs less than 1000 g at birth is unlikely to survive without active medical support and highly skilled nursing. ELBW infants are at increased risk of birth injury, many have respiratory problems and require ventilation, and they need assistance to achieve adequate nutrition. Treatment of infection, anaemia and jaundice is often necessary.

The introduction of intensive care of LBW newborns has been followed by the recognition of a range of complications of monitoring and of treatment. In very immature babies, the margins of safety between effective treatment and iatrogenic injury are often precariously narrow. Preterm delivery itself may be iatrogenic when it follows amniocentesis, undertaken either for prenatal diagnosis [1] or for the management of rhesus disease [2] or when premature operative delivery is undertaken because of severe maternal pre-eclampsia or intrauterine growth retardation.

Some complications are immediately apparent and may be life-threatening; others may not be recognized for several years. We here examine the complications of essential care of the ELBW newborn which are encountered at necropsy examination in the neonatal period and early infancy and look at the sequelae of intensive care amongst survivors during early childhood. Table 20.1 summarizes the commonest iatrogenic lesions observed at necropsy examination in ELBW babies, grouped by age at death.

Birth injury

The very immature baby is at risk of intracranial trauma during vaginal delivery. The cranium is easily deformed as skull bones are thin and poorly mineralized, connective tissue along suture lines is immature and cartilaginous junctions within the occipital bone are wide. Skull fractures and tears of falx and tentorium are uncommon, but cranial deformity is more likely to result in tearing of bridging veins as they cross the subdural space or direct compression of the brain. One form of cranial injury of which the very preterm infant is at risk is occipital osteodiastasis. This type of injury is more commonly found after breech delivery, a relatively frequent mode of presentation for the infant under 34 weeks gestation. Furthermore, a smaller deforming force is probably required in the preterm infant.

Pressure between the internal aspect of the maternal pubic bones and the inferior part of the fetal occipital bone results in internal displacement of the latter and either

Table 20.1 Iatrogenic pathology observed at necropsy amongst 131 babies of birth weight <1000 g by age at death. Necropsies were performed at John Radcliffe Hospital, Oxford between 1975 and 1986 and include babies treated in that intensive care nursery and those referred for post-mortem examination

Age at death	*0–24 h*				*2–7 days*				*8–28 days*			
	M	*F*	*Total*	*Percentage of group (%)*	*M*	*F*	*Total*	*Percentage of group (%)*	*M*	*F*	*Total*	*Percentage of group (%)*
Ventilation												
Laryngeal injury	3	8	11	16	7	9	16	36	7	2	9	45
Tracheal injury	5	5	10	15	4	3	7	16	5	1	6	30
Interstitial emphysema	11	10	21	31	4	9	13	30	3	1	4	20
Pneumothorax	12	4	16	24	5	8	13	30	4	2	6	30
Lung perforation by chest drain	2		2	3	3		3	7		1	1	5
Bronchopulmonary dysplasia					1	1	2	5	11	5	16	75
Large vessel cannulation												
Aortic/iliac thrombosis		1	1	2	8	6	14	32	3	2	5	25
Periumbilical a. haemorrhage	1	2	3	5	2		2	5				
Pulmonary thromboembolism					2	1	3	7	2		2	10
Gangrene of extremities									1	1	2	10
Delivery or resuscitation trauma/hypoxia												
Bruising	13	5	18	27	5	7	12	27	4	1	5	25
Subcapsular haematoma liver	6	4	10	15	3	2	5	11	2		2	10
Haemoperitoneum	2	2	4	6	5		5	11	1		1	5
Skin excoriation	3		3	5	6	3	9	20	2	1	3	15
Total in group	43	24	67	100	22	22	44	100	14	6	20	100

compression or contusion of the cerebellum or tearing of the overlying sigmoid sinus causing subdural haemorrhage [3].

Vaginal breech delivery also predisposes to fractures of long bones, usually the femur, but fractures of the humerus are described when difficulties are encountered in bringing down the arms [4]. Bleeding into the muscles of legs and buttocks results from hypoxic capillary damage and increased hydrostatic pressure in fetal dependent parts whilst awaiting delivery of the head [5]. The blood loss can be considerable and require replacement, and marked hyperbilirubinaemia may occur.

Visceral injuries result from manipulation of the fetal trunk. Hypoxia-induced hypotonia is a contributory factor. The most common injury is subcapsular haematoma of the liver, usually affecting the anterior surface of the right lobe. Posterosuperior tears in the liver capsule close to the emergence of the inferior vena cava may result in severe haemorrhage; rupture of haematomata, producing a haemoperitoneum, is often rapidly fatal. More commonly the hepatic capsule remains intact and the extent of haemorrhage is restricted by increasing pressure within the haematoma. Injuries to the spleen, intestine and mesentery are less frequent.

Ventilation

Complications of ventilation can be conveniently considered in relation to the apparatus and to the mode of administration and composition of ventilating gases.

Apparatus

Orotracheal and nasotracheal tubes are kept in place by the use of adhesive strapping to the face. The epidermis of the preterm infant is thin and poorly keratinized, so cutaneous excoriation is easily produced by frequent changes of tube (Figure 20.1).

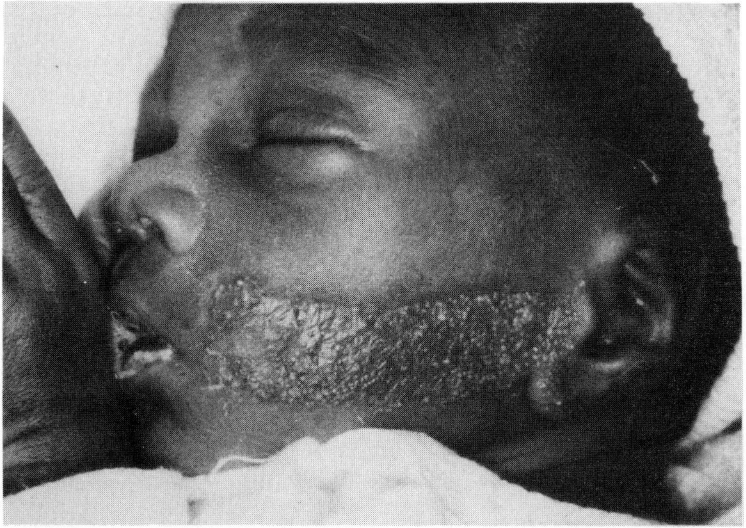

Figure 20.1 Cutaneous excoriation caused by adhesive strapping

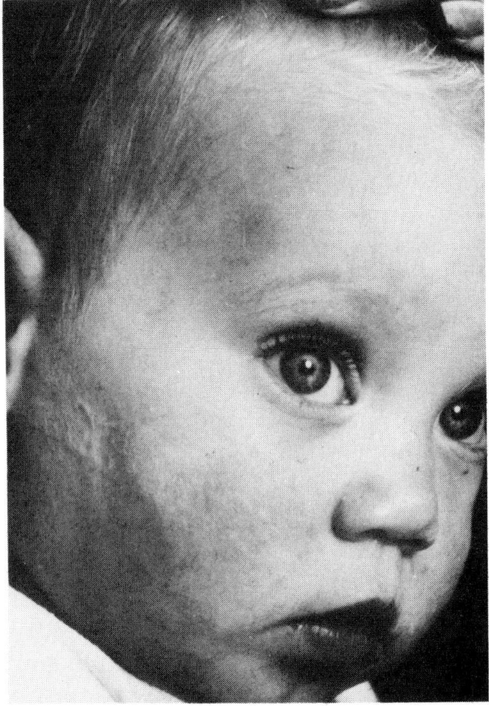

Figure 20.2 Two-year-old with facial scarring from adhesive strapping

This can cause lasting marks which are disfiguring in both light and dark skinned children (Figure 20.2).

Pressure from the tube itself results in local injury at any point along its length. Nasotracheal tubes can cause ulceration at the external nares (Figure 20.3), and in some cases soft tissue injury is accompanied by pressure necrosis of the underlying cartilage which results in permanent disfigurement.

Palatal grooving and central clefts (Figure 20.4) have been reported following the long-term use of orotracheal tubes [6,7] and these can trap milk during feeding and encourage aspiration pneumonitis. The original reports suggested that direct pressure of tube on palate was responsible for the deformity, but Carillo [8] proposed that the continued presence of the tube prevents apposition of tongue and palate and so interferes with the normal spreading and reduction of the postalveolar ridges. Whilst this mechanism would accentuate any secondary palatal grooves, it is unlikely to produce clefts.

Abnormalities of the primary dentition are common in LBW children [9] (Figure 20.5) and it has been suggested that these may be due to gingival pressures from endotracheal tubes [10].

Laryngeal ulceration is a particularly serious side effect of intubation. Ulceration occurs either along the free margin of the vocal cords or in the subglottic region (Figure 20.6). Superficial ulceration is repaired by rapid re-epithelialization following removal of the tube, but deeper ulcers result in necrosis of cartilage [11] or narrowing of the lumen during maturation and subsequent shrinkage of fibrous scars. Laryngeal

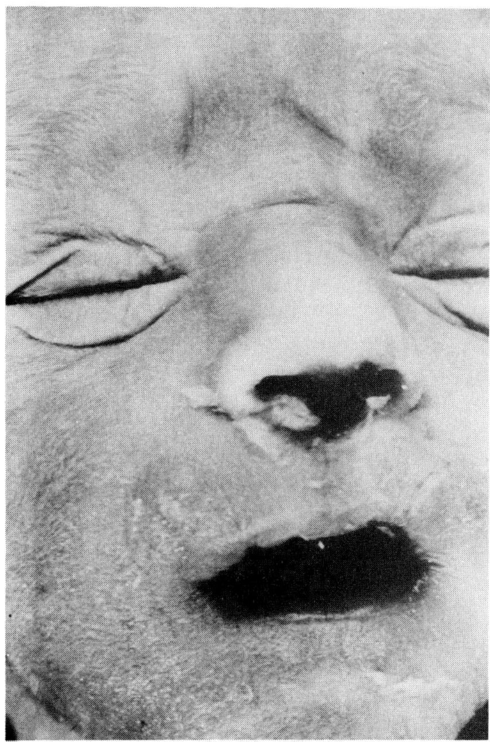

Figure 20.3 Ulcer of nasal skin following nasotracheal intubation [40]

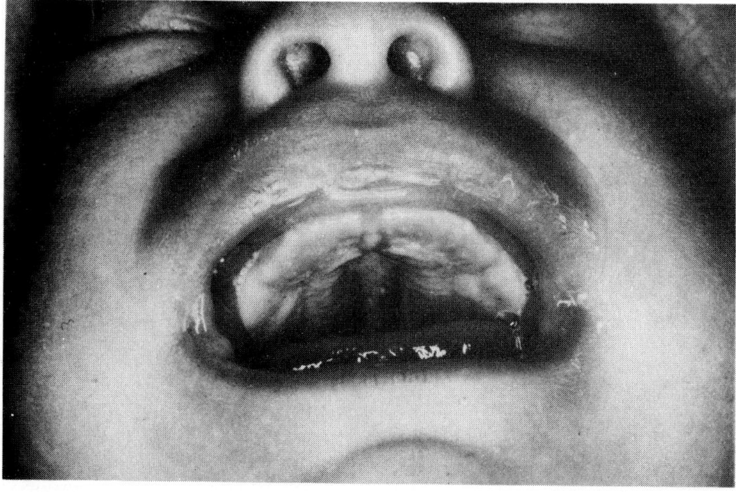

Figure 20.4 Palatal groove following prolonged orotracheal intubation

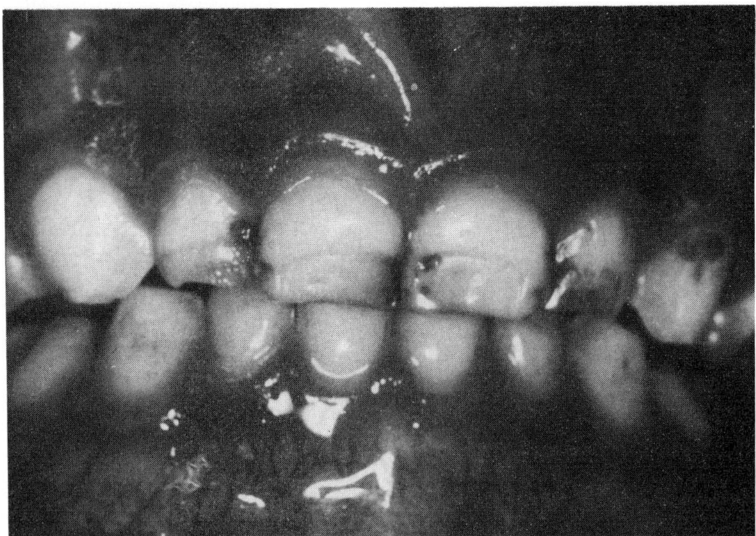

Figure 20.5 Enamel defects of upper incisors in primary dentition [9]

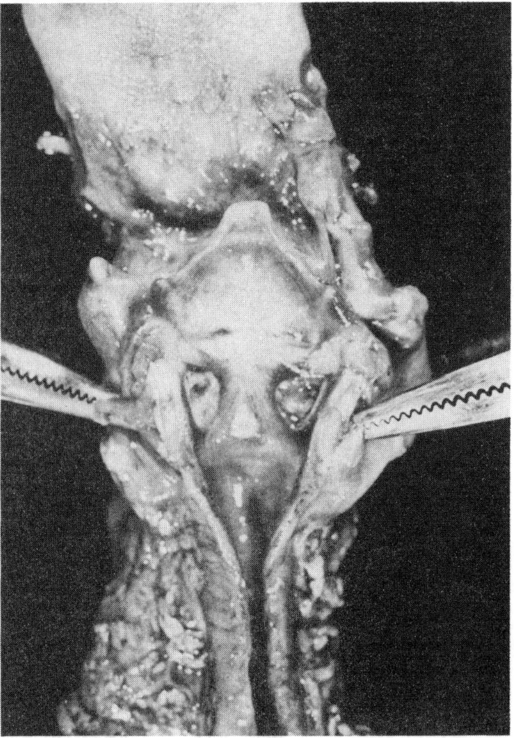

Figure 20.6 Larynx opened posteriorly: ulceration in the midline and to either side below the vocal cords following chronic intubation [40]

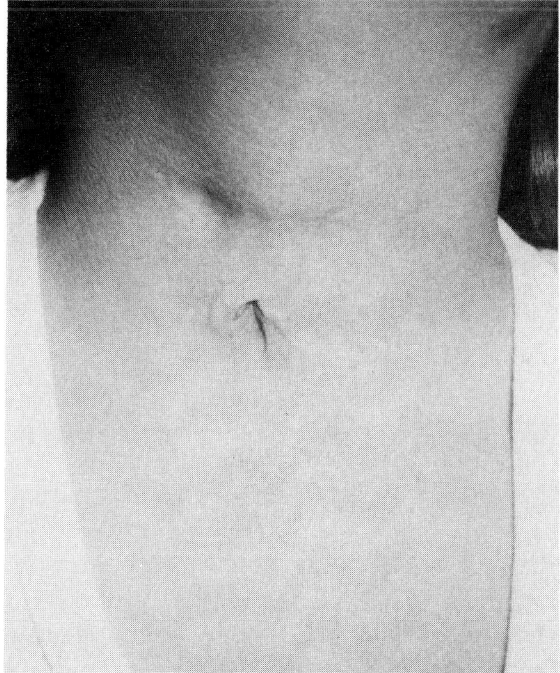

Figure 20.7 Scarring at site of tracheostomy in a six-year-old girl

or tracheal stenosis occurs in about 1.5% of chronically intubated infants [12]; intubation for four weeks or more predisposes to stenosis. Some children require tracheostomy for many years because of laryngeal stenosis and residual scarring is difficult to avoid (Figure 20.7).

Less severe damage to the vocal cords may go unrecorded, but persistent stridor causes anxiety to the parents and attracts distressing comments from outsiders; an abnormal speaking voice may be a grave social disadvantage. Some babies are not able to gain attention by crying, which must be frustrating as well as potentially dangerous.

Tracheal ulceration, usually manifest as focal anterior midline ulcers overlying consecutive cartilaginous rings, is sometimes seen. Squamous metaplasia of the tracheal epithelium is often extensive and involves the whole area of contact between tube and trachea, although epithelium overlying the posterior muscle is usually spared. This change seems to regress rapidly following extubation, but there may be interference with normal bronchial toilet in the period immediately after extubation and this predisposes to infection. Perforation of the trachea [13] or oesophagus [14] are infrequent complications of endotracheal intubation.

Oxygen is sometimes delivered by means of a face mask. This must fit tightly around the mouth and is usually secured by means of a broad (approximately 2 cm) velcro band. Ischaemic necrosis and haemorrhage in the cerebellum have been observed following its use [15]; these are related to inward displacement of the occipital bone.

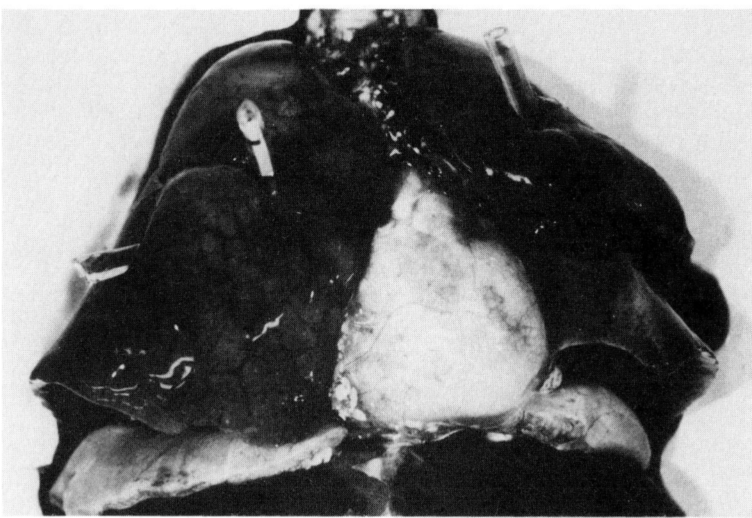

Figure 20.8 Perforation of the lung by chest drain

Pressure of ventilating gases

Interstitial emphysema is a common complication of ventilation of immature lungs. Gas accumulates initially in the interstitial connective tissue around intrapulmonary bronchi and vessels and along interlobular septa. From this situation gas can collect beneath the pleura where it can be seen as small blebs.

Accumulation of gas also occurs in the interlobar fissures and at the hila. Rupture of the pleural surface produces pneumothorax. Eventually such defects close spontaneously. From hilar accumulations gas may track up into the mediastinum and thence to subcutaneous tissues over the head and neck, where its crepitant quality is readily apparent. Gas may accumulate within the pericardial sac, occasionally giving rise to tamponade, or track downwards into retroperitoneal tissues where it may mimic pneumoperitoneum occurring in the course of necrotizing enterocolitis.

Pneumothorax is a common complication of ventilation in the very preterm infant. Estimates of its frequency vary widely and are closely related to both the admissions policy of a particular unit and the maximum ventilatory pressures used. Lindroth *et al.* [16] observed pneumothorax in 20% of babies receiving intermittent positive pressure ventilation in their unit. A frequent complication of management of this life-threatening event is perforation of the lung by a chest drain (Figure 20.8), particularly if a rigid introducer is used. Such perforation can provoke considerable haemorrhage without injury to large vessels because of the gross pulmonary congestion which is usually present. Injury to major vessels or other mediastinal structures is unusual. The authors have seen major haemothorax when an intercostal artery was torn during introduction of a chest drain. There was extensive retropleural and intramuscular haemorrhage as well.

An anterior chest drain scar is not only unsightly but may affect female breast development. Whenever possible the axilla is a preferable site as this ensures that the scar is hidden and the risk to the breast is removed.

Composition and delivery of gas mixtures

Bronchopulmonary dysplasia (BPD) is a frequent and serious complication of ventilation. Its cause continues to be disputed. All of the histological features of BPD can be produced in animals by administration of increased oxygen concentrations at atmospheric pressures [17]. Edwards, Dyer and Northway [18] were able to induce pulmonary changes comparable to BPD by ventilating with air at the same pressure. In the human infant a relationship to gas pressures and length of ventilatory cycle has been described [19]. Interstitial oedema secondary to elevated pulmonary arterial pressure [20] may also be important.

The histological appearances of BPD were first described by Northway, Rosan and Porter [21]. Some of the features originally described are now rarely seen. Squamous metaplasia of intrapulmonary bronchi, for instance, is now uncommon. It was only seen in patients who died before 20 days of age.

Oxygen monitoring

Recognition of an association between administration of oxygen-rich mixtures and retrolental fibroplasia in preterm infants (retinopathy of prematurity) [22] led to the introduction of methods of monitoring oxygen levels to maintain them within the confines of adequacy and safety. Intermittent sampling from peripheral arteries is less satisfactory than continuous monitoring because of limitation of the number of samples by availability of sampling sites and the inaccuracy of results obtained when a baby is disturbed by the procedure.

Temporal artery sampling was largely discontinued following reports of contralateral hemiplegia during the ensuing months due to cerebral infarction [23]. Radial artery sampling is sometimes followed by carpal tunnel syndrome due to haematoma [24], or gangrene of the forearm (Figure 20.9) but minor bruising is often the only sequel [25]. However, in the longer term extensive scarring and depigmentation of the forearm (Figure 20.10), particularly against a sun tan, may cause embarrassment.

Indwelling aortic cannulae which permit withdrawal of regular blood samples or have an oxygen detecting electrode incorporated into the tip have been used for systemic oxygen monitoring. Use of such cannulae in ELBW infants is always a cause of concern as their presence produces a marked reduction in the cross-sectional area of the vessel. In addition, intimal injury is common and predisposes to thrombosis. Minor thrombosis is a frequent complication of chronic aortic cannulation [26]; major thrombosis results in gangrene of lower limbs (Figure 20.11), ischaemic necrosis of the buttocks and external genitalia or visceral infarction. The risk and degree of thrombosis is related to the duration of cannulation, whether the cannula is used for intravenous alimentation, site of hole (side-hole cannulae have a dead space at the tip) and, finally, the position of the cannula. Aortic aneurysm is an uncommon complication and appears to be related to concomitant septicaemia [27,28]. Hypertension is an infrequent but serious late complication and is responsible for the majority of cases of hypertension seen in children in the UK and USA. Peripheral artery cannulation is now being more often used thus reducing major complications, although serious local ischaemia can occur. The magnitude of the complications of invasive methods of oxygen monitoring has stimulated the development of non-invasive monitoring techniques. The use of transcutaneous oxygen electrodes has produced only minor, transient erythema.

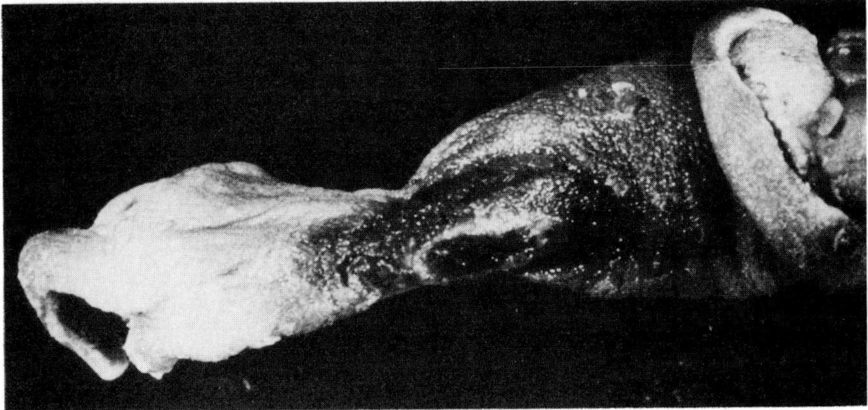

Figure 20.9 Gangrene of forearm necessitating amputation following radial then brachial artery sampling [40]

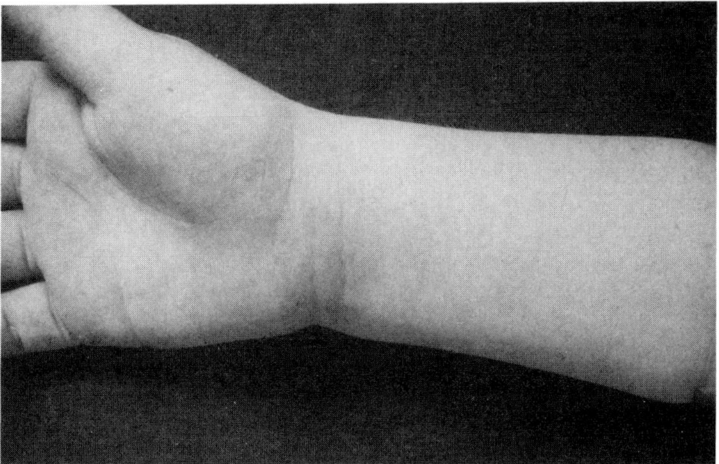

Figure 20.10 Scarring and depigmentation of forearm following multiple radial artery sampling in the neonatal period at six years

Umbilical venous cannulation

Umbilical vein cannulation was undertaken initially for exchange transfusions in the treatment of rhesus disease. Later it was used for blood sampling and intravenous alimentation as it is technically easier than umbilical arterial catheterization. The rate

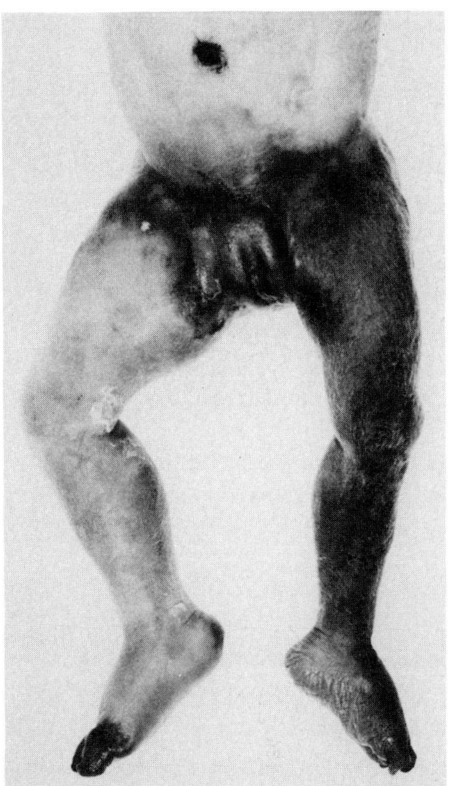

Figure 20.11 Gangrene of the lower limbs and genitalia following massive aortic thrombosis

of complications resulting from thrombosis around or beyond the catheter is very high (Figure 20.12). Pulmonary thromboembolism and hepatic vein or inferior vena cava thrombosis are frequent; massive hepatic necrosis is also recorded and portal hypertension is a late complication [29], and perforation of the heart has also been reported [30]. Necrotizing enterocolitis has been recognized as a complication of this procedure for many years [31,32].

Drugs and their administration

Side effects of drugs do not pose as great a problem in the neonatal period as they do in adults, perhaps because of the restricted range of drugs prescribed in the neonatal period. The side effects of some drugs are predictable; tolazoline with its histamine-like structure, used in the neonate to reduce pulmonary hypertension, provokes gastric ulceration, sometimes accompanied by massive haemorrhage. Gentamicin is toxic to the auditory nerve.

The method of administering drugs may cause damage. Some antibiotics such as

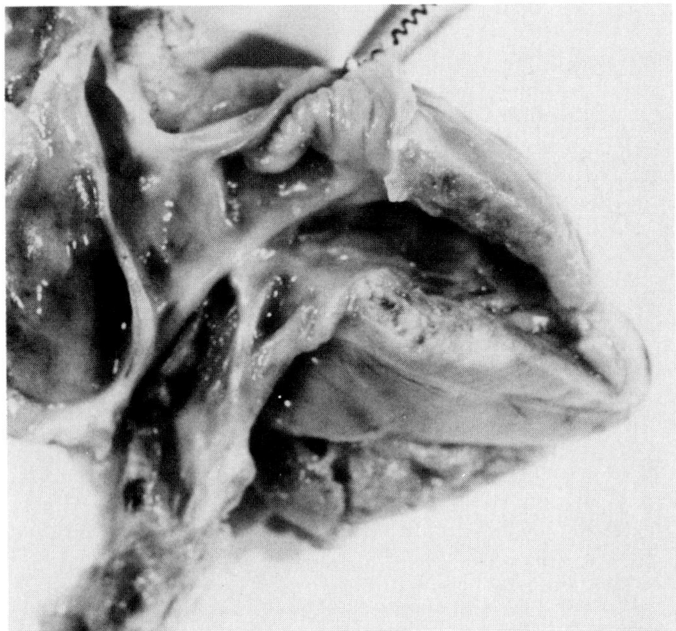

Figure 20.12 Heart from right side: a cylindrical thrombus is present in the inferior vena cava and extends through the foramen ovale [40]

nafcillin give rise to soft tissue necrosis should extravasation of the infusion occur [33]. Extravasation of calcium gluconate has resulted in dystrophic calcification around the drip site (Figure 20.13). Quadriceps contracture is an unusual but well recognized complication of intramuscular injections in the thigh [34]. An abscess at the site of an intramuscular injection has led to osteomyelitis and deformity [35]. Intravenous alimentation is more hazardous in the VLBW baby than in mature infants and is in part related to immaturity of the reticuloendothelial system and liver. Pulmonary lipid thromboembolism has been reported following the administration of lipid emulsions as a bolus [36] and subsequently when administered continuously [37]. Pulmonary infarction was reported by the latter group. Lipid is present throughout the reticuloendothelial system and work in animals indicates compromised handling of microorganisms which might be an additional hazard in the ELBW infant whose immune competence is incompletely developed.

Amino acid infusions induce cholestasis and portal fibrosis [38]. This usually reverses after cessation of infusion but occasionally there is progression to cirrhosis. Cholelithiasis has been described when frusemide has been given at the same time as amino acid infusions: the drug enhances calcium secretion into the biliary tract [39].

Topical applications

The skin of the VLBW infant is poorly keratinized and is thus readily permeable. This permeability allows absorption of constituents of topical applications (see Chapter 9).

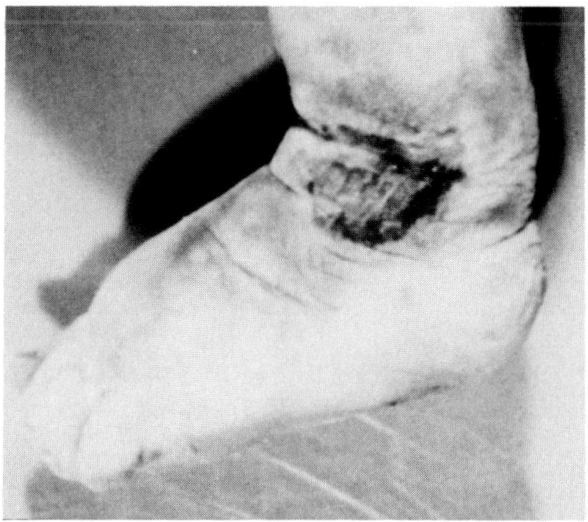

Figure 20.13 Ulceration and dystrophic calcification around a venepuncture site following extravasation of calcium gluconate

Conclusion

The price of intensive care of ELBW babies who survive may be iatrogenic damage which can, at worst, produce lasting physical or emotional handicap and at least a social embarrassment. Constant vigilance is essential if the long-term happiness of these ELBW survivors is not to be marred by some avoidable action on the part of the caretakers in the early weeks.

References

1. Medical Research Council (1978) An assessment of the hazards of amniocentesis. *Br. J. Obstet. Gynaecol.*, **85** (Suppl. 2), 1–41
2. Brinsmead, M. W. (1976) Complications of amniocentesis. *Med. J. Aust.*, **1**, 379–385
3. Wigglesworth, J. S. and Husemeyer, R. P. (1977) Intracranial birth trauma in vaginal breech delivery: the continued importance of injury to the occipital bone. *Br. J. Obstet. Gynaecol.*, **84**, 684–691
4. Wigglesworth, J. S. (1984) Intrapartum and early neonatal death: the interaction of asphyxia and trauma. In *Perinatal Pathology*, W. B. Saunders, Philadelphia, pp. 93–112
5. Ralis, Z. A. (1975) Birth traumas to muscles in babies born by breech delivery and its possible fatal consequence. *Arch. Dis. Child.*, **50**, 4–13
6. Duke, P. M., Coulson, J. D., Santos, J. I. and Johnson, J. D. (1976) Cleft palate associated with prolonged orotracheal intubation in infancy. *J. Pediatr.*, **89**, 990–991
7. Erenberg, A. and Nowak, A. J. (1984) Palatal groove formation in neonates and infants with orotracheal tubes. *Am. J. Dis. Child.*, **138**, 974–975
8. Carrillo, P. (1985) Palatal groove formation and oral endotracheal intubation. *Am. J. Dis. Child.*, **139**, 589–590
9. Fearne, J., Bryan, E., Elliman, A. and Elliman, A. (1985) Enamel defects in deciduous dentition of low birth weight infants. Presented to the Paediatric Research Societies in Europe, Munich, 1985
10. Moylan, F. M. B., Seldin, E. B., Shannon, D. C. and Todres, I. D. (1980) Defective primary dentition in survivors of neonatal mechanical ventilation. *J. Pediatr.*, **96**, 106–108

11. Gould, S. J. and Howard, S. (1985) The histopathology of the larynx in the neonate following endotracheal intubation. *J. Pathol.*, **146**, 301–311
12. O'Neill, J. A. Jr (1984) Experience with iatrogenic laryngeal and tracheal stenoses. *J. Pediatr.* Surg., **19**, 235–238
13. Reynolds, E. O. R. and Taghizadeh, A. (1974) Improved prognosis of infants mechanically ventilated for hyaline membrane disease. *Arch. Dis. Child.*, **49**, 505–515
14. Clarke, T. A., Coen, R. W., Feldman, B. and Papile, L. (1980) Esophageal perforations in premature infants and comments on the diagnosis. *Am. J. Dis. Child.*, **134**, 367–368
15. Pape, K. E., Armstrong, D. L. and Fitzhardinge, P. M. (1976) Central nervous system pathology associated with mask ventilation in the very low birthweight infant: a new aetiology for intracerebellar haemorrhages. *Pediatrics*, **58**, 473–483
16. Lindroth, M., Svenningsen, N. W., Ahlstrom, H. and Jonson, B. (1980) Evaluation of mechanical ventilation in newborn infants. *Acta Paediatr. Scand.*, **69**, 143–149
17. Bonikos, D. S., Bensch, K. G., Ludwin, S. K. and Northway, W. H. (1975) Oxygen toxicity in the newborn. The effect of prolonged 100% O_2 exposure on the lungs of newborn mice. *Lab. Invest.*, **32**, 619–635
18. Edwards, D. K., Dyer, W. M. and Northway, W. H. (1977) Twelve years' experience with bronchopulmonary dysplasia. *Pediatrics*, **59**, 839–845
19. Taghizadeh, A. and Reynolds, E. O. R. (1976) Pathogenesis of bronchopulmonary dysplasia following hyaline membrane disease. *Am. J. Pathol.*, **82**, 241–258
20. Brown, E. R., Stark, A., Sosenko, I., Lawson, E. E. and Avery, M. E. (1978) Bronchopulmonary dysplasia: possible relationship to pulmonary edema. *J. Pediatr.*, **92**, 982–984
21. Northway, W. H. Jr., Rosan, R. C. and Porter, D. Y. (1967) Pulmonary disease following respirator therapy of hyaline membrane disease. Bronchopulmonary dysplasia. *N. Engl. J. Med.*, **276**, 357–368
22. Ashton, N. Ward, B. and Serpell, G. (1954) Effect of oxygen on developing retinal vessels with particular reference to the problem of retrolental fibroplasia. *Br. J. Ophthalmol.*, **38**, 397–432
23. Simmons, M. A., Levine, R. V., Lubchenco, L. O. and Guggenheim, M. A. (1978) Warning: serious sequelae of temporal arterial catheterisation. *J. Pediatr.*, **92**, 284
24. Koenigsberger, M. R. and Moessinger, A. C. (1977) Iatrogenic carpal tunnel syndrome in the newborn infant. *J. Pediatr.*, **91**, 443–445
25. Adams, J. M. and Rudolph, A. J. (1975) The use of indwelling radial artery catheters in neonates. *Pediatrics*, **55**, 261–265
26. Wesstrom, G., Finnstrom, O. and Stenport, G. (1979) Umbilical artery catheterization in newborns. I. Thrombosis in relation to catheter type and position. *Acta Paediatr. Scand.*, **68**, 575–581
27. Rajs, J., Finnstrom, O. and Wesstrom, G. (1976) Case report. Aortic aneurysm developing after umbilical artery catheterization. *Acta Paediatr. Scand.*, **65**, 495–498
28. Colclough, A. B. and Barson, A. J. (1981) Infantile aortic aneurysm complicating umbilical arterial catheterisation. *Arch. Dis. Child.*, **56**, 795–797
29. Lauridsen, U. B., Enk, B. and Gammeltoft, A. (1978) Oesophageal varices as a late complication to neonatal umbilical vein catheterization. *Acta Paediatr. Scand.*, **67**, 633–636
30. Purohit, D. M. and Levkoff, A. H. (1977) Pericardial effusion complicating umbilical venous catheterization. *Arch. Dis. Child.*, **52**, 520
31. Corkery, J. J., Dubowitz, V., Lister, J. and Moosa, A. (1968) Colonic perforation after exchange transfusion. *Br. Med. J.*, **ii**, 345–349
32. Orme, R. L. E. and Eades, S. M. (1968) Perforation of the bowel in the newborn as a complication of exchange transfusion. *Br. Med. J.*, **iv**, 349–351
33. Tilden, S. J., Craft, C., Cano, R. and Daum, R. S. (1980) Cutaneous necrosis associated with intravenous nafcillin therapy. *Am. J. Dis. Child.*, **134**, 1046–1048
34. Lloyd-Roberts, G. C. and Thomas, T. G. (1964) The etiology of quadriceps contracture in children. *J. Bone Joint Surg.*, **46B**, 498–502
35. Elliman, A. M., Bryan, E. M. and Elliman, A. D. (1986) Low birth weight babies at three years of age. *Child Care, Health Dev.*, **12**, 287–311
36. Barson, A. J., Chiswick, M. L. and Doig, C. M. (1978) Fat emulsion in infancy after intravenous fat infusions *Arch. Dis. Child.*, **53**, 218–223

37. Levene, M. I., Wigglesworth, J. S. and Desai, R. (1980) Pulmonary fat accumulation after Intralipid infusion in the preterm infant. *Lancet*, **ii**, 815–818
38. Peden, V. H., Witzleben, C. L. and Skelton, M. A. (1971) Total parenteral nutrition. *J. Pediatr.*, **78**, 180
39. Whitington, P. F. and Black, D. D. (1980) Cholelithiasis in premature infants treated with parenteral nutrition and frusemide. *J. Pediatr.*, **97**, 647–649
40. Keeling, J. W. (1981) Iatrogenic disease in the Newborn, *Virchows Archiv. (Pathol. Anat.)*, **394**, 1–29

Chapter 21

Nursing procedures and chest physiotherapy

Kathrine L. Peters

In critical care, it strikes me that the issues are three: realism, dignity and love.

Jacob Javits (1986)

Introduction

Modern society and technology has enabled great advances to be made in neonatology. Infants who would not have survived ten years ago are not only alive, but their quality of survival has greatly improved [1]. Three factors have contributed a great deal to the decreasing birth weight at which infants are surviving. First, through advancing technology, equipment has been adapted to and developed for smaller and less mature infants; second, the skills, and third, the attitudes of caretakers have also changed.

Care of ELBW babies severely taxes the creative and emotional stamina of caregivers [2]. While the basic needs of ELBW infants are the same as larger infants – oxygenation and ventilation, warmth, nourishment, and protection from harm – nursing care of ELBW infants must be adjusted in order to accommodate the inherent differences due to short gestational age. These infants exhibit, in addition to their obvious miniscule size, poorly developed organ systems which must develop and mature in the artificial, highly technical environment of the NICU. The aim of this chapter is to closely examine routine nursing and diagnostic procedures and infants' responses to those procedures. In addition, suggestions will be made to help the caretaker in reducing the stress presented by these procedures.

Infant responses to handling

The extremely immature nervous system of ELBW infants leads to poor tolerance of all forms of stimulation. This is well documented in a recent study in our NICU of four infants of less than 1000 g who were continuously monitored to examine the duration, nature and frequency of infant handling. In addition, the infants' physiological responses to that handling were analysed. The infants, whose mean birth weight was 898 g (range 820–960 g), were studied at an average age of 5.5 (range 1–8) days. Physiological responses were assessed by changes in the following parameters which were recorded on an eight-channel industrial recorder:

(1) Heart rate (HR);
(2) Mean arterial blood pressure (BP);
(3) Transcutaneous partial pressure for carbon dioxide (tc$P\text{CO}_2$);

(4) Transcutaneous partial pressure for oxygen (tcPo_2);
(5) Oxygen saturation (Sao_2);
(6) Intracranial pressure (ICP).

All measurements were non-invasive with the exception of the BP which had previously been ordered by the physician in charge of the infant's care. The responses were measured as changes in the parameter that occurred from a baseline calculation of 30 s prior to the procedure. Whenever the recorder was at the bedside, a research nurse noted when the infant or the equipment was touched and how long it lasted. The average duration of the recordings was 249 (range 195–290) min.

During this short space of 3–4 h it was found that the infants were disturbed an average of 35 (range 32–41) times in addition to 19 (range 11–24) changes in the Fio_2 delivered to the infants. An average of 30.7% (range 16.3–43.6%) of the observation time was spent in infant handling. The different types of stimulation – 20 in all – are listed in Tables 21.1 and 21.2. In addition, a note was made of each infant's responses to a sudden loud noise in the environment.

Despite the fact that there were only four babies included in this sample, a general idea of responses of ELBW infants to stimulation can be inferred from these data. For the most part, stimulation (even TLC) resulted in a decrease in tcPo_2 and Sao_2 and an

Table 21.1 Different types of stimulation studied: nursing care procedures

Procedure	*Mean duration* (s)
Buttocks care	27.5
Position change	45.6
Chest physiotherapy	553.5
Instill endotracheal tube	7.4
Suction endotracheal tube	75.0
Oral suction	52.3
tcPo_2/tcPco_2 probe	14.7
Adhesive removal	16.0
Bladder expression	5.0
Mouth care	54.8
TLC (tender loving care)	309.0
Sudden noise	5.7

Table 21.2 Different types of stimulation studied: diagnostic procedures

Procedure	*Mean duration* (s)
HR and RR (auscultation)	125.0
BP by Doppler	160.3
Rectal temperature	77.8
Arterial blood gases	113.8
Heel prick	64.8
Weighing	630.0
Ultrasound	1126.0
X-ray	208.0
Doctor's examination	111.7

Table 21.3 Significant correlations among variables

Procedure	*Variable*	*Variable(s)*
HR and RR (auscultation)	Duration	↑HR
BP by Doppler	Duration	Peak ICP
Heel prick	Duration	↑BP
Instillation of endotracheal tube	Duration	↑Sao_2
Oral suctioning	Duration	↑BP
Mouth care	Duration	↑O_2
TLC	Duration	↑O_2, ↑BP
Sudden noise	Duration	↑HR, ↑Sao_2, ↑BP
Buttocks care (negative correlation)	↑O_2	↑BP

increase in ICP. While the HR and BP changes were not consistent in any one direction, wide swings from the baseline were detected. Significant correlations between the duration of the procedures and various parameters were also noted (Table 21.3). The longer the time required to perform the procedure, the greater the detrimental effect noted in the infants. In addition, while most procedures were quite short in duration, the infants responded for up to 4 min following completion of the task. The nurse performing the task, however, remained at the bedside for an average of only 1.3 min.

Chest physiotherapy and suctioning

Because of the immaturity of the respiratory system, the ELBW infant often exhibits respiratory distress in ways which are vastly different from their larger, more mature counterparts [3]. In many cases these infants initially show little or no overt lung disease, yet must be supported by intubation, ventilation and supplemental oxygenation [4]. The routine use of physiotherapy and frequent suctioning must be questioned. These tiny infants have very little reserves with which to withstand the vigorous handling required for these procedures. Benefits of physiotherapy for ELBW infants have yet to be established and therefore should only be performed when indicated. Because poorly developed lungs collapse quickly when disconnected from the distending pressure of conventional ventilators, consideration must be given to the use of in-line suctioning adapters to reduce the time off the ventilator and away from the O_2 source [5]. Pre-oxygenation, by increasing the Fio_2 to at least 0.15 higher than the infant's resting Fio_2 should help reduce the amount of hypoxia associated with suctioning [6]. Fanconi and Duc have suggested the use of muscle paralysis to minimize significant increases in ICP noted during suctioning thus stabilizing cerebral perfusion pressure by preventing dangerous decreases [6]

Oxygenation: O_2, apnoea and monitoring

Providing O_2

Care must be taken to ensure that the infant receives the required amount of O_2 at all times. Monitoring the Fio_2 delivered to the infant will help to ensure constancy of that

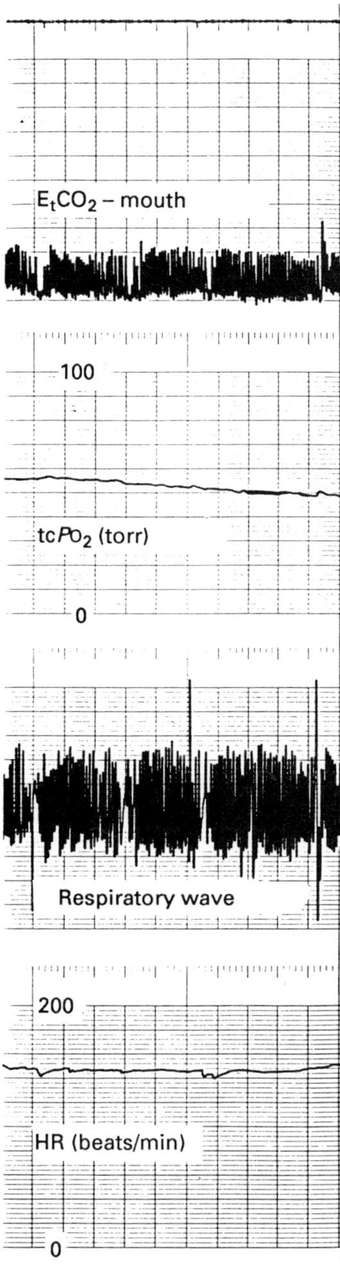

Figure 21.1 This four-channel recording depicts mouth breathing in an 800 g infant girl at 10 days of age. The end-tidal capnography (E_tco_2) sampling tube was placed at the side of the mouth so as to avoid detection of CO_2 expelled from the nares

flow, especially during procedures. In spite of these devices, however, the neonate can be inadvertently exposed to great fluctuations in FiO_2 with resultant undesired variations in $tcPO_2$ [7]. Despite earlier therories to the contrary, it is becoming more evident that neonates are, at times, capable of mouth breathing [8,9]. It is therefore beneficial to ensure that the environment of the infant requiring ventilation using nasal prongs or a nasopharyngeal tube contains the same FiO_2 as prescribed for the prongs. Figure 21.1 is a recording of an 800 g infant in whom this phenomenon is demonstrated using end-tidal capnography.

Apnoea

End-tidal capnography has also been very helpful in diagnosing a respiratory problem more specific to this weight group than larger babies – that of obstructive

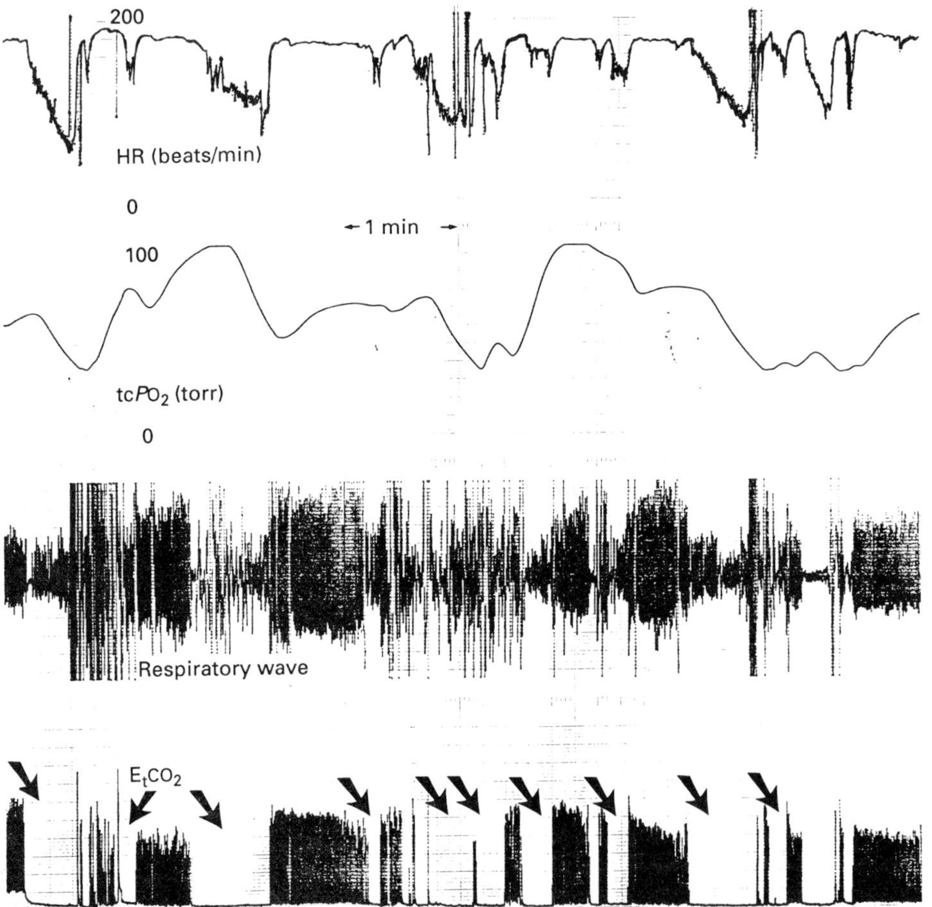

Figure 21.2 Arrows in this four-channel recording of a 580 g infant point out apnoeas which are purely obstructive or mixed in character. Note the profound drops in HR and $tcPO_2$ which accompany the apnoeas

apnoea. Continuous monitoring using end-tidal capnography has revealed that many bradycardic, cyanotic spells reported by the nurses as 'not accompanied by apnoea' are in fact resulting from obstructive apnoea. In a recent study in which infants' cardiorespirographs, end-tidal CO_2 tension level (E_tCO_2), and SaO_2 and/or tcPO_2 were continuously recorded by a multi-channel computer, we have determined that 54% of all apnoeas exhibited by small infants are either purely obstructive or mixed in nature [10]. Figure 21.2 is a recording of a spontaneously breathing 580 g infant suffering from frequent obstructive apnoeas. Unfortunately, careful postioning of the infant (prone or placement of a small roll under the neck when the infant is supine) failed to entirely alleviate the problem. Figure 21.3 shows the response of the same infant following insertion of a nasopharyngeal tube to ensure an open airway. This form of treatment, however, is not entirely without side effects and should not be entered into lightly [7].

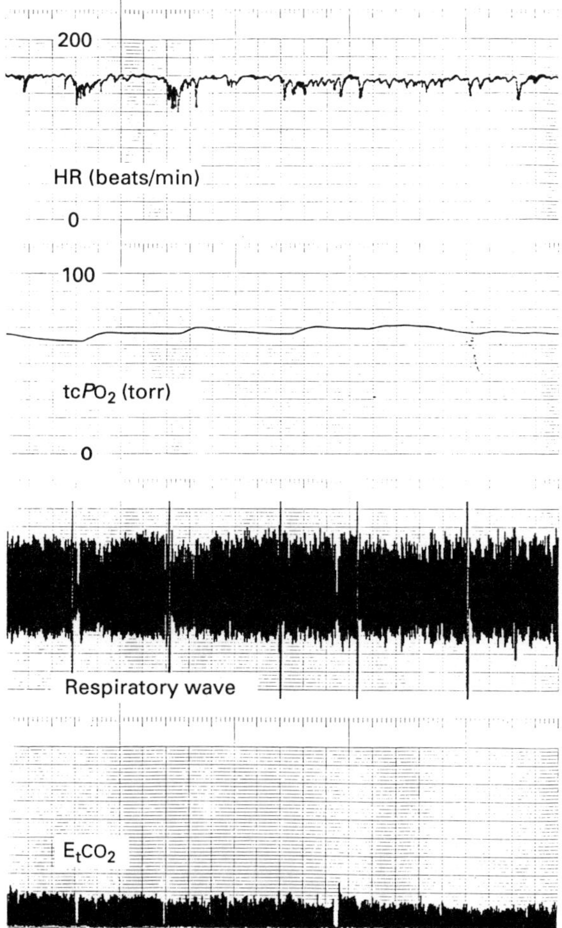

Figure 21.3 This trace was taken from the same 580 g infant as in Figure 21.2 following the insertion of a nasopharyngeal tube. The central apnoeas exhibited are tolerated much better than the apnoeas noted when the airway was partially or completely obstructed

Monitoring oxygenation

The recent introduction of pulse oximetry has been a welcome addition for NICU staff. However, the information imparted by these machines must be interpreted with caution. Recent studies in our unit have established that these monitors are extremely motion-sensitive, resulting in inaccurate readings for as much as 25–30% of monitored time [11]. Caretakers must be cautioned to always visually assess the monitor wave contour, if available, and the infant prior to any intervention when alerted by this device. As the saturation depends on the pulsatile nature of the HR, the numerical readout should be within 10 beats/min of the infant's actual HR in order to be accurate.

Oxygenation and saturation levels should be more tightly controlled in the ELBW infant. Caretakers must be aware that the presence of high concentration of fetal haemoglobin (HbF) in the neonate's bloodstream may interfere with the accuracy of saturation monitors [12]. In addition, it has been demonstrated that the presence of fetal haemoglobin in the IL 282 co-oximeter produces an artefactually high concentration of carboxyhaemoglobin which is directly proportional to the amount of HbF present and this fact must be taken into account when interpreting oxygen saturation [13]. In view of the $\pm 2\%$ error and the slope of the haemoglobin dissociation curve, pulse oximeters are not adequate hyperoxia monitors. While the addition of an upper acceptable limits alarm has been helpful, pulse oximeters should not be used for long periods of time in ELBW infants without using an additional probe to monitor $Pa\text{O}_2$. This will help prevent hyperoxic injury by alerting the caregiver to situations in which the infant is receiving too much oxygen despite what appears to be a satisfactory saturation level.

Skin care during monitoring

All non-invasive monitors, while having the advantage of imparting valuable information about the ELBW without exposing them to the risks of invasive monitors must, however, be attached in some way to the infant. Skin breakdown thus becomes a serious problem. The use of a pectin-based barrier such as Hollihesive or a synthetic polyurethane film or spray such as Op-Site (Smith & Nephew, Lachine, Quebec) has greatly reduced this problem [14,15]. Electrodes whose adhesive responds to water saturation by losing its adhesive quality, thus allowing for painless removal, have recently appeared in NICU's Sentry Silver Sircuit Electrodes or Limbtrodes (Sentry Medical Products, Santa Ana, California). In addition, the adhesive quality is restored by the application of one or two drops of water thus allowing for numerous reapplications of these more expensive electrodes.

The ELBW infant is at a greatly increased risk of toxicity from substances applied to the skin. Caretakers must therefore be cautioned against the use of any substance such as alcohol which, while easing the removal of conventional adhesive electrodes and tapes, will be absorbed by the ELBW's extremely porous epidermis.

While transcutaneous O_2 and CO_2 monitoring have provided much needed continuous information regarding the oxygenation and ventilation of the infant, there is a price to be paid. The requirement that the probe is heated in order to function correctly necessitates frequent probe changes and, consequently, handling of the infant. While this procedure in itself is hazardous to the neonate (Table 21.1), the infant's poorly developed skin may also be severely damaged by this procedure. The epidermis may literally be lifted off with the adhesive ring, leaving the neonate at greater risk to water loss and sepsis – one of the main causes of death amongst ELBW infants in our unit. A recent study has reported that use of a spray-on copolymer acrylic dressing (Op-Site) can aid in the reduction of skin damage caused by the electrode and its adhesive ring [15]. The tiny size of the infant also limits the number of sites available for transcutaneous probe placement. Because the probes rely heavily on heat and perfusion to function accurately, there is a delay (albeit less than in the more mature neonate) in read-out, leading to possible over- or under-oxygenation. One advantage of the ELBW's poorly developed skin, however, lies in the fact that the skin permeability is increased, thus allowing use of lower probe temperatures.

Nursing care and diagnostic procedures

It must be noted that measuring vital signs exposes the ELBW infant to needless noxious stimulation (Tables 21.1 and 21.2). If the monitors attached to the infant are calibrated and applied correctly, the information they impart may be more accurate than that gathered by nurses using a stethoscope, Doppler BP machine, and rectal thermometer. From direct observation in our NICU, on average the HR change elicited by measuring HR and RR by auscultation was + 19.3 beats/min. The change in directly measured mean arterial BP resulting from measuring BP using a Doppler ranged from –5 to + 10 mmHg.

The effective use of monitoring equipment aids greatly in prevention of neonatal complications. Because these infants are in a continual state of development and it is not possible to determine the exact effects of lack of or excessive amounts of stimulation, one must closely examine the limits provided for monitors. The inability of the fetal and hence ELBW neonate heart to significantly increase stroke volume leads to a fall in cardiac output with a fall in HR [16]. This fall in turn may lead to a fall in BP and perfusion to tissues. The common practice of placing the bradycardia level at 100 beats/min is therefore not safe for these tiny neonates whose mean heart rate is often higher than their larger more mature counterparts [17]. The bradycardia level for each infant must be individually determined on a 12–24-hourly basis as a fraction of the infant's baseline resting heart rate. As a 25% fall in HR is acceptable for more mature infants, caretakers should be notified when the ELBW infant's HR falls to greater than 25% from its own baseline.

Results of a recent study in our unit have pointed out that the neonatal monitors must be redesigned if they are to be used effectively in the NICU for care of ELBW infants. At least 54% of significant apnoeas are missed by nursing staff using conventional monitors with static bradycardia alarm levels when compared to a computer program written to detect apnoeas based on a HR drop of 25% from the previous 30 s baseline and/or a decrease in $Sa\text{O}_2$ of 10% or tc$P\text{O}_2$ of 5 torr [9]. As the condition of the ELBW infant changes from moment to moment, so too must the alarm levels on the equipment monitoring his/her condition. The cardiac alarm should be floating so that it is based on a fraction of the preceding 60–120 s of heart rate input.

One continuous monitor which has not received enough use in the care of ELBW infants is the electronic weigh scale. As shown in Table 21.2, the weighing of infants is hazardous. While a great deal of time would be saved by using this device, the protection of the neonate from such a procedural insult as weighing the infant using conventional means cannot be overstated. The electronic scales come in two forms. One allows the infant to be nursed on top of the scale and the other remains outside the isolette and weighs the infant who is placed in a sling constructed for that purpose. If such scales are not available, caretakers must carefully examine the need to expose the neonate to frequent periods of stress required in weighing by removing him/her from the O_2 and heat source more than once every 24–48 h. Caretakers must learn to use other indicators such as urine output and skin turgor to assess the fluid and electrolyte balance of a relatively stable ELBW infant.

Environmental concerns

It has been established that the NICU is an extremely unfavourable environment in which to live – brightly lit 24 h a day, noisy, with constant interventions throughout the day [18]. Glass *et al.* [19] suggest that prolonged exposure to damaging ambient nursery illumination may be one of the contributing factors in the aetiology of retinopathy of prematurity. This may mean protecting the developing infant's eyes from continual light exposure through the use of eye shields or decreasing the amount of ambient light to which the infant is exposed.

Extensive analyses of NICU environments further indicate that premature infants respond to a great deal of the sensory stimulation inherent in intensive care nurseries. It is uncertain if high intensity noise exposure contributes to sensorineural hearing loss in the premature infant but it has been demonstrated that there are definite negative physiological changes associated with auditory stimulation in the NICU (Table 21.3). Infants may experience frequent sleep disruptions and expend a great deal of energy responding to loud noises with jerky, flailing movements. Early in life, however, these responses seem to be largely on a physiological rather than perceptual level suggesting little, if any, benefit to maturing sensory systems. Infants exposed to high noise levels when medical rounds approach the bedside have more apnoea and bradycardia during that time [20]. It is advisable for the physician to refrain from examining the infant during such a time of high stress in light of the knowledge of the infant's physiological responses to such an examination (Table 21.2). Such rounds should be used to closely evaluate each procedure and medication order used in the care of the individual patient in order to decrease infant disturbances to a minimum. Caretakers must learn to become more observant of the condition of the infant in their care without touching him.

Contrary to earlier beliefs, social interaction (tender loving care, TLC) can produce as much, if not more, stress to the ELBW infant as can painful procedures such as a heelprick (Table 21.1). The prolonged duration of TLC adds to the negative effect of this procedure (Table 21.3). Nurses must therefore be prepared to limit the amount of social interaction presented to the infant if it produces a negative effect until the infant can better tolerate this stimulation.

While two methods of providing a neutral thermal neonatal environment have been suggested for ELBW infants, neither is without drawbacks [21]. Our current solution to the initial problem of stabilizing the condition of the ELBW infant lies in the use of 'nesting beds' (plexiglass heat shields used upside down and lined with sheepskin) in conjunction with the open, overhead radiant warmer beds. This concept is based on assessments of radiant energy and insensible water losses by infants nursed in radiant warmer beds [22]. The use of these beds for provision of acceptable personal space for the developing ELBW infant has been studied by Hull and Wheldon [21]. While they provide a limited area in which the neonate is cared for, they also provide for better body alignment. Because the bottom of the bed is slightly rounded, the infant's shoulders are kept in a more neutral position which aids in the development of coordination of moving the infant's hands to the midline position. The nesting bed is lined with sheepskin in order to provide warmth and tactile stimulation while reducing the possibility of the development of decubitus ulcers. The sheepskin may also have an added feature in sound absorption. The application of a glove attached to a respirator on the outside wall of the nesting bed serves to provide kinaesthetic stimulation to the infant, without intrusion into his space. Concentrations of O_2 and humidity (provided to overcome the dehydrating effects of overhead warming beds) in the nesting bed are controlled by the application of a cling-type plastic wrap over the top of the bed. This transparent barrier also acts as a deterrent to unnecessary disruptions to the infant. If such disruptions seem to continue, caretakers must seriously consider the use of reverse isolation to protect the ELBW infant. If one must face the prospect of donning a mask, gown and gloves prior to touching the infant, the number of unnecessary disruptions to the infant has been noted in our unit to fall dramatically. We are currently evaluating the differences between the nesting bed and double-walled incubator environments with relation to light and noise levels and number and frequency of caretaker disruptions to the infant.

In light of the above information, caretakers must closely examine their procedures and the infants' environments to decrease the amount of stimulation presented to ELBW babies. It appears that these tiny infants have difficulty coping with even one stimulus at a time. Therefore, each intervention must be examined for its effect on the infant and modified to produce the least amount of stress and prescribed for infants on an individual basis only when the benefit outweighs the risk. In addition a more holistic approach is required for care of the ELBW infant. Caretakers must learn to integrate the knowledge imparted to them about *all* the systems of the neonate – not just one at a time. The more frequent use of a multichannel computer, monitor or recording device will provide the caretaker with a more global understanding of the infant's current physiological status. Computers can be programmed to display any number of the infant's physiological parameters all at the same time. This display provides the caretaker with a complete picture of the infant's responses to procedures and enable intervention to offset the infant's deterioration to occur before global resuscitation is necessary.

In addition to promoting thermal stability and adequate ventilation, oxygenation and perfusion, the nurse needs to provide a safe environment for the ELBW infant. Prevention of environmental stressors that may cause or potentiate deterioration should be one of the prime objectives for nursing care for these infants. Als *et al.* [23] have suggested that careful evaluation of the infant's behavioural and physiological responses to stimuli in the NICU can provide a basis on which to individualize nursing care and significantly improve both medical and developmental outcome of the ELBW infant. By reducing the stress presented to the infant or helping him to retain homeostasis prior to and during the procedure, fewer resuscitative efforts will be required. This again necessitates careful observation of the infant's responses prior to, during and after the intervention.

Data from psychobiological literature outlining the prenatal development of sensory systems reveal that sensory responses are certainly possible in infants born as early as 25–26 weeks gestation [24–26]. If the ELBW infant survives the perinatal period, there is a new environment to contend with where sensory stimuli are drastically different from those encountered *in utero*. While the NICU environment may be undeniably stressful, it has yet to be established that exposure to this environment at a time that is normally spent *in utero* results in permanent harm to the developing central nervous system. There is, however, an emerging body of evidence indicating a relationship between the effects of NICU environmental factors and the medical developmental states of premature infants [27].

Studies show that some premature ELBW infants exhibit alterations in sensory functioning representing possible delays in sensory development on follow-up examination [28,29]. At present it is not possible to be certain about the cause of the observed delays, but the desire to achieve normal sensory and intellectul outcome remains very strong. As the age of viability becomes increasingly younger, infants will be spending longer periods of time in the NICU and the risks of impairment may increase accordingly. Thus it becomes even more important to delineate the exact course of postnatal sensory development and to determine which aspect of the environment, if any, can seriously alter this course.

Conclusion

Neonatal intensive care units were designed to sustain life and enhance the possibility of intact infant survival. A growing awareness of the potential iatrogenic risks inherent in highly technical medical care has begun to occur among caretakers. These aspects must now be taken together to focus efforts towards change of the NICU environment as well as the study of inherent aspects of nursery care.

References

1. Hack, M., Fanaroff, A. A. and Merkatz., I. R. (1979) The low-birth-weight infant – evolution of a changing outlook. *N. Engl. J. Med.*, **301**, 1162–1169
2. Armentrout, D. (1986) Attitudes/beliefs/feelings held by neonatal nurses toward the care and management of fetal-infants. *Neonatal Network*, **5**, 23–29
3. Kling, P. (1986) Respiratory distress syndrome in the tiny baby. *Neonatal Network*, **4**, 7–13
4. Cunningham, M. D. and Desai, N. S. (1986) Methods of assessment and findings regarding pulmonary function in infants less than 1000 grams. *Clin. Perinatol.*, **13**, 299–313
5. Gunderson, L. P., McPhee, A. J. and Donovan, E. F. (1986) Partially ventilated endotracheal suction: use in newborns with respiratory distress syndrome. *Am. J. Dis. Child.*, **140**, 462–465
6. Fanconi, S. and Duc, G. (1987) Intratracheal suctioning in sick preterm infants: prevention of intracranial hypertension and cerebral hypoperfusion by muscle paralysis. *Pediatrics*, **79**, 538–543
7. Peters, K. L. (1988) Nursing care of babies receiving oxygen and ventilatory support. In *Routines in Neonatal Care* (ed. R. Cooke), Blackwell Scientific Boston
8. Rodenstein, D. O., Perlmutter, N. and Stanescu, D. C. (1985) Infants are not obligatory nasal breathers. *Am. Rev. Respir. Dis.*, **131**, 343–347
9. Fanaroff, A. A. (1985) Oral breathing in newborn infants. *J. Pediatr.*, **107**, 465–469
10. Muttitt, S., Tierney, A. and Finer, N. N. (1988) The diagnosis of apnea: nurses versus computers. Manuscript submitted, 1987
11. Barrington, K. J., Finer, N. N. and Ryan, A. (1988) An evaluation of pulse oximetry as a continuous monitoring technique in the NICU. Manuscript submitted, 1987
12. Jennis, M. S. and Peabody, J. L. (1987) Pulse oxymetry: an alternative method for the assessment of oxygenation in newborn infants. *Pediatrics*, **79**, 524–528
13. Ryan, C. A., Barrington, K. J., Vaughan, D. and Finer, N. N. (1986) Directly measured oxygen saturation in the newborn infant. *J. Pediatr.*, **109**, 526–529

14. Lund, C., Kuller, J. M., Tobin, C., Lefrak, L. and Frank, L. (1986) Evaluation of a Pectin-based barrier under tape to protect neonatal skin. *J. Obstet. Gynaecol. Neonat. Nurs.*, Jan/Feb, 39–44
15. Evans, N. J. and Rutter, N. (1986) Reduction of skin damage from transcutaneous oxygen electrodes using a spray on dressing. *Arch. Dis. Child.*, **61**, 881–884
16. Rudolph, A. M. and Haymann, M. A. (1973) Control of the foetal circulation. In *Foetal and Neonatal Physiology* (eds R. S. Comline, K. W. Cross, G. S. Dawes and P. W. Nathanielsz), Cambridge University Press, London
17. Cabal, L. A., Larrazabal, C. and Siassi, B. (1986) Hemodynamic variables in infants weighing less than 1000 grams. *Clin. Perinatol.*, **13**, 327–338
18. Gottfried, A. W. and Hodgman, J. E. (1984) How intensive is newborn intensive care? An environmental analysis. *Pediatrics*, **74**, 292–294
19. Glass, P., Avery, G. B., Subramanian, K. N. S., Keys, M. P., Sostek, A. M. and Friendly, D. S. (1985) Effect of bright light in the hospital nursery on the incidence of retinopathy of prematurity. *N. Engl. J. Med.*, **313**, 401–404
20. Gaiter, J. L., Avery, G. B., Temple, C. J., Johnson, A. A. S. and White, N. B. (1981) Stimulation characteristics of nursery environments for critically ill preterm infants and infant behavior. In *Intensive Care in the Newborn*, Vol. III (ed. L. Stern), Masson, New York
21. Hull, D. and Wheldon, A. (1986) Open or closed incubators. *Arch. Dis. Child.*, **61**, 108–109
22. Baumgart, S. (1982) Radiant energy and insensible water loss in the premature newborn infant nursed under a radiant warmer. *Clin. Perinatol.*, **9**, 483–503
23. Als, H., Lawthorn, G., Brown, E. *et al.* (1986) Individualized behavioral and environmental care for the very low birth weight preterm infant at high risk for bronchopulmonary dysplasia: neonatal intensive care unit and developmental outcome. *Pediatrics*, **86**, 1123–1132
24. Bradley, R. and Mistretta, C. (1975) Fetal sensory receptors. *Psychol. Rev.*, **55**, 352–383
25. Humphrey, T. (1978) Function of the nervous system during prenatal life. In *Perinatal Physiology* (ed. U. Stave), Plenum, New York
26. Bench, J. (1978) The auditory response. In *Perinatal Physiology* (ed. U. Stave), Plenum, New York
27. Peabody, J. P. and Lewis, K. (1985) Consequences of newborn intensive care. In *Infant Stress Under Intensive Care* (eds A. W. Gottfried and J. L. Gaiter), University Park Press, Baltimore
28. Friedman, S., Jacobs, B. and Werthman, M. (1981) Sensory functioning in pre- and full-term infants. In *Pre-term Birth and Psychological Development*, (eds S. Friedman and M. Sigman), Academic Press, New York
29. Newman, L. (1981) Social and sensory environment of low birth weight infants in a special care nursery. *J. Nerv. Ment. Dis.*, **169**, 448–455

Chapter 22

Preparation for home

Jean Boxall

Babies of less than 1000 g often go home at an age of 3–4 months but still under 2000 g in weight, immature and not yet due to be born.

At the time the parents would have been preparing for the new baby, attending parentcraft classes, painting the bedroom and generally nesting, the mother of an early baby is either confined to bed in an antenatal ward, or the family is undergoing the stresses and strains of visiting a very small person in a neonatal intensive care unit [1]. Both the parents and nurses are therefore unable even to think about preparation for home and parentcraft.

Most other babies are born to families who have had time to adjust to the idea of a new member. The parents have also received several months support from their community midwife. Many have got to know the team of people who will be with them at the time of the birth and during the weeks following birth. One of the most frightening yet thrilling times for a family is the first few days after they have their new baby at home. One mother described her feelings as 'happily terrified'. The majority of parents of mature infants will have had other babies, or be attending parentcraft classes, or at least will have had time to prepare for this event. They will have obtained information on baby care from their own families, by reading books and magazines, or through personal communication with their midwife or health visitor [2]. When a baby is born very early, unless the parents have had a previous small baby, everything is different. They need special help, as is given to those who are adopting a baby [3].

In the UK, if the full term baby is born at home the midwife will visit at home for ten days, and in some instances up to one month after birth. The health visitor will also visit the baby at home for ten days. The majority of UK babies are born in hospital but the mothers and babies are transferred home within a few days of birth and they also benefit from the same postnatal support. Many countries throughout the world have similar support systems but they are all created to suit the majority of term or near term births. The families who have LBW babies not only have to cope with the exposure to newborn intensive care which is both frightening and stressful, they also do not get the same support as the parents of term infants. A study in Exeter identified this problem (Figure 22.1). A few specialist preterm community teams do exist, but the numbers of LBW infants are small and many live in areas where these teams are not available.

To overcome this problem for these vulnerable babies the systems designed for the term infants ideally could be adjusted to their special needs. For instance, in the UK the midwife may visit up to 28 days after the birth. If this was reworded to say up to 28 days after the expected date of delivery, then 24-hour community support on going

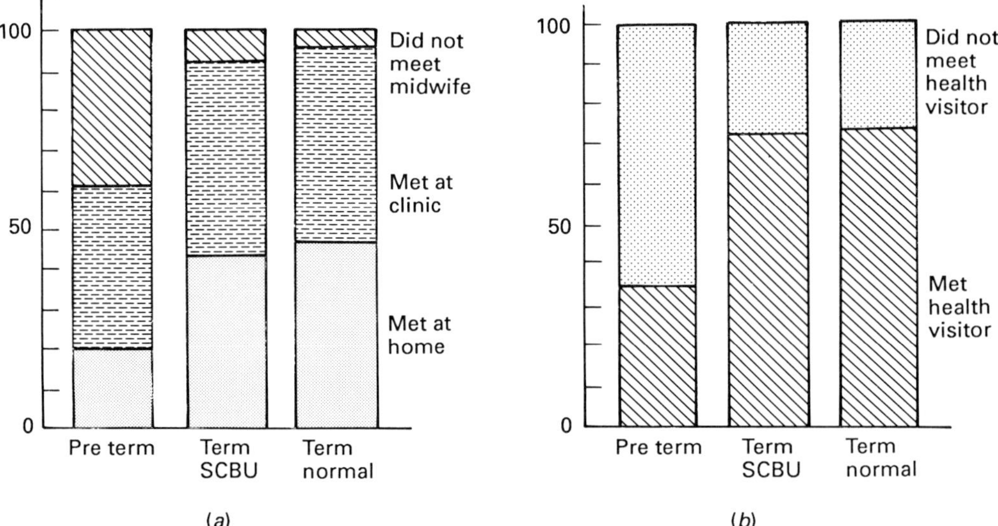

Figure 22.1 Exeter survey: timing of meeting with (*a*) community midwife and (*b*) health visitor before birth [4]

home would be available to all babies regardless of gestation, except those infants with long-term hospital stays for medical reasons.

After the birth the grandparents and other family members and friends also may be afraid to be normal and so do not provide the gifts which help to create the baby's own special appearance and environment. There are several ways that these problems can be overcome:

(1) Preparation for being parents.
(2) Antenatal parentcraft.
(3) Staff awareness of the need for preparation for home in neonatal intensive care units and intermediate care.
(4) Transfer of care to the parents when the baby is in the low dependency part of the unit.
(5) Support after discharge home.

Preparation for being parents

This should occur naturally in a population where there are large families. Children take part in sibling baby care from when they are replaced as the youngest. In a society where families are small this needs to be replaced with education.

Parentcraft teaching is often offered to the less able girls in school. The boys and brighter girls do not often get this aspect of sex education. Maternity units and neonatal units can influence this learning by loaning out videos and slides to schools. Many neonatal intensive care units receive charity funds from groups such as schools, Girl Guides and Scouts. This can provide an excellent opportunity for the staff to speak to young people and in some instances they may even show a few around the unit. A video or slide show is one way in which the local young population can be introduced to the fact that a minority of babies are born very small and can survive, and the need for learning parentcraft in preparation for the future.

Antenatal parentcraft

Unfortunately most parents of very small babies have not attended relevant parentcraft teaching [4]. Even if they have had previous mature infants they may not know how different a very small baby will be and yet how similar.

A video made in Exeter – *Your Special Baby* – was used to introduce the neonatal unit parents to the concepts of neonatal intensive care and special care. A survey carried out amongst a group of parents following the birth of a baby admitted to the neonatal unit suggested that they would have preferred to see the video as part of their parentcraft classes. The session would be optional, as it does show babies receiving ventilation. Conversely there is a part showing twins of 25 weeks gestation visiting the unit when aged one year. The video needs to be shown before 24 weeks. Although only a minority of babies are born very small, at least if a family is subjected to this experience they will have been introduced to the subject. Also their friends who are having babies who go to term will at least be able to understand some of the dilemmas of these parents. Through recent personal communication with several parents who have had LBW babies, one of the problem areas has been the antenatal ward. They have felt intensely bored if admitted, and would have liked to know what would happen if their baby was born before 28 weeks. Several assumed their baby would be born dead. Conversely, antenatal ward staff inevitably wish to keep the mother's mind on rest, relaxation and keeping her baby.

A careful balance has to be kept between the two needs. It helps if the neonatal unit staff can visit mothers in the antenatal ward [5]. Family visits to the neonatal unit may be arranged and parentcraft sessions organized. Videos and a parents' library can be helpful. The midwives in these wards should encourage the family to continue to prepare for the baby's birth.

From the Exeter study several problems were identified for parents of early gestation infants during the antenatal period and after the birth [4]. Three groups of parents were sent postal questionnaires. All the mothers were primigravida and the babies were singletons.

(1) Preterm: infants of 32 weeks gestation or less who were admitted to SCBU.
(2) T-SCBU: term infants admitted to the SCBU for one week or less.
(3) T-MAT: term infants receiving normal care in maternity ward.

The results are shown in Table 22.1.

Table 22.1 Results of questionnaire on parentcraft before delivery

	Preterm (n = 18)	*T-SCBU* (n = 20)	*T-MAT* (n = 15)
Started antenatal classes on preparation for labour (%)	10 (55)	20 (100)	14 (93)
Able to attend baby care classes	2 (11)	18 (90)	14 (93)

Preparation for home

Both staff and parents are too frightened to tempt providence and to think of the baby going home, yet during this time such projects as preparing the infant's room or getting new accommodation should be initiated. The unit social worker should become involved with the family early. This will enable her to get to know the family. If the child survives she will have time to mobilize the necessary agencies such as housing.

Many parents are shocked by the fact that the baby is born alive. They also find his appearance very different to the fat cuddly baby they expected [4]. They may later describe him and say he looked like a skinned rabbit, or a blob covered in wires, or a very small doll covered in spaghetti. Many small babies will tolerate a 'cuddle' but even this feels different. One mother burst into tears and said 'I can't feel him. He felt like a bunch of feathers and had no substance'.

Despite all these difficulties it is vital that the nursing staff take an optimistic and realistic approach to the baby and his family, as in most good units over 50% of these infants will go home. Many nurses are afraid to mention home at this time. Conversely the parents are often wondering how they will cope if the baby does survive, but are afraid to mention their worries.

When the numbers of babies nursed in the Neonatal Unit in Exeter were compared with the numbers of patients ventilated in the District General Hospital Adult Intensive Care Unit similar figures emerged; 1.6% of all SCBU admissions weighing less than 1000 g compared with 1% of the District General Hospital admissions were ventilated on intensive care. Their survival rates for 1984 and 1985 were 48% compared with 44% [6].

These figures may help neonatal staff to realize that although these babies are the longest stay, highest dependency group, increasing numbers will eventually go home. Neonatal nurses can have as optimistic an attitude to outcome as do their colleagues in the adult field and similarly to their patients' families.

At this early stage the family can become involved in normal baby care. Even very small babies need booties. Some may wear hats, jackets and other clothes [7]. If the mother is not feeling well enough, grandmothers, aunts and friends should be encouraged to help to knit and sew. Neonatal units should have patterns available for the family to buy or borrow. These should not be referred to as dolls' patterns, which is insulting to some parents.

A useful aid to creating rest patterns for incubator babies [8], which could influence later sleep patterns at home, is a 'snooze cover' (personal communication, Karen Schriener, University Hospital, Portland, Oregon).This is a dark blue cover which can be placed over, or partly over, the incubator. The upper side is appliqued with a moon and stars to indicate this is rest time and that the baby should not be disturbed. A creative relative or friend might make a personal cover for the baby. The parents could indicate the pattern of rest and activity they wish for their baby.

Another helpful item for these parents can be charts showing the earliest, average and latest age that babies have been ready for home from the unit according to weight and gestation. This will probably vary from unit to unit according to the population and local policies and support services. The nurses on units caring for small babies could look at their ages of discharge home and update these annually and produce prediction charts.

In Exeter this was done using the nursing kardex as the record. During the exercise it was observed that the babies below 1500 g who were in the unit the longest time also had the greatest percentage of homes not ready to accept them at the time they were ready for home. Some of the reasons for the home not being ready were simple and could have been avoided if the staff had foreseen them. The following list shows the reasons given for the home not being ready in the Exeter study:

(1) No suitable accommodation.
(2) Lack of heat.
(3) The bedroom had not been decorated.
(4) The layette was not ready.
(5) Grandmother or the mother's help was not ready.
(6) Mother wished to stay in a parents' room to establish breast feeding, but father could not arrange time off work to care for siblings.
(7) The family just did not feel ready (expressed by concerns over family colds or tummy upset).

Identification of family strengths and weaknesses

Most patients admitted to hospital have both medical and social needs documented on the nursing records. This is social information and is often difficult to obtain in newborn intensive care and may not be possible for a few days. One way round this is to design a separate questionnaire for parents where they can state their needs in their own words. Less able or foreign families will require help with this. On the sheet should be such questions as 'Have you met your health visitor?' If the answer is no, the nurse should give the mother the health visitor's name and address. Housing, transport or financial difficulties, if ticked, should be referred to the social worker. Even what colour clothes the mother prefers her baby to wear can be asked. This simple question will show the family that the staff are already considering their baby to be a person.

The recording of the names of the brothers and sisters helps staff to greet them in a friendly way. Ideally the sheet should be kept under the other record charts by the baby so they are easily available to both medical and nursing staff, but not where other parents can read them. The form may not be completed at first but it can be updated; on this sheet questions should be asked about what if anything the family would like help with, e.g. making up feeds, bathing, development, keeping baby warm.

In the Exeter parentcraft survey, several questions were asked regarding what worried parents most on going home. There was no difference in the three groups regarding feeding, bowels, fear of cot death and other questions, except for three items, stated by the preterm parents:

(1) Keeping baby warm.
(2) Milestones.
(3) Baby being fragile.

The home is often not satisfactory for term infants: it is even more crucial that parents should learn what is appropriate for the preterm baby [9]. A few parents will wish to provide their own baby clothes, so facilities for washing them should be provided. This may be the start of their preparation for taking over care.

There should be a collection of books on preterm care and baby care for parents to borrow, together with suitable videos and albums showing the development of previous preterm infants. There is now a children's book available called *Special Care Babies* [10] which could also be helpful to the less able parents who find adult reading matter beyond their abilities. This mentions preparing home for the baby.

Transfer to low dependency care

This should be a happy event for parents, but many have said how frightening it is. The nursing staff should be aware of their fears and be supportive and encouraging in their attitudes; changes such as transferring a baby to a cot or removing monitors should be done when mother is visiting if possible.

At the time a baby goes into a cot the nurses who have given intensive care to the baby in physical terms should now turn their attention to mother and final preparation for home. Some babies are ready for home when they would have been 35 weeks gestation, others are later; most are home before they were due to be born. The mother should be involved with making care plans which will suit her own life style. Sleeping patterns at night can be established if a day and night programme of care is used. Ideally the mother should spend as much time as she can with her baby; she may move into a parent's room. Flexibility in accommodation needs to be considered; a toddler or father may need to be accommodated as well when the family takes over care.

Criteria for discharge home should not be just weight dependent, but general guidelines for nurses should be:

(1) The baby is medically fit for home.
(2) He can maintain his temperature in a cot.
(3) The parents can provide adequate heat at home.
(4) The family feels confident enough to care for the child at home over 24 h.
(5) The midwife, health visitor or social worker are satisfied that the home is suitable for the care of a small baby.

The more involved parents are with caring for their infants throughout his stay, the earlier the baby will go home. The health visitor should be welcomed to visit the unit to meet the family if she has not already done so. If preparation for home has been adequately undertaken over the preceding weeks, no problem should arise. Many units now discharge babies smaller and earlier. Many babies are home when they weigh only 1700–2000 g (Figure 22.2) [11]. This means normal newborn clothes are too large. A loaning system for premature baby clothes in the form of a clothes library is helpful [12].

An album containing names, addresses and photographs of other preterm families can be used as a means of giving parents a local contact to meet or telephone and exchange feelings and ideas. This can be introduced earlier but seems to be most needed at the time of discharge.

Support at home

Most families usually prefer to take their babies home at the weekend. The father is then home and mother is not on her own for the first two days. The health visitor or social worker may prefer this to be on a weekday so they can visit. The community

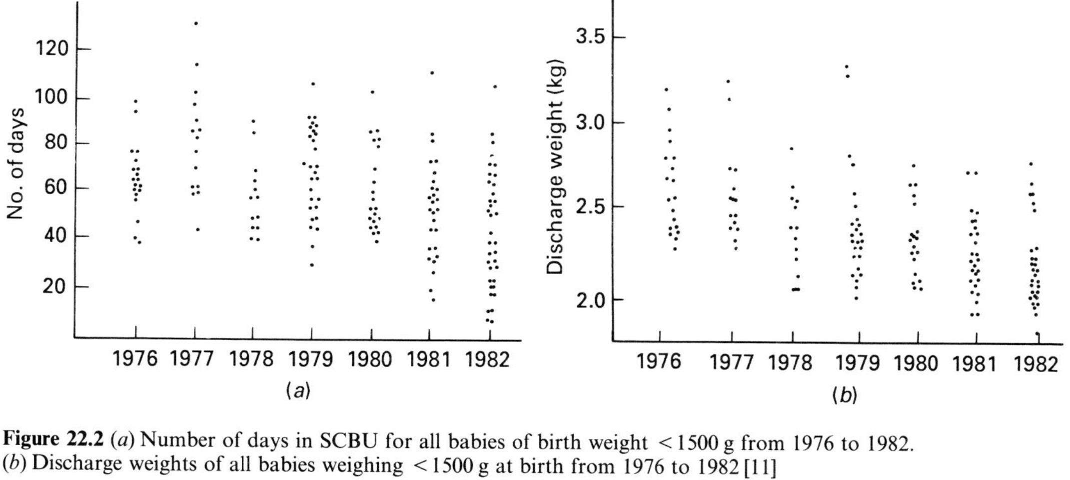

Figure 22.2 (*a*) Number of days in SCBU for all babies of birth weight <1500 g from 1976 to 1982. (*b*) Discharge weights of all babies weighing <1500 g at birth from 1976 to 1982 [11]

Table 22.2 Answer to question: 'Who could best help you when baby goes home?'

	Preterm (n = 18)	*T-SCBU* (n = 20)	*T-MAT* (n = 15)
Midwife	0	7	6
Health visitor	5	4	3
SCBU nurse	11	2	0
Relative/friend	1	3	4
Other	1	3	3

service may need to involve the on-call midwife out of office hours unless there is a preterm baby team. Table 22.2 indicates that term parents would like the midwife and health visitor to help while preterm parents would prefer a neonatal nurse. When asked who they went to for help when first home, the Exeter preterm parents said the health visitor, or that they contacted the neonatal unit. This indicates that parents will feel happier if they can telephone or visit the unit if they have a minor problem when the health visitor is not available [13]. The neonatal unit and local health visitors should support this need and recognize each others' strengths. If the child health record has been started the nurse can enter such a visit so the health visitor is aware of the problem present.

In conclusion, one mother who first met her health visitor on going home, commented that it was difficult to get to know this stranger when she already knew her midwife who could not visit. Her final comment was 'I felt a tremendous feeling of pride in having this precious little person, he was a baby for longer, I had more time to get to know him before he was a toddler'.

References

1. Redshaw, M. E., Rivers, R. P. A. and Rosenblatt, D. B. (1985) The need for visiting. In *Born Too Early*, Oxford University Press, Oxford, pp. 65–80
2. Guillemin, J. H. and Holmstrom, L. L. (1986) Mixed blessings, intensive care for newborns. In *Parents and Newborn Intensive Care*, 1st edn, Oxford University Press, Oxford and New York, p. 171
3. Fraser, J. (1987) Parenthood education for adaptive parents. *Midwives Chronicle*, September, p. 276–278
4. Boxall, J. and Hunter, S. (eds) (1987) Born too soon for parentcraft. In *Midwife, Health Visitor, Community Nurse* (eds J. Boxall and S. Hunter), Newbourne Publications
5. Boxall, J. (1987) The role of the nurse in mother–baby interaction. In *Midwife, Health Visitor, Community Nurse* (eds J. Boxall and S. Hunter), Newbourne Publications
6. Searle, J. F. (1985) Outcome of mechanical ventilation. *Ann. R. Coll. Surg.*, **3**, 187–189
7. Eiser, C., Town, C. and Tripp, J. (1985) Dress and care of infants in health and illness. *Arch. Dis. Child.*, **60**, 465–470
8. Mann, N. P., Haddow, R., Stokes, L., Goodley, S. and Rutter, N. (1986) Effect of night and day in newborn nurseries. *Br. Med. J.*, **293** (6557): 1265–1267
9. Davies, D. P. and Derbyshire, F. M. (1984) Discharging preterm babies from neonatal units. In *Parent–Baby Attachment in Premature Infants* (eds A. Davis, M. P. M. Richards and N. R. C. Roberton), Croom Helm
10. Althea *Special Care Babies.* Illustrated by Nicola Spoor, Dinosaur Publications

11. Boxall, J. (1984) Changing patterns of neonatal nursing care. In *Neonatal Intensive Care – A Dilemma of Resources and Needs*, Spastics Society
12. Boxall, J. (1986) A clothes library. *Nippers Newsletter*, p. 10
13. Glover, B. and Hodson, C. (1985) Going home. In *You and Your Premature Baby*, 1st edn., Sheldon Press, London, p. 83

Video 'Your Special Baby'

Available for hire from Neonatal Nurses Association (Coordinator: Mrs Timson), 107 Arnald Road, Basford, Nottingham NG5 1NI, UK
For purchase from Chris Morris, Line-up, Freshford, Bath BA3 6BY, UK.

Snooze covers

Available from Tiddlywinks, 7 Banks Avenue, Golcar, Huddersfield HD7 4L, UK.

Chapter 23

The social and emotional needs of the parents and baby

M. P. M. Richards

Introduction

While there is general agreement among clinicians and nursing staff that the birth and early months of life of an ELBW baby are often stressful for parents, the amount of research on the problem is very limited and much of what is available relates to very small samples. To add to our difficulties we need to be rather cautious in generalizing from findings from one centre to another as much may depend on the ways in which staff relate to parents, as well as such factors as attitudes in the community towards very small babies and their problems in the community. It is tempting to fill in the gaps in our knowledge from the results of studies of larger preterm babies on the assumption that the issues and problems for the ELBW baby and parents will be much the same in kind, though more frequent and more serious. Up to a point this strategy is probably not too misleading; however, it must remembered that there are differences in the patterns of association with social and demographic variables for the larger and smaller preterm babies.

The parents' perspective

Like many of the crises of parenting, one of the difficulties of the situation of the birth of an ELBW baby is that at a time when great emotional demands are likely to be made of parents they are often already in a stressed state. The early birth and the small baby are, in themselves, factors that often stress parents. Apart from the point that an earlier than expected birth may upset all sorts of practical arrangements, it may mean that parents are not psychologically ready for the birth. For a mother there may be a sense of failure and inadequacy at being unable to carry a pregnancy to term and perhaps guilt at having done things which she feels may have caused the preterm delivery or the slow rate of fetal growth. A women's capacity as a mother is still often seen as a basic part of her nature and the ability to grow a fetus adequately may seem to a mother herself as the fundamental part of that capacity [1–3]. Reactions will vary widely, however, not only because of differing attitudes towards motherhood but also because in some situations a mother may have had some prior warning of the likelihood of an ELBW baby. While one might expect that prior warning and specific preparation for a preterm delivery are likely to ameliorate the stress of such birth, there appears to be no direct evidence for this.

Parents may have an image of the baby they would like to have and so part of what they have to face at the birth is the grief of the loss of that expected fantasy baby. This grief may make it hard to relate to the VLBW baby.

Among the feelings of any pregnancy for both mothers and fathers there is often anxiety that all may not go well. There may be fears and fantasies of producing a damaged child. In recent years a growing number of screening and diagnostic techniques such as amniocentesis and ultrasound are being deployed as part of medical care in pregnancy. While we still await systematic studies of how these influence feelings in pregnancy, we do know that in some situations their use may increase anxiety [4].

The final point to be considered in this brief discussion is the birth itself. Caesarian section is commonly employed for the delivery of very preterm babies. There is accumulating evidence that some mothers are less responsive to their babies and feel more negative in general about the birth after a caesarian section [5]. So, in brief, all is not likely to be equal at the birth of an ELBW baby; not only may the mother be recovering from a surgical delivery, but she and her partner will often have troubled feelings of failure, guilt and anxiety and perhaps a sense that their worst fears and fantasies of pregnancy have been realized.

The ELBW baby

Any ELBW baby is likely to be moved straight from the delivery room to a neonatal unit. If the mother is conscious she may have a chance to hold the baby briefly or at least have a glimpse before the baby is carried off. The baby she sees will not be the conventional image of the newborn so prominent in the photographs in baby books. For some the first sight will be in the neonatal unit with the baby in an incubator, attached to various monitoring devices and perhaps on a ventilator. Appearances matter. While the work does not specifically relate to ELBW babies, we know that parents of preterm and other babies receiving specialized neonatal care are very concerned about their babies' appearance [6,7]. It is easy to understand why this may be particularly important for parents of ELBW babies. These babies do not correspond to the stereotype of the desirable newborn, but appearance is more or less all that parents and other relatives have to go on. Because the baby cannot be freely held and is a poor partner in social interaction, appearance has a special importance. This also goes for the wider family whose members might expect to visit and hold a newborn full term baby at home but are likely to have to make do with a photograph and the parents' description for a baby that remains in a neonatal unit. In this connection, it is important to note that there may be negative images of preterm babies in the community. In one study in which mothers were given strange babies, reactions were more guarded and negative when the mother was told (falsely) that the babies had been born prematurely [7].

During the time that an ELBW baby is in a neonatal care unit, the parents have two crucial psychological issues to deal with: the containment of their anxiety about the baby's survival and prognosis, and the building of a social relationship with him or her. Of course, the two issues may be linked as some parents may manage their fears and anxieties by remaining distant until they feel confident that their child will survive. This is an important point to bear in mind when discussing visiting with parents. As well as the obvious practical difficulties which may arise because of such things as travel costs and the need to care for older children at home, there may be psychological issues to resolve. Indeed, some regard regular visiting as a sign that these have been successfully worked through.

Parents vary widely in their understanding of the complications of extremely low birth weight and the likely prognosis. Most will, at least at times, fear the worst – but what constitutes the worst is not the same for all. For some survival seems to be all that matters, but for others the thought of a severely damaged baby is worse than a death. These are very difficult issues for most parents (and, indeed, paediatricians and nurses) to confront openly even between themselves, let alone with those who have responsibility for the care of their child. Most parents have great need to talk about their baby's problems and (not surprisingly) studies in neonatal units show that they are not always satisfied with the time available to see the paediatrician [8]. Despite the need to talk, they may find it very hard to ask for more time, not least because they may fear that such discussion time takes the staff away from caring for their baby. Some units have found it of great help to have someone with counselling or psychotherapy skills available to talk to parents (and to staff) [9].

Increasingly, the attitude amongst staff in neonatal units is that they should be straightforward and full in the explanations offered to parents – 'honest but not cruel' as one writer has put it [10]. Often parents will need to go over the same ground several times before they can accept and understand what is being said. Often the uncertainty of the developmental process may lead to difficulties. Not unnaturally parents want to know about the longer term prognosis – how will she do at school, will he be of normal height and so on – and they may find it hard to accept that precise answers cannot be given and feel that the uncertainty is because something is being hidden from them.

But the psychological work with parents suggests that for many, but not all, parents full information and the opportunity to talk are not enough. Some parents wish to be fully involved in all important decisions about the care of their child and, if the situation arises, about the withdrawal of some forms of treatment [11,12]. There has been some resistance to policies of this kind, not least on the grounds that most parents do not have sufficient knowledge and understanding of the relevant technical questions. However, others have found that it is usually possible to convey the basic issues involved in clinical situations and though, once again, we are badly in need of some systematic study of the question, there are indications that the grieving process is eased for parents who felt that they were involved in the important decisions [13].

The great bulk of the psychological research carried out on the parent–child relationship of preterm babies has centred on the possible effects of early separation or, as it has come to be known, on the question of bonding. As specialized units for neonatal care grew up, there was growing disquiet among some parents and professionals about the possible consequences of the parent–infant separation. These concerns became focused on the concept of bonding originally proposed by Klaus and Kennell [14]. Drawing on some research on animal species as well as on human data, these authors suggested that mothers enter a sensitive period after delivery during which they are particularly able to form a relationship with their baby. They further suggested that if mother and baby were separated during this sensitive period, which was hypothesized to last about two days, there may be long-term, if not permanent, difficulties in subsequently forming a satisfactory relationship. Many studies have been carried out to test these ideas and there have been several theoretical discussions of the concepts involved [15–18]. The general consensus is that while there may be some short-term effects of early separation, there are powerful recuperative processes so that separation *per se* does not seem to have long-term effects. Nevertheless, most parents dislike forced separation; this and the short-term effects that have been demonstrated make the avoidance of separation a high priority in neonatal care. Indeed, the evidence goes further than this and indicates that more is required than the avoidance of separation and that active steps should be taken to engage parents in as much caretaking of their baby as they may feel comfortable with. This involvement appears to reduce the short-term effects of separation that have been described, such as a feeling of lack of confidence in being able to cope with the baby and a distance and strangeness in the relationship. In recent years, units have gained considerable experience with a wide range of techniques and practices designed to foster good relationships and reduce the inevitable stresses created by an admission to a neonatal unit [19]. These not only include parents but also siblings and grandparents.

As these kinds of programmes have developed, research interest and accompanying practice have focused on a somewhat different issue – the behaviour of preterm babies and the difficulties of building satisfactory relationships with them. The analysis of the growth of social relationships of full term infants and their caretakers has demonstrated the importance of mutuality in the interactions. Even from the first days after birth, the infant's behaviour has a structure that is relatively predictable so that the caretaker can mould her behaviour around what the infant is doing. This, in turn, provides a predictable social world for the infant. For the caretaker, the sense that the infant can respond in some way to what she is doing seems to be a crucial step in the early formation of their relationship.

The extent to which an infant's behaviour is structured (and there is a possibility of interactive behaviour) is related to gestational age. So, quite simply, preterm babies make very poor social partners. Their behaviour is unpredictable and disorganized and it is very difficult for the parent to get any sense of being engaged in a social relationship. Direct observation of preterm babies with their parents demonstrates differences in interaction which may persist for some weeks, if not months, after birth [20]. While it is important not to overstress differences of this kind, parents often need support and the reassurance that, with time, satisfactory relationships will develop. Especially in the United States, various home visiting programmes have been developed, some of which have specifically set out to enhance parent–infant interaction. However, though it is somewhat difficult to generalize, the more broadly based programmes of support such as are offered by health visitors in the UK, seem as effective as those with more specific aims [21,22]. Given the relatively high rates of problems indexed by such measures as hospital readmissions that ELBW babies and their parents experience at least for the first couple of years, there is a case for follow-up studies which would investigate more fully the psychological problems that might arise in this period. [23]

The emotional needs of the ELBW baby

Despite the considerable interest among psychologists in bonding and the early parent–infant relationship of preterm and other LBW babies, there has been little interest in the emotional needs of the babies themselves in the neonatal period. While it is possible to point to a whole number of features of this early environment which set it apart from that of a full term baby, it is another matter to assess the significance of these differences.

An incubator seems to operate as a psychological, as well as physical, barrier for parents and caretakers [8]. The baby's crying is difficult to hear and this, together with features of the way in which nursing care is usually organized, means that there is a lack of correlation between the infant's behaviour and that of the caretakers [24]. Again, compared with the normal situation, a very large number of different caretakers are likely to be involved and none of them is likely to learn in detail about a baby's individual characteristics. There are also aspects of the physical environment such as the general noise level and the repeated sharp sounds that are heard when a hard object is placed on an incubator. Light levels may be high and vary little by day or night. There may be a very high rate of medical intervention including procedures that might well be painful [25]. For tube-fed babies there is the lack of sucking experience. Here there is evidence that the provision of a teat to suck on during a tube feed may be associated with higher rates of weight gain [26]. However, this study, like the many others that have tested a wide range of intervention from stroking, through rocking water beds to the provision of piped music, has not involved ELBW babies. This is a major research need at present.

Studies are required of the physical and social environment of these babies and of ways in which these may be enhanced. In particular, it needs to be established if the use of potentially stressful and painful procedures can be reduced or their effect ameliorated. Of course, the issue of pain in immature babies is a controversial one. However, there is sufficient evidence to suggest that it cannot be assumed that preterm babies lack pain perception and the use of pain relieving techniques may improve the medical prognosis [27].

Multiple births

A final issue that requires brief mention is that of multiple births which figure prominently among ELBW babies. While the evidence, such as it is, about the social relationships of LBW twins is relatively reassuring [28], the same may not be true for higher multiples. The birth of three or more infants, even in relatively ideal situations, may cause extreme stress for parents. When the babies are all of VLBW it is likely that these problems are multiplied (F. Price, unpublished work, Child Care and Development Group, University of Cambridge) and it should be remembered that such births are becoming more frequent.

Conclusion

It is disappointing that with the great strides that have been made in the medical care of the ELBW baby, there has not been a corresponding growth of our knowledge of social and psychological matters. Most of what can be said has still to be based on extrapolations from studies of heavier babies. While these do provide a general understanding, much more work is needed to see what specific problems may accompany the birth of a baby weighing less than 1000 g.

References

1. Silcock, A. (1984) Crises in parents of prematures. An Australian study. *Br. J. Dev. Psychol.*, **2**, 257–268

2. Yu, V. Y. H. (1977) Caring for parents of high-risk infants. *Med. J. Aust.*, **2**, 534–537
3. Richards, M. P. M. (1986) Psychological aspects of neonatal care. In *Textbook of Neonatology* (ed. N. R. C. Roberton), Churchill Livingstone, Edinburgh, pp. 20–24
4. Fearn, J., Hibbard, B. M., Lawrence, K. M., Roberts, A. and Robinson, J. O. (1980) Screening for neural-tube defects and maternity anxiety. *Br. J. Obstet. Gynaecol.* **89**, 218–221
5. Marut, J. S. and Mercer, R. T. (1979) The Caesarean birth experience: implications for nursing. *Nurs. Res.*, **28**, 260–266
6. Goodman, J. R. and Sauve, R. S. (1985) High risk infant: concerns of the mother after discharge. *Birth*, **12**, 235–242
7. Stern, M. and Hildebrandt, A. (1986) Prematurity stereotyping: effects on mother–infant interaction. *Child Dev.*, **57**, 308–315
8. Jacques, N. C. S., Hawthorne-Amick J. T. and Richards, M. P. M. (1983) Parents and the support they need. In *Parent–Baby Attachment in Premature Infants* (eds J. A. Davis, M. P. M. Richards and N. R. C. Roberton), Croom Helm, London, pp. 100–128
9. Bender, H. and Swan-Parente, A. (1983) Psychological and psychotherapeutic support of staff and parents in an intensive care baby unit. In *Parent–Baby Attachment in Premature Infants* (eds J. A. Davis, M. P. M. Richards and N. R. C. Roberton), Croom Helm, London, pp. 165–176
10 Bogdan, R., Brown, M. A. and Foster, S. B. (1982) Be honest but not cruel: staff parent communications on a neonatal unit. *Human Organisation*, **41**, 6–16
11. Whitelaw, A. (1986) Death as an option in neonatal intensive care. *Lancet*, **ii**, 328–331
12. Harrison, H. (1986) Neonatal intensive care: parents' role in ethical decision making. *Birth*, **13**, 165–175
13. Stimson, R. and Stimson, P. (1983) *The Long Dying of Baby Andrew*, Little Brown, Boston
14. Klaus, M. H. and Kennell, J. H. (1976) *Maternal-Infant Bonding*, C. V. Mosby, St. Louis
15. Campbell, S. B. G. and Taylor, P. M. (1980) Bonding and attachment: theoretical issues. In *Parent–Infant Relationships* (ed. P. M. Taylor), Grune and Stratton, New York, pp. 3–23
16. Herbert, M., Sluckin, W. and Sluckin, A. (1982) Mother-to-infant 'bonding'. *J. Child Psychol. Psychiatry*, **23**, 205–217
17. Richards, M. P. M. (1983) The myth of bonding. In *Progress in Child Health* (ed. J. A. Macfarlane), Churchill Livingstone, Edinburgh, pp. 113–120
18. Goldberg, S. (1983) Parent–infant bonding, another look. *Child Dev.*, **54**, 1355–1382
19. J. A. Davis, M. P. M. Richards and N. R. C. Roberton (eds) (1983) *Parent–Baby Attachment in Premature Infants*, Croom Helm, London
20. Goldberg, S. and Divitto, B. A. (1982) *Born Too Soon*, Freeman, San Francisco
21. Barrera, M. E., Rosenbaum, P. L. and Cunningham, C. E. (1986) Early home intervention with low birth-weight infants and their parents. *Child Dev.*, **57**, 20–33
22. McCormick, M., Bernbaum, S., Stemmlet, M. and Farran, A. (1984) The LBW infant goes home: impact on the family. *Pediatr. Res.*, **18**, 109
23. Ford, G., Rickards, A., Kitcher, W. H., Ryan, M. M. and Lissenden, J. V. (1986) Relationship of growth and psychoneurologic status of 2-year-old children of birthweight 500–999 g. *Early Hum. Dev.*, **13**, 329–337
24. Prince, J., Firlej, M. and Harvey, D. (1978) Contact between babies in incubators and their caretakers. In *Separation and Special Care Baby Units* (eds F. S. W. Brimblecombe, M. P. M. Richards and N. R. C. Roberton), *Clin. Dev. Med.*, No. 68, Heinemann Medical Books, London
25. Murdock, D. R. and Darlow, B. A. (1984) Handling during neonatal care. *Arch. Dis. Child.*, **59**, 957–961
26. Ignatoft, E. and Field, T. (1982) Effects of non-nutritive sucking during tube-feeding on the behaviour and clinical course of ICU preterm neonates. In *Infant Behaviour and Development in Perinatal Risk and Newborn Behaviour* (eds L. P. Lipsitt and T. M. Field), Ablex, Norwood, pp. 107–116
27. Anand, K. J. S., Sippell, W. G. and Aynsley-Green, A. (1987) Randomised trial of Fentanyl anaesthesia on preterm babies undergoing surgery: effects on the stress response. *Lancet*, **i**, 62–65
28. Goldberg, S., Perrotta, M., Minde, K. and Corter, C. (1986) Maternal behaviour and attachment in low-birth-weight twins and singletons. *Child Dev.*, **57**, 34–46

Chapter 24

Outcome

Ann L. Stewart*

Introduction

As more and more ELBW infants survive demands for information about their long-term outcome increase. Society questions the ethics of the survival of such tiny infants, and financial constraints mean that the cost effectiveness should be examined. Thirty years ago similar questions were asked about infants who weighed less than 1500 g. Since then the lower limit for survival has moved down, until it is now realistically quoted as 500 g in specialist centres in Europe, North America and Australasia; and attention has been focused particularly on the infants who weigh less than 1000 g. The first published report devoted exclusively to these tiny infants was made in 1972 by Alden *et al.* [1]. There were few further reports until after 1980 when the survival improved dramatically [2]. This chapter will review these reports with the specific intention of providing information to answer two questions:

(1) What sort of citizens do ELBW infants grow into?
(2) What impact do these infants have on society, particularly health care and educational resources?

The question of cost effectiveness will be considered in another chapter. The first question is asked primarily by parents, although the society from which these parents come also asks such questions collectively in a broader way. Society asks the second question, too, both directly and through economic constraints imposed on the allocation of resources. This chapter will not attempt to review the information obtained from study of these infants concerning, for example, the development of the brain or the cause of brain damage.

Source material

Twenty-six reports were reviewed [1,3–27], including five [23–27] which exclusively concerned the tiniest infants who weighed less than 800 g. All of these reports were published after 1972 and referred to infants born after 1965. They were chosen because they were the only ones which gave information about both neonatal (28-day) and long-term mortality as well as morbidity, including the number of infants

* Supported by The Medical Research Council

Table 24.1 Outcome for ELBW infants born since 1965

Reference no.	*Location*	*Year*	*No.*	*Died (%)*	*Disabled (%)*	*Able-bodied (%)*
1	Washington[c]	1965–70	161	88	4	8
3	London (UCH)	1966–70	60	83	2	15
4	Wisconsin	1968–72	98	72	6	22
5	Toronto	1974	97	54	8	38
3	London (UCH)	1971–75	88	67	5	28
6	Hershey	1973–76	69	65	6	29
7	Illinois[c]	1974–76	100	77	4	19[b]
8	Philadelphia	1974–77	77	74	3	23[b]
9	Rome	1974–77	40	70	5	25
10	London (UCH)	1976–77	61	59	8	33
11	Syracuse[c]	1976–78	134	70	7	23
12	New York	1977–78	54	56	7	37
13	Melbourne	1977–80	107	45	11	44
14	Hamilton[a]	1977–80	255	56	10	34
15	London (UCH)	1978–80	67	70	4	26
16	Melbourne[a,c]	1979–80	351	75	6	19
17	Toronto (WCH)	1979–80	106	33	11	66
18	Chapel Hill	1980	56	48	14	38
19	Providence[c]	1977–81	247	70	7	23[b]
20	Hammersmith	1979–81	67	58	6	36[b]
21	Mersey (UK)[a]	1979–81	202	77	3	20
15	London (UCH)	1981–82	52	54	15	31
22	Melbourne	1981–82	83	52	14	34

[a] Population-based studies
[b] Loss to follow-up greater than 5%
[c] Birth weight less than 1000 g

Table 24.2 Outcome for infants weighing <800 g born since 1974

Reference no.	*Location*	*Year*	*No.*	*Died (%)*	*Disabled (%)*	*Able-bodied (%)*
23	Toronto	1974–78	158	76	5	19
10	London (UCH)[c]	1975–77	20	65	15	20
			(41)	(56)	(12)	(32)
24	Buffalo	1977–79	147	56	9	35[b]
25	San Francisco[c]	1975–80	60	63	3	34[b]
26	Seattle	1977–80	95	81	2	17
13	Melbourne[c]	1977–80	26	58	15	27
			(81)	(41)	(10)	(49)
14	Hamilton[a]	1977–80	142	73	9	18
			(113)	(35)	(12)	(53)
17	Toronto (WCH)[c]	1979–80	39	51	18	31
			(67)	(22)	(7)	(71)
18	Chapel Hill	1980	17	76	6	18
			(39)	(36)	(18)	(46)
15	London (UCH)[c]	1978–82	40	85	7	8
			(79)	(52)	(10)	(38)
27	Cleveland[c]	1982–84	41	73	7	20

[a] Population-based study
[b] Loss to follow-up greater than 5%
[c] Birth weight less than 751 g
Figures in parentheses refer to infants weighing above 751 g or 800 g in same study

Table 24.3 Outcome for ELBW survivors born since 1965

Reference no.	*Location*	*Year*	*No.*	*Disabled (%)*	*Able-bodied (%)*
1	Washington[c]	1965–70	20	35	65
3	London (UCH)	1966–70	10	10	90
4	Wisconsin	1968–72	27	22	78
5	Toronto	1974	45	18	82
3	London (UCH)	1971–75	29	14	86
6	Hershey	1973–76	24	17	83
7	Illinois[c]	1974–76	33	12	88[b]
8	Philadelphia	1974–77	20	10	90[b]
9	Rome	1974–77	12	17	83
10	London (UCH)	1976–77	25	20	80
11	Syracuse[c]	1976–78	40	25	75
12	New York	1977–78	24	17	83
13	Melbourne	1977–80	59	20	80
14	Hamilton[a]	1977–80	113	23	77
15	London (UCH)	1978–80	20	15	85
16	Melbourne[a,c]	1979–80	89	22	78
17	Toronto (WCH)	1979–80	71	17	83
18	Chapel Hill	1980	29	28	72
19	Providence[c]	1977–81	75	24	76[b]
20	Hammersmith	1979–81	28	14	86[b]
21	Mersey (UK)[a]	1979–81	46	15	85
15	London (UCH)	1981–82	24	29	71
22	Melbourne	1981–82	40	30	70
		Average disability rate = 20%			

[a] Population-based studies
[b] Loss to follow up greater than 5%
[c] Birth weight less than 1000 g

followed up, the methods of ascertainment used and details of the impairments included when defining an adverse outcome. Follow-up had been continued until the end of the first year of life in all the studies. The median value for the minimum age at final assessment was two years, but final assessments were made at ages ranging from ten months to seven years of age.

Adverse outcome was clearly and consistently defined in all of the reports. Affected infants had neuro-developmental impairments which caused disability and required specific interventions or management (analogous to 'special needs' as defined in the UK Education Act, 1981) [28]. These impairments were usually serious and permanently disabling. In addition, in 12 reports [6,11–14,19,20,23–27] infants were described as having *minor* neuro-developmental abnormalities when they had defined deviations from normal development, according to age-specific standards, without disability requiring intervention at the age of assessment. In these studies it was possible to calculate the total numbers of infants whose development was in any way abnormal; and by contrast, the numbers of infants whose development could be regarded as completely normal – at least at the age of assessment. Unfortunately these 12 reports were in the minority, so it was only possible to examine all the data for trends in the proportions of mortality, serious disability and survival without disability – referred to as able-bodied. The results have been tabulated with long-term mortality, disability and able-bodied survival calculated as proportions of the total number of live births enrolled in the study (Tables 24.1 and 24.2) and with disability and able-bodied survival calculated as proportions of the total number of long-term

Table 24.4 Outcome for survivors weighing <800 g born since 1974

Reference no.	*Location*	*Year*	*No.*	*Disabled (%)*	*Able-bodied (%)*
23	Toronto	1974–78	38	21	79
15	London (UCH)[c]	1975–77	7	43	57
24	Buffalo	1977–79	65	20	80[b]
25	San Francisco[c]	1975–80	22	9	91[b]
26	Seattle	1977–80	18	11	89
13	Melbourne[c]	1977–80	11	36	64
14	Hamilton[a]	1977–80	39	33	67
17	Toronto (WCH)[c]	1979–80	19	37	63
18	Chapel Hill	1980	4	25	75
15	London (UCH)[c]	1978–82	6	50	50
27	Cleveland[c]	1982–84	11	27	73
		Average disability rate = 23%			

[a] Population-based study
[b] Loss to follow-up greater than 5%
[c] Birth weight less than 751 g

survivors (Tables 24.3 and 24.4). The results for the tiniest infants weighing less than 800 g are shown separately (Tables 24.2 and 24.4).

Discussion

Quality of the source material

Although 26 fully documented reports were found for review, only three [14,16,21] were population-based. The remainder were from specialist centres where selection for admission was likely to have occurred. All the studies were small, reflecting the low proportion of ELBW among live births. According to the most recent UK population study [21], these infants represented approximately 3 per 1000 live births in the region under consideration during the years 1979–1981. More recently UK birth weight specific data have been reported [29] which indicate that the proportion of births weighing less than 1000 g in England and Wales in 1982 was lower, at 2.6 per 1000 live births (or 2.4 per 1000 for birth weights of less than 1000 g, in accordance with WHO criteria for birth weight groupings). This may represent a true population difference between one region in the UK and the country as a whole. It, however, may be the result of variation in reporting policy throughout the country. For example, Dunn [2] showed that the numbers of ELBW notifications in one UK Health District (Avon) increased from 0.8 per 1000 to 4 per 1000 live births in the three years following the adoption of a policy of offering full intensive care to these infants. During the same period, registration in England and Wales ranged from 1–2 per 1000 live births.

Variation in notification policy, both in the official guidelines issued and in their implementation, is probably the most important factor accounting for differences in ELBW study populations. It is extremely difficult to document for ethical reasons, yet it affects the interpretation of all data concerning ELBW infants. For example, it may be argued that ELBW infants will only be referred to specialist centres for care when they are in good condition, thus producing a bias in the notification of these infants towards under-reporting and favourable results. In contrast, specialist centres themselves will regard as potentially viable even the tiniest infants born within their own units, regardless of condition, which will bias notifications of ELBW in the opposite direction. Until attitudes to care and notification policies for ELBW are standardized, these considerations will affect the composition of study samples and must be borne in mind when interpreting results. They must not, however, be used as an excuse to disregard the results of all studies of ELBW infants.

The results of the reports reviewed here indicated in general that the proportions of dead, disabled and able-bodied ELBW infants were consistent between specialist centres at any one time; and the results of one [14] of the three population-based studies were in keeping with those from the specialist centres for the same years. This finding was noted previously among VLBW infants [10,30] and has been interpreted as meaning that the outcome for such infants depends predominantly upon expertise available at the time. In the case of the ELBW infant, it also may be argued that the results apply to the infants registered as live births at the time; this at least provides an indication of what can be achieved, given the notification policy prevailing at the time and place under consideration.

Outcome

During the 20 years under review, infant mortality (total deaths from birth to end of follow-up period) fell consistently and significantly ($P<0.005$) among the ELBW infant subjects of the published reports (Table 24.1). The proportion of able-bodied survivors rose correspondingly ($P<0.005$) but the proportion of disabled survivors calculated as a proportion of the total live births remained constant. This trend was not noted among the tiniest infants weighing less than 800 g, so it appears that it was accounted for entirely by changes in the outcome for the larger infants who weighed 751–1000 g (Table 24.2). This was confirmed in the six reports [10,13–15,17,18] which gave information on both infants weighing below and above 751 or 800 g.

These changes resulted in significantly more able-bodied survivors but, because there was no change in the proportion of disabled survivors, actual numbers of disabled children must have risen. It is this aspect which has caused particular concern among those responsible for health and educational services. Although the proportion of disabled children is small when considered as a percentage of total live births, it averages 20% for all ELBW survivors (Table 24.3) or 23% of those who weigh less than 800 g (Table 24.4) in the 20 years covered by this review. These values are larger than those (10–15%) generally quoted for the heavier infants who weigh up to 1500 g (VLBW) in the same time period. However, they confirm the observation originally made by Orgill *et al.* [13] that among ELBW infants only mortality increases as birth weight decreases; the outcome for ELBW survivors is the same, however low the birth weight.

Impact of ELBW infants on the community

In order to investigate the impact that changes in mortality and survival of ELBW infants may have on a community, specimen calculations have been made, using the results of the most recent UK population-based study [21] and two specialist centre studies [15,22] (Tables 24.5 and 24.6). Because reliable figures for the total numbers of ELBW infants born in the UK in a year were not available, certain assumptions have had to be made. In whatever way the values were calculated, the numbers of disabled

Table 24.5 Proportions per 10 000 live births of disabled and able-bodied ELBW infants, calculated on the basis of the results of one population-based [21] and two specialist centre studies [15,22]

1980	Mersey [21] (1979–81)	London (UCH) [15] (1978–82)
Base population (live births)	60 771	36 000[a]
ELBW live births	202	119
ELBW survivors	7/10 000	12/10 000
Disabled	1/10 000	3/10 000
Able-bodied	6/10 000	9/10 000
1982	**London (UCH) [15] (1981–82)**	**Melbourne [22] (1981–82)**
Base population (live births)	15 644[a]	24 969[a]
ELBW live births	52	83
ELBW survivors	15/10 000 (24)	16/10 000 (40)
Disabled	5/10 000 (8)	4/10 000 (12)
Able-bodied	10/10 000 (16)	12/10 000 (28)

[a] Calculated on the assumption that the ELBW infants studied represented 33.24/10 000 of the population from which they were drawn, as in the Mersey population-based study [21].
Figure in parentheses refer to actual numbers of infants

Table 24.6 Estimated numbers of disabled and able-bodied ELBW infants surviving in England and Wales in 1980 and 1982, derived from the results of one population-based [21] and two specialist centre studies [15,22]

1980	Mersey [21]		London (UCH) [15]	
	A[a]	B[b]	A[a]	B[b]
ELBW survivors	460	501	789	807
Disabled	66	65	197	196
Able-bodied	394	436	590	611
Disabled as % of total[c]	0.2%	0.2%	0.6%	0.6%
1982	**London (UCH) [15]**		**Melbourne [22]**	
	A[a]	B[b]	A[a]	B[b]
ELBW survivors	937	705	1000	736
Disabled	312	230	250	215
Able-bodied	625	475	750	521
Disabled as % of total[c]	1%	0.75%	0.8%	0.7%

[a] Calculated per 10 000 live births from total of 656 234 in 1980 and 625 931 in 1982 [29].
[b] Calculated per 100 ELBW live births from an estimated (33.24/10 000 live births) total of 2180 for 1980 and a reported (29) total of 1533 for 1982.
[c] Calculated per 100 total seriously (2%) and moderately (3%) disabled children expected per year, estimated at 32 032 (5% of 640 654 survivors) for 1980 and 30 630 (5% of 612 605 survivors) for 1982 [29]. Estimates for % disabled children expected in England and Wales derived from Alberman [39].

children were small and represented not more than 1% of the disabled children expected in England and Wales in the year under consideration. For every disabled child, more than two able-bodied ones survived, suggesting that an appreciable number of families would be joined by healthy new members without undue cost to the community in terms of the resources needed to care for a disabled child. This does not take account of the actual cost of saving these children – but that has to be offset against the cost of a lifetime of care for a disabled child, which seems a likely alternative if perinatal care is inadequate. Death is not the automatic alternative to healthy survival and this must not be forgotten.

Quality of life for ELBW infants

In virtually all the reports reviewed here, outcome in survivors was judged on the basis of assessments made at young ages – between one and three years. These assessments are likely to identify accurately children with serious, disabling impairments; and these disabilities are likely to be permanent [31]. However, it is unlikely at such young ages that the types of assessment used would provide accurate information on the prevalence of minor impairments which may not have much effect on the function of young children. Such impairments may affect learning once the child is of school age. Although there is now evidence [32] that many children who present in school with learning difficulties may be recognized in the early months of life with neurological impairments, no data of this kind were presented in the studies reviewed here. Twelve of the reports gave figures for 'minor' disabilities, and three [3,25,26] gave intellectual quotient (IQ) values for some older children; but none gave the results of, for example, cognitive assessments for all the survivors nor of the school performance. Some early studies of VLBW survivors [33,34] gave IQ values for ELBW infants separately. These studies concerned infants born before there was an appreciable improvement in ELBW mortality and may well not represent the current status of such infants. One report [33] indicated that birth weight within the range 500–1500 g was not an important determinant of IQ. Another [34] showed a significant different between the mean values for infants weighing above and below 1000 g; but both studies included very few ELBW infants. A more recent study [35] attempted to assess the cognitive development of a group of ELBW infants at around ten years of age. Unfortunately almost half of the children could not be traced so the results are of little value.

In a more recent study of very preterm infants born 1979–81 at University College Hospital London [36], the mean McCarthy General Cognitive Index of 21 of the 25 ELBW survivors without congenital defects was 96 ± 17 (range 62–125). These values did not differ significantly from the values for the larger infants weighing 1001–1500 g, 99 ± 15 (range 61–130). The proportion of seriously disabled survivors in the two groups also was similar at 3/25 (12%) for the ELBW group and 9/95 (9%) for the larger infants. However, in addition seven of the 25 ELBW children had difficulties with learning because of either a moderately low General Cognitive Index between 70 and 80 (5), or minor neurological impairments (3) or both (1). Four of these seven children were already receiving special educational provisions by the age of four years and the remaining three were expected to need them once they entered full-time education. Thus 40% of the ELBW group had some form of disability, leaving 60% who were developing normally.

All the ELBW infants in the University College Hospital study had ultrasound brain imaging in the early days of life. Seven of the 10 children who showed definite or presumed evidence of hypoxic ischaemic injury on their brain scans by the time they left hospital had neuro-developmental impairments when assessed at four years. By contrast, just three of the 15 ELBW infants who did not have evidence of hypoxic ischaemic injury on their brain scans had an adverse outcome at the age of four years ($P < 0.05$). This tends to confirm that ELBW infants do have the potential for normal development, particularly if hypoxic ischaemic brain injury can be avoided. It also indicates that the same relation exists between the findings on neonatal ultrasound brain scanning and outcome at four years, as has been reported for very preterm infants at 12–18 months of age [37]. Prediction of long-term outcome on the basis of ultrasound brain scanning is therefore feasible in these tiny infants. As methods for detecting hypoxic ischaemic damage are developed [38], prediction should improve and allow the identification of infants with very large probabilities of serious neurodevelopmental impairments to be recognized at an early stage and thus allow management to be carried out on a more rational basis.

References

1. Alden, E. R., Mandelkorn, T., Woodrum, D. E., Wennberg, R. P., Parks, C. R. and Hodson, W. A. (1972) Morbidity and mortality of infants weighing less than 1000 grams in an intensive care nursery. *Pediatrics*, **50**, 40–49
2. Dunn, P. M. (1985) Fetal viability: a perinatal viewpoint. In *Preterm Labour and its Consequences* (eds R. Beard and F. Sharp), Royal College of Obstetricians and Gynaecologists, London, pp. 295–301
3. Stewart, A. L., Turcan, D. M., Rawlings, G. and Reynolds, E. O. R. (1977) Prognosis for infants weighing 1000 g or less at birth. *Arch. Dis. Child.*, **52**, 97–104
4. Grassy, R. G., Hubbard, C., Graven, S. N. and Zachman, R. D. (1976) The growth and development of low birth weight infants receiving intensive neonatal care. *Clin. Pediatr.*, **15**, 549–553
5. Pape, K. E., Buncic, R. J., Ashby, S. and Fitzhardinge, P. M. (1978) The status at two years of low-birth-weight infants born in 1978 with birth weights of less than 1001 g. *J. Pediatr.*, **92**, 253–260
6. Rothberg, A. D., Maisels, M. J., Bagnato, S., Murphy, J., Gifford, K. and McKinley, K. (1983) Infants weighing 1000 grams or less at birth: developmental outcome for ventilated and non-ventilated infants. *Pediatrics*, **71**, 599–602
7. Bhat, R., Raju, T. K. N. and Vidyasagar, D. (1978) Immediate and long-term outcome of infants less than 1000 grams. *Crit. Care Med.*, **6**, 147–150
8. Kumar, S. P., Anday, E. K., Sacks, L. M., Ting, R. Y. and Delivoria-Papadopoulus, M. (1980) Follow-up studies of very low birth weight infants (1250 grams or less) born and treated within a perinatal center. *Pediatrics*, **66**, 438–444
9. Picece Bucci, S., Colarizi, P., Di Tullio, F. *et al.* (1979) Prognosi a distenza di bambini con peso alla nascita di 1500 g o meno. *J. Ital. Pediatr.*, **5**, 583–591
10. Stewart, A. L., Reynolds, E. O. R and Lipscomb, A. P. L. (1981) Outcome for infants of very low birth weight: survey of world literature. *Lancet*, **i**, 1038–1041
11. Ruiz, M. P. D., LeFever, J. A., Hakanson, D. O., Clark, D. A. and Williams, M. L. (1981) Early development of infants of birth weight less than 1000 grams with reference to mechanical ventilation in newborn period. *Pediatrics*, **68**, 330–335
12. Driscoll, J. M., Driscoll, Y. T., Steir, M. E. *et al.* (1982) Mortality and morbidity in infants less than 1001 grams birth weight. *Pediatrics*, **69**, 21–26
13. Orgill, A. A., Astbury, J., Bajuk, B. and Yu, V. Y. H. (1982) Early development of infants 1000 g or less at birth. *Arch. Dis. Child.*, **57**, 823–827
14. Saigal, S., Rosenbaum, P., Stoskopf, B. and Sinclair, J. C. (1984) Outcome in infants 501 to 1000 g birth weight delivered to residents of the McMaster Health Region. *J. Pediatr.*, **105**, 969–976
15. Stewart, A. L. (1987) Unpublished data
16. Kitchen, W., Ford, G., Orgill, A. *et al.* (1984) Outcome in infants with birth weight 500 to 999 g: a regional study of 1979 and 1980 births. *J. Pediatr.*, **104**, 921–927
17. Hoskins, E. M., Elliot, E., Shennan, A. T., Skidmore, M. B. and Keith, E. (1983) Outcome of very low-birth weight infants born at a perinatal center. *Am. J. Obstet. Gynecol.*, **145**, 135–139
18. Kraybill, E. N., Kennedy, C. A., Teplin, S. W. and Campbell, S. K. (1984) Infants with birth weights less than 1000 g. *Am. J. Dis. Child.*, **138**, 837–842
19. Walker, D.-J.B., Feldman, A., Vohr, B. R. and Oh, W. (1984) Cost-benefit analysis of neonatal intensive care for infants weighing less than 1000 grams at birth. *Pediatrics*, **74**, 20–25

20. Skouteli, H. N., Dubowitz, L. M. S., Levene, M. I. and Miller, G. (1985) Predictors for survival and normal neurodevelomental outcome of infants weighing less than 1001 grams at birth. *Dev. Med. Child Neurol.*, **27**, 588–595
21. Powell, T. G., Pharoah, P. O. D. and Cooke, R. W. I. (1986) Survival and morbidity in a geographically defined population of low birthweight infants. *Lancet*, **i**, 539–543
22. Yu, V. Y. H., Wong, P. Y., Bajuk, B., Orgill, A. A. and Astbury, J. (1986) Outcome of extremely low birthweight infants. *Br. J. Obstet. Gynaecol.*, **93**, 162–170
23. Bennett Britton, S., Fitzhardinge, P. M. and Ashby, S. (1981) Is intensive care justified for infants weighing less than 801 g at birth? *J. Pediatr.*, **99**, 937–943
24. Buckwald, S., Zorn, W. A. and Egan, E. A. (1984) Mortality and follow-up data for neonates weighing 500 to 800 g at birth. *Am. J. Dis. Child.*, **138**, 779–782
25. Hirata, T., Epcar, J. T., Walsh, A. *et al.* (1983) Survival and outcome of infants 501 to 750 g: a six-year experience. *J. Pediatr.*, **102**, 741–748
26. Bennett, F. C., Robinson, N. M. and Sells, C. J. (1983) Growth and development of infants weighing less than 800 g at birth. *Pediatrics*, **71**, 319–323
27. Hack, M. and Fanaroff, A. A. (1986) Changes in the delivery room care of the extremely small infant (< 750 g): effects on morbidity and outcome. *N. Engl. J. Med.*, **314**, 660–664
28. UK Education Act, 1981
29. Office of Population Censuses and Surveys (1982, 1983, 1984) Monitor DH3 82/3, 83/3, 84/6. HM Stationery Office, London
30. Koops, B. L., Morgan. L. J. and Battaglia, F. C. (1982) Neonatal mortality risk in relation to birth weight and gestational age: update. *J. Pediatr.*, **101**, 969–977
31. Stewart, A. L., Costello, A. M. deL., Hamilton, P. A. *et al* (1989) Relation between neurodevelopmental status at one and four years in very preterm infants. *Dev. Med. Child Neurol.* (in press)
32. Amiel-Tison, C., Dube, R., Garel, M. and Jequier, J. C. (1984) Outcome at age 5 years of full term infants with transient neurologic abnormalities in the first year of life. In *Intensive Care in the Newborn*, Volume IV (ed. L. Stern), Masson, New York, pp. 247–257
33. Francis-Williams, J. and Davies, P. A. (1974) Very low birthweight and later intelligence. *Dev. Med. Child Neurol.*, **16**, 709–728
34. Stewart, A. (1983) Severe perinatal hazards. In *Developmental Psychiatry* (ed. M. Rutter), Guildford Press, New York, p. 15
35. Nickel, R. E., Bennett, F. C. and Lamson, F. N. (1982) School performance of children with birth weights of 1000 g or less. *Am. J. Dis. Child.*, **136**, 105–110
36. Costello, A. M. de L., Hamilton, P. A., Baudin, J. *et al* (1988) Prediction of neurodevelopmental impairment at four years from beam ultrasound appearance of very preterm infants. *Dev. Med. Child Neurol.*, **30**, 711–722
37. Stewart, A. L., Reynolds, E. O. R., Hope, P. L. *et al.* (1987) Probability of neurodevelopmental disorders estimated from ultrasound appearance of brain in very preterm infants. *Dev. Med. Child Neurol.*, **29**, 3–11
38. Wyatt, J. S., Delpy, D. T., Cope, M., Wray, S. and Reynolds, E. O. R. (1986) Quantification of cerebral oxygenation and haemodynamics in sick newborn infants by near infrared spectrophotometry. *Lancet*, **ii**, 1063–1066
39. Alberman, E. (1982) The epidemiology of congenital defects: a pragmatic approach. In *Paediatric Research: A Genetic Approach* (eds M. Adinolfi, P. Benson, F. Giannelli and M. Seller), Heinemann, London pp. 1–12

Chapter 25

The cost of intensive care

Richard W. I. Cooke

Introduction

In an ideal world with infinite resources for health care, many health professionals believe that it would not be necessary to consider the cost of caring for sick and ELBW infants; but, in reality, we are forced to do this. In making decisions about resource allocations we reveal something of our attitudes toward our patients, their parents, and our own feelings about disability in later life. In this chapter we will examine the methods by which the costs of care have been examined, how they compare with the costs of other forms of medical care, and to what extent we are able to and are justified in limiting them.

In the earlier days of intensive care for LBW babies, intensive treatment for the infant under 1000 g was rarely attempted. The very high mortality with the techniques which were available, and the generally low expectations of parents and doctors, meant that no real dilemma existed. Gradually as results improved there was an enthusiasm to extend attempts at intensive care further down the birth weight scale until the first gloomy follow-up reports caused a reappraisal. At about the same time units undertaking intensive care for the ELBW infant became all too aware of the very extended periods of care required by some survivors, particularly those who had developed chronically disabling disorders such as bronchopulmonary dysplasia and post-haemorrhagic hydrocephalus. In countries without a free health service the costs of this care had to be borne mainly by the hospital or university, as the parents could rarely meet the enormous bills generated. Intense interest in the actual costs of care developed as a result.

Costs

In 1959 Baumgartner, Jacobziner and Pakter [1] reported that the cost of neonatal intensive care for US hospitals was about $25 per day, but it is unlikely that this included many infants of less than 1000 g or represented a level of intensive care that we would recognize today. By 1978 escalating costs and, in particular, the inability of hospitals to collect these from parents of very premature patients, caused a reappraisal of the attitude that 'no cost is too great' when caring for the ELBW infant.

Pomerance *et al.* [2] showed that the costs (adjusted for a 94% collection rate) were $450 per day for survivors and $825 per day for non-survivors. Total costs were lower for non-survivors at $14 236 compared to $40 287 for survivors. The high rate of later disability in these infants was recognized in that the authors also quote a total cost per 'normal' survivor of $88 058. They conclude: 'It is our belief that the cost of living for infants weighing less than 1000 g at birth is justifiable. Society, however, must be the ultimate judge, for society must pay the bill and reap the benefits and the heartaches as well.' The approach to costs in this paper did not try to take into account any of the long-term costs of care for the disabled, their loss of income and increased hospital usage in later years, and so an economic appraisal of the value of neonatal intensive care was not possible.

In the same year, however, Marsh, Coleman and Jung [3] drew attention to the serious stress being placed on families who had to meet medical costs of infants of less than 1000 g admitted to intensive care. In the following year there was a report of the costs of neonatal intensive care which included the extra considerable transport costs experienced in Denver, Colorado [4]. Day costs for survivors under 1000 g were $340 and average total costs $24 150. They noted large debts written off by the hospital, and some parents were sued by debt collection agencies. Costs compared favourably with those for adult intensive care, although the survival rate was three times higher. Nevertheless, the highest charges were paid by the parents of the babies with the worst outcomes who were usually the smallest.

Phibbs, Williams and Phibbs [5] in 1981, when using a multiple regression analysis to investigate the sources of the high costs in neonatal intensive care, found that three measures of risk – low birth weight, mechanical ventilation and surgical intervention – explained a significant proportion of the variation in individual costs. Variations between institutions in costs of caring for newborns previously published were due to differences in case mix.

In looking for ways in which to contain hospital costs, Pomerance, Schifrin and Meredith [6] examined the theoretical reductions in costs that might be produced by the extension of gestation by admission of mothers in premature labour and the use of tocolysis. By identifying hospital costs for preterm infants they noted a linear relationship between cost of survival and gestational age. Between 29 and 34 weeks this cost average $772 per day. Since the cost of admitting the mother to hospital was $310 per day the difference represented a saving of $462 per day ('womb-rent') if that admission resulted in a prolongation of gestation. It was also pointed out, however, that if such an admission resulted in a 24 week gestation fetus being born at 25 weeks the effect would be in the opposite direction. The former would almost certainly die within a short time, but the latter would live expensively with a high chance of long-term sequelae. Although ths argument has been repeated elsewhere, evidence that effective tocolysis of preterm labour is possible or even desirable from a fetal point of view in the infant under 1000 g is lacking.

Most recently Hack and Fanaroff [7] have recorded their anxieties about the morbidity costs and outcome of infants under 750 g in Cleveland, Ohio. They noted increasing numbers of very immature infants whose prolonged and extremely complex courses resulted in many poor outcomes and an average cost of care of $158 800 (range $72 110–524 110). Many of the mothers were socio-economically disadvantaged, young, unsupported and black. Some did not wish to or were unable to care for their infants after discharge and there were late deaths. The authors conclude that 'the implications and cost-benefit ratios of extending the trend whereby intensive care is applied to progressively smaller immature infants must be seriously considered in order for definitive guidelines to be devised'.

In Europe interest in the costs of neonatal intensive care was not apparent until nearly ten years after discussions had begun in the US. This was probably due in part to the slower development of such units in Europe and to the effects of socialized health care making costs less immediately evident. In Paris in 1984, a study [8] showed costs to be related mainly to duration of stay which averaged 71 days for infants less than 1000 g. These costs were increased most by the development of bronchopulmonary dysplasia or necrotizing enterocolitis in survivors. In the UK in the same year day costs were found to be £235 for intensive care, £122 for high-dependency care, and £43 for special care [9]. The average cost for a survivor under 1000 g was £10 000, but for a non-survivor £800, reflecting the short duration of care for the latter also seen in previous US costings. More enthusiastic efforts with very immature babies have resulted in increased costs for those that eventually die in the UK in a way similar to the recent Cleveland experience with infants under 750 g.

A similar UK costing study to that of Newns *et al.* [9] was published in 1986 from Liverpool [10]; it showed very similar day costs when corrected for inflation, but markedly dissimilar costs for non-survivors. They cost nearly as much as the survivors; presumably, they survived longer as a result of more energetic care. It is clear that medical policies concerning the approach to the tiniest babies may radically alter the overall costs of a service without necessarily substantially altering outcome. Such factors need to be taken into account when comparing costings. In the same study the relationship between cost and birth weight was examined, as almost all similar studies have shown a negative correlation between the two. A significant correlation was seen but this was found to be largely an artefact produced by grouping the data in 100 g groups before calculating the correlation. When a correlation was sought using data from individual patients, the correlation, whilst still statistically significant, was very small ($r^2 = 0.04$). This indicates that most of the variance was due to factors other than birth weight. All other studies to date have calculated correlations with grouped data thus exaggerating the effect of weight on cost and outcome.

In a detailed review in 1981, Sinclair *et al.* [11] pointed out that although some of the individual interventions in neonatal intensive care programmes had been evaluated scientifically, their overall effectiveness had not. Such non-experimental evidence that existed derived from referral units and did not describe the effect on the actual population served. They believed that the greatest priority for a full economic evaluation was the care of the VLBW infant because of the very high financial outlay involved and the ethical issues this raised. They also pointed out that 'there was no firm evidence that measures of the use of neonatal intensive care adequately reflect the desire, need, or demand for these services. Indeed it is possible that the supply of neonatal intensive care determines its use, rather than the converse'.

Walker *et al.* [12] performed a cost-benefit analysis on the care of 247 infants of less than 1000 g admitted to a single unit over a five year period. Using follow-up data in conjunction with hospital and estimated future therapeutic care required by disabled children, total lifetime costs were estimated. An inverse correlation between cost and weight was obtained ranging from $362 992 per survivor at 600–699 g to $40 647 at 900–999 g. Estimates were then made at current rates of lifetime earnings and these ranged from $0 for the lowest weight group to $77 084 for the highest. Only in the 900–999 g group did lifetime earnings exceed costs of lifetime care.

In a subsequent publication [13], the authors point out the many limitations of their study, and that they have not considered any intangible benefits or what alternatives might reasonably be followed. To answer some of these questions they produced a further cost-benefit analysis for all infants less than 1500 g born in a geographically defined area (Rhode Island) during two periods, 1974–75 and 1979–80. In the former period intensive care was in its initial stages but considered to be established in the later period. Costs per survivor over the two periods remained essentially the same, but lifetime earnings increased largely because of an increase in normal survivors. When costs and benefits were compared an excess of benefit over cost of $1 390 000 in the former period and $3 706 000 in the latter was observed although this difference was not statistically significant. When, however, the sub-groups of infants of under 1000 g were examined, the benefits to costs were –$74 310 in the earlier period but –$378 774 in the later period. Because of the relatively small numbers in this ELBW category the 'losses' they produced were absorbed by the gains in the larger group. Nevertheless, increased intensive care for the infant under 1000 g produced an increased lifetime deficit for the region.

These findings reflect those of the most detailed study to date by Boyle *et al.* [14] from Ontario in Canada. They evaluated the economic aspects of neonatal intensive care using outcomes and costs of care before and after the introduction of a regional neonatal intensive care programme in Hamilton-Wentworth County. Two periods, 1964–69 and 1973–77 were compared. Health outcomes were expressed in terms of both life years gained and quality-adjusted life years (QUALY) gained. The latter were produced using a range of utility values for different health states derived by interviewing parents of school children in the area. These ranged from 1 for perfect health to 0 for dead. As some states were perceived as worse than death by some parents the range of values extended to –0.39. Hospital costs and long-term costs and estimated lifetime earnings were obtained. Cost effectiveness, cost utility, and cost-benefit analyses were performed. A 5% discount rate to allow for inflation was used. For infants weighing less than 1000 g, each additional survivor produced by intensive care cost $102 500 and $9 300 per life year gained. When utility values were included a cost of $22 400 per QUALY was derived. For infants under 1000 g the net economic loss produced by intensive care was $16 100 per live birth. When sub-groups by weight below 1000 g were examined, the results were even worse with a net economic loss of $25 500 for infants of between 750 and 999 g (smaller infants still were less costly as they lived for a shorter time and the few survivors did better). The authors suggested that similar methodologies to theirs should be used to evaluate other therapeutic interventions so that direct comparisons could be made which would allow more rational use of health care resources. They have published [15] some approximate comparisons in terms of cost (US$ 1983) per QUALY: antepartum anti-D prophylaxis, $1220; screening for congenital hypothyroidism, $6300; postmenopausal oestrogen therapy, $27 000; coronary single vessel by-pass for angina, $36 000; hospital haemodialysis, $54 000. Using data from their 1983 study and comparing it with a period ten years earlier, Sandhu *et al.* [10] were able to produce similar QUALY costs for neonatal care of infants under 1500 g in the UK. The costs were £1500 as compared with recently quoted UK costs per QUALY of £750 for hip replacement and £3000 for renal transplantation (unpublished).

It seems, however, that although we are a little nearer to knowing the cost in financial terms of caring for very small infants, it does not necessarily help the clinician to make daily decisions. Many object to the consequentialist approach to clinical and ethical problems which QUALYs seem to imply, i.e. the greatest good for the greatest number. This is seen to legitimize discrimination between patient groups. The QUALY is a useful tool to determine cost effectiveness, but a relatively poor one for cost-benefit. The health economist feels the need for a mechanism in health care provision whereby the planners may be assisted in improving value for money in the face of an increasing demand for health care with limited resources. The QUALY may provide this. It is very important that the methodology is the same when comparisons are made, and so far this has not often proved to be the case.

The clinician's problem is not so much the provision of resource, but the effects at an individual level of its restriction. There is a fear that excessive expenditure on the tiny infant with a poor prognosis may deflect funds from the care of the more numerous larger infants who stand a better chance of a good outcome if treated well. The clinician seeks a set of rules that might be a guide in making non-treatment or selective treatment decisions. Can the QUALY do this? Rules should make meaningful distinctions between classes of patients to be treated or not. With the complex and multiple diagnoses, rules based on a single characteristic such as birth weight will never be adequate or fair. It is necessary to balance equity with efficiency in resource allocation. One day of ventilator care each, or random allocation of care would both be equitable but very inefficient. Clinical decision making involves these balances, and knowledge of costs may help the clinician in assessment of the efficiency side of the equation.

References

1. Baumgartner, L., Jacobziner, H. and Pakter, J. (1959) A critical survey of the New York program for the care of premature infants. *J. Pediatr.*, **54**, 725–729
2. Pomerance, J. J., Ukrainski, C. T., Ukra, T., Henderson, D. H., Nash, A. H. and Meredith, J. L. (1978) Cost of living for infants weighing 1000 g or less at birth. *Pediatrics*, **61**, 908–910
3. Marsh, L. A., Coleman, T. D. and Jung, A. L. (1978) Financial impact to families of less than 1000 g babies admitted to an NICU. *Pediatr Res.*, **12**, 374–376
4. McCarthy, J. T., Koops, B. L., Honeyfield, P. R. and Butterfield, L. J. (1979) Who pays for neonatal intensive care? *J. Pediatr.*, **95**, 755–762
5. Phibbs, C. S., Williams, R. L. and Phibbs, R H. (1981) Newborn risk factors and costs of neonatal intensive care. *Pediatrics*, **68**, 313–321
6. Pomerance, J. J., Schifrin, B. S. and Meredith J. L. (1980) Womb rent. *Am. J. Obstet. Gynecol.*, **137**, 486–490
7. Hack, M. and Fanaroff, A. A. (1986) Changes in the delivery room care of the extremely small infant (<750 g): effects on morbidity and outcome. *N. Engl. J. Med.*, **314**, 660–664
8. Monset-Couchard, M., Jaspar, M. L., Bethmann, O. and Relier, J. P. (1984) Cout de la prise en charge initiale des enfants de poids de naissance inferieur ou egal à 1500 g en 1981. *Arch. Fr. Pediatr.*, **41**, 579–585
9. Newns, B., Drummond, M. F., Durbin, G. M. and Culley, P. (1984) Costs and outcomes in a regional neonatal intensive care unit. *Arch. Dis. Child.*, **59**, 1064–1067
10. Sandhu, B., Stevenson, R. C., Cooke, R. W. I. and Pharoah, P. O. D. (1986) Cost of neonatal intensive care for very-low-birthweight infants. *Lancet*, **i**, 600–602
11. Sinclair, J. C., Torrance, G. W., Boyle, M. H., Horwood, S. P., Saigal, S. and Sackett, D. L. (1981) Evaluation of neonatal-intensive-care programs. *N. Engl. J. Med.*, **305**, 489–493
12. Walker, D.-J. B., Feldman, A., Vohr, B. R. and Oh, W. (1984) Cost-benefit analysis of neonatal intensive care for infants weighing less than 1000 grams at birth. *Pediatrics*, **74**, 20–25
13. Walker, D.-J. B., Vohr, B. R. and Oh, W. (1985) Economic analysis of regionalised neonatal care for very low-birth-weight infants in the State of Rhode Island. *Pediatrics*, **76**, 69–74
14. Boyle, M. H., Torrance, G. W., Sinclair, J. C. and Horwood, S. P. (1983) Economic evaluation of neonatal intensive care of very-low-birthweight infants. *N. Engl. J. Med.*, **308**, 1330–1337
15. Torrance, G. W. and Zipursky, A. (1984) Cost-effectiveness of antepartum prevention of Rh immunisation. *Clin. Perinatol.*, **11**, 267–281

Index

Abortion, 2
  threatened, 3
Acidosis
  bilirubin toxicity and, 122
  effects of, 27
  respiratory distress syndrome and, 28
Acquired immunodeficiency syndrome (AIDS), 176
Active expiratory reflex, 81
Age
  glomerular filtration rate and, 214
  see also Gestational age
Alertness, assessment of, 241
Alkalosis, 68
Allo-immune thrombocytopenia, 183
Alpha tocopherol, 168
Alphacalcidol in rickets, 160
Alveoli, immaturity of, 24
Ambroxol reducing severity of RDS, 36
Amino acid solutions, 141
  dangers of, 300
Aminophylline, 70
Amniocentesis, 6
Anaemia
  central venous oxygen tension and, 173
  copper deficiency, 167
  megaloblastic, 170
  pathophysiology of, 163
  role of iron, 166
  vitamin E deficient, 168
Anencephaly, 6
Antepartum haemorrhage, 16
Anticoagulants, 180
Antigen detection, 191
Anxiety, 3
Aortic aneurysm, 297
Aortic cannulation, thrombosis from, 297
Aortic coarctation, 202
Aortic stenosis, 202
Apgar scores, 51
Apnoea
  monitoring, 109
  respiratory distress syndrome and, 27
Arterial oxygen saturation, 164
Arterial pressure, 109, 110
Artificial Lung Expanding Compound, 37
  see also Surfactant
Asphyxia, 196
  Apgar scores, 75
  assessment of, 51
  bilirubin toxicity and, 122
  brain injury and, 228, 229
  causing periventricular haemorrhage, 55
  incidence of, 28
  perinatal, 52
  sequelae of, 57
  ventilation and, 52
Aspiration, role in chronic lung disease, 90

Basal metabolic rate, 143
Behaviour, assessment of, 234, 235
Betamethasone preventing RDS, 14, 32, 33, 34
Betamimetics postponing labour, 13
Bicarbonate concentrations, 216
Bilirubin
  affecting brain, 229, 232
  crossing blood–brain barrier, 123
  free, 122
  toxicity, 120
    adjunctive methods of treatment, 129
    exchange transfusion in, 124, 128
    management of, 124
    manifestations of, 121
    pathology of, 122
    phototherapy in, 126
    risk factors, 122
Birth
  effect on skin maturation, 95
  injury, 289
  multiple, 329
Birth weight, 1
  maternal age and, 10
  parity affecting, 11
  pneumothorax and, 78
  social class and, 11
Bleeding in pregnancy, 3
Blood, normal parameters, 163

Blood–brain barrier,
  bilirubin crossing, 123
  protecting from toxic substances, 232
Blood clotting factors, 179
Blood coagulation, changes in, 185
Blood flow, disturbances of, 185
Blood gases
  measurement of, 51
  monitoring, 110
  values during artificial ventilation, 68
Blood gas analyser, 66
Blood platelets, 179
  transfusions, 183
Blood pressure
  cerebral perfusion and, 277
  control in lung, 27
  transducer systems of measurement, 66, 110
Blood transfusion, 171–178
  AIDS transmitted by, 176, 177
  complications, 173
  cytomegalovirus infection from, 174, 175
  exchange, 128
    complications, 174
    in bilirubin toxicity, 124
  indications for, 171, 172
  metabolic problems, 174
  in small quantities, 176–177
  transmission of infection, 175
  walking donor system, 176
Blood vessels, wall abnormalities, 184
Body weight, glomerular filtration rate and, 211
Bone disease, 91
Brain
  birth injury, 289
  blood flow
    measurement, 228
    monitoring, 114
  blood supply, 228
  capillary permeability, 227
  circulation, development of, 226
  development of, 226–228, 251
  haemorrhage, 113, 116
  infarction, 231
  injury
    bilirubin toxicity, 120, 121
    causes of, 228
    hypoxic, 113, 116, 338
    toxic, 232
  intraventricular haemorrhage, *see* Periventricular haemorrhage
  metabolism, 116
  monitoring, 113, 116
  parenchymal haemorrhage, 231
  parenchymal unilateral cystic lesions, 273
  venous system, 227
Brain stem, respiratory neurones, 27
Breech presentation, 16, 17, 19, 21
Bronchopulmonary dysplasia, 86, 169, 203, 208, 340
  complicating ventilation, 296
  cost of intensive care and, 342
Bronchopulmonary dysplasia–*cont.*
  incidence and aetiology, 87
  steroid treatment, 89
  treatment of, 88
  water loss and, 99

C-reactive protein, 195
Caesarean section
  considerations, 17
  for breech presentation, 17
  indications for, 21
  infection indicating, 16
  maternal views on, 22
  mortality rates, 22
  periventricular haemorrhage and, 229
  respiratory distress syndrome following, 17, 26
Calcium, 155
  absorption, 156
Capillary damage in RDS, 52
Capnography, 308
Carbohydrate in intravenous feeding, 142
Carbon dioxide tension
  during ventilation, 69
  monitoring, 112, 117
    skin surface, 112
  periventricular haemorrhage and, 56
Cardiac output, 52, 226, 228
Cardiorespiratory monitoring, 107
Carnitine, 143
Catheters
  infection in, 147
  PVC, potential dangers of, 178
  thrombosis from, 185
Central nervous system, assessment of function, 124
Central venous oxygen tension, 173
Cerebral circulation, development of, 226
Cerebral cortex, development of, 251
Cerebral haemorrhage, 113, 116, 228
Cerebral palsy, 232
Ceruloplasmin, 167
Cervical incompetence
  causing low birth weight, 12
  causing preterm labour, 4, 5
  treatment of, 12
Cervix
  cone biopsy, 5
  infection of, 4
Chest
  changes in, 109
  physiology, 306
Chest wall, compliant, 27
Cholelithiasis, 125, 148
Cholestasis, 125
Choreoathetosis, 232
Chorion vessels, 184
Cigarette smoking
  causing premature labour, 3
  RDS and, 30
Community, impact of ELBW infants on, 335

Congenital heart disease, 200, 208
Congenital malformations, 9, 17
Convulsions, treatment of, 273
Copper, 167
  deficiency, 144, 167
Cor pulmonale, 203, 208
Counter immunospectrophoresis, 191
Cranial ultrasonography, 261–273
Crigler-Najjar syndrome, 123
Crying, 329
Cyanosis, 200, 201
Cystic periventricular leucomalacia, 247
Cytomegalovirus infection, 243, 263
  from blood transfusion, 174, 175

Delivery
  breech, 16, 17, 18, 21
  causes of, 2
  mode of, 16–22
    mortality rates and, 19
    RDS and, 30
  techniques, 17
  use of forceps, 21
  vaginal, 16
  vertix presentation, 17, 18, 19, 21
    head compression in, 20
  See also Caesarean section
Depression, 3
Dexamethasone preventing RDS, 33, 34
Dialysis in renal failure, 220
Diazepam in convulsions, 276
Diet, respiratory distress syndrome and, 25
Disability, 332, 333, 335, 336
Discharge of patient, 321
Disseminated intravascular coagulation, 180, 181
Dopper echocardiography, 202
Doppler ultrasound, 114
Down's syndrome, 3
Drugs
  absorption of, 102
  dangers of administration, 300
  in resuscitation, 60
  side effects of, 299
Ductus arteriosus, *See under* Persistent ductus arteriosus

Echocardiography, 202
Eclampsia, 182
Electrocardiographic monitoring, 107, 202
Electroencephalogram, 235
  abnormality of, 257
  changes in with age, 255
  delta brush, 256
  maturation of, 252
  normal, 250
  seizures, 259
Electrodes
  immature skin and, 103
  kuraya gum, 103, 107
Emotional needs of parents and baby, 325
Emphysema, interstitial, 295

Encephalopathy, 260
  post-icteric, 121, 122
Endocarditis, infective, 200, 209
Endotracheal tubes, 59
Energy supplements, 138
Environmental concerns, 312
Eosinophilia, 148
Erythrocyte sedimentation rate, 197
Erythropoiesis, 165
Erythropoietin, 163
Ethamsylate, 230
Eyes, assessment of, 234, 241

Feeding, 134–140
  assessment of, 241
  development of gastrointestinal tract and, 135
  early enteral, 137
  intravenous, 141–154
    benefits of, 146
    carbohydrate content of solution, 142
    catheters for, 145
    complications, 146, 300
    composition of solutions, 141
    fat content of solution, 142
    fluid and energy intake, 143
    infection of catheter, 147
    metabolic complications, 147
    mineral and trace elements in, 143
    monitoring, 146
    protein content of solutions, 141
    techniques, 145
  late enteral, 138
  metabolic milieu and, 136
  nitrogen requirements, 137
  protein and energy supplements, 138
  protein requirements, 138
  requirements of infant, 134
Fetal haemoglobin, 165, 310
Fetal size, ultrasonic estimation of, 233
Fetus
  abnormality, 6
  growth of, 11
  weight, calculation of, 12
Fibrinolytic system, 180–181
  changes in, 185
Fluid balance, 100
  management of, 99
Fluid therapy, 143
  in bronchopulmonary dysplasia, 88–89
  in congestive heart disease, 203
Folic acid, 169
Follow-up, 65
  long-term, 20
Fractures
  birth, 289, 291
  spontaneous, 159
Free bilirubin theory, 123

Gastrointestinal tract
  feeding and, 135
  mucosal macromolecular permeability of, 136

Gentamicin
  neurotoxicity of, 232
  renal clearance, 214
Gestation, length of, 1
Gestational age
  calculation of, 1
  effect on EEG, 255
  estimation of, 233
  RDS and, 24
  transepidermal water loss and, 96
Glomerular filtration, 213–215, 221
Glomerular filtration rate, 211
Glucocorticoids stimulating surfactant, 31
Glucose-6-phosphate deficiency, 123
Graft versus host disease, 175
Growth, quality of, 135

Haematinics, 166
Haematology, 163–189
Haemoglobin
  developmental changes in, 164
  fetal, 165
Haemoglobin concentration, 163, 166, 172
  blood transfusion and, 172, 173
Haemolysis, 168, 174
Haemolytic anaemia, 168
Haemorrhagic disease of newborn, 181
Haemostasis, 179
  developmental, 179
  hepatic maturity and, 181
Handling, infant's response to, 304
Head
  ultrasonography
    diagnosis by, 262
    purpose of, 262
    technique, 261
    value of, 273
Hearing, assessment of, 234, 242
Heart disease, 200–210
  clinical examination, 200
  investigations, 201
  range of, 202
  secondary, 208
Heart failure, 203
Heparin, 186
Hepatitis, post-transfusion, 175
Holoprosencephaly, 263
Home
  care in
    family involvement, 319
    preparation for, 316–324
    transfer to, 321
Human immune deficiency virus (HIV), 90
  transmission, 176
Human milk, 137, 138
  protein content, 171
  sodium in, 216
Humidification
  in artificial ventilation, 70, 74
  in incubators, 101
  use of, 66
Humidity, transepidermal water loss and, 98
Hyaline membrane disease, *see under* Respiratory distress syndrome
Hydrocephalus
  following periventricular haemorrhage, 246, 267
  post-haemorrhagic, 230, 340
  ultrasonic diagnosis, 263
Hydrocortisone preventing RDS, 32, 33
Hyperbilirubinaemia, 196
  adjunctive methods of treatment, 129
  brain damage from, 121
  exchange transfusion in, 128
  management of, 124
  neurological assessment in, 124
  pathology of, 122
  treatment, 126
  See also under Jaundice
Hypercalcaemia, 157
Hypertension, 16
Hypocalcaemia, 156
Hypocapnia, 68
Hypophosphataemia, 157
Hypoplastic left heart syndrome, 208
Hypotension, 55, 228
Hypothermia
  in incubators, 101
  respiratory distress syndrome and, 28
Hypoxia
  causes of, 54
  effects of, 27

Iatrogenic disease, 289–303
Inappropriate ADH secretion, 217
Incidence of ELBW births, 1
Incubators
  humidity in, 101
  radiant warmers in, 102
  water loss and, 101
Indomethacin
  in persistent ductus, 207
  renal function and, 218, 221
Infant mortality, 335
Infection, 190–199
  in bronchopulmonary dysplasia, 89
  causing preterm labour, 4
  in chronic lung disease, 90
  diagnosis of, 190
    C-reactive protein in, 195
    evaluation of methods, 192, 193
    limulus lysate test, 194
    non-cultural, 191
    physiological methods, 195
  from blood transfusion, 175
  risk of, 190
  RDS and, 30
  thrombosis and, 185
Inositol preventing RDS, 25, 36
Intensive care
  cost effectiveness, 331, 340–344
  cost of, 340–344
  effectiveness of, 342

Interstitial emphysema, 295
Intestines
  absorption, 136
  transit of contents, 136
Intracranial hypertension, 280
Intracranial pressure, 279
  monitoring, 113
Intralipid, 143
Intrauterine growth retardation, 6–7
  delivery and, 16
  haematological manifestations, 182
Intravascular catheters causing thrombosis, 185
Intraventricular haemorrhage, 196, 273
  germinal layer and, 229
  neurological profiles, 246
  vitamin E and, 169
  See also Periventricular haemorrhage
Intubation
  causing laryngeal ulceration, 292
  causing tracheal ulceration, 295
  in resuscitation
    advantages of, 58
    reasons for, 57
Iron, 166
  supplements, 167
Ischaemic hypoxic encephalopathy, 260

Jaundice, 120–133, 243
  cholestatic, 148
  development of, 120
  free bilirubin theory, 123
  management of, 124
  obstructive, 125
  phototherapy, 126
  physiology of, 120
  risk factors, 122
  toxicity of, 120
  See also under Hyperbilirubinaemia

Kernicterus, 120, 122, 232
  free bilirubin and, 123
Kidney, 211–225
  congenital abnormalities of, 219
  function, 211
  glomerular filtration, 213, 221
  role of, 212
  sodium excretion, 218
  tubular function, 215
  water metabolism, 216, 217, 218
  See also under Renal
Kuraya gum electrodes, 103, 107

Labour
  postponement by betamimetics, 13
  preterm, *see* Preterm labour
  transfer during, 13
Laryngoscopy, 58, 59
Larynx, ulceration of, 292
Lecithin–sphingomyelin ratio, 14, 28
  surfactant and, 25
Leucomalacia, prevention by ventilation, 55
Lewin's air-filled multi-compartment mattress, 109
Limulus lysate test, 194
Listeria infection, 192
Liver
  carcinoma, 148
  erythropoiesis in, 165
  maturity, haemostasis and, 181
Lumbar punctures, 280
Lung
  air leak *see* Pulmonary air leak
  clearance of fluid, 26
  development of, 87
  expansion of, RDS and, 27, 28
  immature structure, RDS and, 24
  fat accumulation in, 147
  maturation, hormones influencing, 31, 36
  perforation by drain, 296
  perfusion, ventilation and, 54
  retained secretions, 90
Lung disease
  chronic, 70, 86–93
    aspiration and, 91
    bronchopulmonary dysplasia and, 86
    causes of, 86
    definition of, 86
    following pulmonary air leak, 79
    incidence of, 87
    long-term prognosis, 91
    prevention and treatment, 91
    role of infection, 90
    Wilson–Mikity syndrome and, 89–90
  in respiratory distress syndrome, 68
  with low compliance, 68

Magnetic resonance spectroscopy, 116
Maternal age, birth weight and, 10
Maternal smoking, respiratory distress syndrome and, 30
Megaloblastic anaemia, 170
Membranes
  premature rupture of, 4
  prolonged rupture, 29
Meningitis, 191, 196
Milk, human, 137, 138
  protein content, 171
  sodium in, 216
Mineral metabolism, 155
Minerals and trace elements in intravenous feeding, 143
Mineral supply, maternal, 155
Monitoring, 106–119
  apnoea, 108, 308
  arterial pressure, 109
  blood gases and pH, 110
  cardiorespiratory, 107
  cerebral, 113
  cerebral blood flow, 114
  cerebral metabolism, 116
  intracranial pressure, 113
  intravenous feeding, 146

Monitoring–*cont.*
  kuraya electrodes, 107
  multiple sensors, 116
  oesophageal, 108, 117
  oxygen, 297, 306, 310
  sensors, 106
  skin care during, 310
  design, 311
Morbidity, 332, 333
Mortality
  from asphyxia, 51
  rates, 9, 335
    caesarean section, 22
    from pulmonary air leak, 79
    mode of delivery and, 19
    of breech presentation, 19
    of vertex presentation, 20
    respiratory distress syndrome, 44
    surveys, 332, 333
Movement, assessment of, 238
Multiple births, 329
Muscle tone, assessment of, 235, 244

Naloxone, 60
Necrotizing enterocolitis, 100, 146, 169, 178, 218, 299
  periventricular leucomalacia following, 231
Neonatal deaths, 9
Neonatal reflexes, 241
Nervous system, 226–288
  abnormalities, 226–232
    aetiology of, 226
  clinical evaluation, 233–250
  development of, 243–244
  disorders of, 273
  evaluation of, 233
    systemic, 234
  impairments of, 337
Nesting beds, 312
Neural tube defects, 6
Neurological profiles, 243
  of specific insults, 246
Neurological sequelae of RDS, 57
Nitroblue tetrazolium test, 197
Nitrogen requirements, 137, 141
Nursing
  environmental concerns, 312
  infant response to handling, 304
Nursing care, 304
  diagnostic procedures and, 311
  monitoring, 306
  oxygenation, 306
  stimulation from, 305

Obstetrical management, 9–15
Occipital osteodiastasis, 289
Oedema in heart disease, 200
Oesophagus, monitoring via, 108, 117
Osteopenia, 147, 157, 159
Oxygen
  arterial saturation, 164
  availability of, 164
  delivery to tissue, 165, 166
  monitoring, 297
  toxicity, 88
  transcutaneous monitoring, 66
Oxygenation, 306
  during ventilation, 69
  monitoring, 310
Oxygen tension
  central venous, 173
  measurement sensors, 110
  monitoring, 112, 117
    skin surface, 112

Paraldehyde for convulsions, 275
Parenchymal haemorrhage, 231
Parent–child relationship, 327
Parentcraft, 318
Parents
  involvement of, 327
  perspective, 325
  preparation of, 316
    antenatal, 318
  social and emotional needs, 325–330
  support for, 316, 321
  understanding, 327
Peak inspiratory pressure, pulmonary air leak and, 80
Peritoneal dialysis, 220
Peritonitis, 221
Perivascular haemorrhage, hydrocephalus following, 340
Periventricular cerebral atrophy, 267
Periventricular haemorrhage, 18, 44, 50
  aetiology of, 229
  association with pulmonary leak, 79
  blood loss in, 277
  caesarean section protecting from, 229
  hydrocephalus following, 230, 267
  hypotension and, 228
  neurological profiles, 246
  prevention of, 229
  prevention by ventilation, 55
  respiratory distress syndrome and, 55
  treatment of, 276
  ultrasonography in, 267
  ventricular dilatation and, 277
  vertex presentation and, 20
Periventricular leucomalacia, 50, 230–231
  cystic, 247
Persistent ductus arteriosus, 200, 202, 203–207
  bronchopulmonary dysplasia and, 88
  defective closure, 184–185
  haemodynamics, 204
  respiratory distress syndrome and, 27, 34
  surfactant effect on, 44
  symptoms and signs, 204
  treatment, 205

Pertussis, 90
pH
  monitoring, 110
  surfactant and, 53
Phenobarbitone for convulsions, 274
Phenytoin in convulsions, 276
Phospholipid glycerol levels, 14
Phosphorus, 155, 156
Phototherapy, 124, 126, 127
Physiology of ELBW infant, 135
Physiotherapy, 70
Placenta
  erythropoietin crossing, 163
  steroids crossing, 32
Platelets, 179
  transfusions, 183
Pneumothorax, 44
  birth weight and, 78
  complicating ventilation, 296
  pulmonary air leak and, 83
  in respiratory distress syndrome, 55
Polyhydramnios, 6
Post-haemorrhagic ventricular dilatation, 277
  shunt surgery for, 280
  treatment, 279
Posture, assessment of, 235
Pregnancy
  bleeding in, 3
  multiple, 5
  termination of, 2
Prematurity, metabolic bone disease of, 91
Preterm labour, 2
  background, 10
  complicated, 3
  prevention of, 10
  stress causing, 3
  uncomplicated, 3
Prognosis, 65, 331–339
  surveys, 331–334
Prostaglandins, 2
  effect on capillaries, 228
  intraventricular haemorrhage and, 229
Prostaglandin synthetase inhibitors, 207
Protein, 171
  exudation in RDS, 26
  in intravenous feeding, 141
  requirements, 138
  synthesis, 171
  turnover, 137
Pulmonary air leak, 78–85
  aetiology of, 79
  association with periventricular haemorrhage, 79
  incidence of, 78, 82, 83
  mortality and morbidity, 79, 83
  peak inspiratory pressure and, 80
  prevention of, 81
  ventilation in, 80, 81
Pulmonary atresia, 202, 208
Pulmonary blood pressure, 27
Pulmonary hypoplasia, 30
Pulmonary interstitial emphysema, 78, 83
  see also Pulmonary air leak
Pulmonary oedema, 88
Pulmonary perfusion, ventilation and, 54
Pulmonary stenosis, 207
Pulmonary thromboembolism, 299
Pulse oximetry, 310
Purpura, 184

Quality of life, 337
Quality of life years, 343

Red blood cell antigens, 174
Red cell mass, blood transfusion and, 172
Reflexes, 241
Renal failure, acute, 219, 221
Renal function, 211–225
  indomethacin and, 218, 221
  respiratory distress and, 218, 219
  standardizing measurements, 211
Respiratory audit, 72, 74
Respiratory depression, 29
Respiratory distress, in heart failure, 200
Respiratory distress syndrome (RDS), 9, 50, 180
  acidosis and, 28
  ambroxal and, 36
  apnoea in, 27
  association with periventricular haemorrhage, 55
  brain and, 229
  compliant chest wall and, 27
  definition of, 23
  dietary factors, 25
  eclampsia and, 29
  exogenous surfactant theory, 37
  factors affecting, 23
  fluid balance and, 99
  following caesarean section, 17, 26
  gestational age and, 24
  hypothermia and, 28
  hypoxic capillary damage and, 52
  immature lung structure and, 24
  infection and, 30
  lung expansion and, 28
  lung fluid clearance and, 26
  measuring severity of, 39, 75
  mode of delivery and, 30
  neurological sequelae, 57
  patent ductus arteriosus and, 27, 34
  physiotherapy and, 306
  pneumothorax in, 55
  prevention of, 23–49
    antenatal steroids, 32, 35
    betamethasone, 14, 32, 33, 34
    dexamethasone, 33, 34
    follow-up, 45
    inositol and, 25, 36
    tocolysis and, 35
  prolonged rupture of membrane and, 29
  prostacyclin and, 228
  protein exudation in, 26

Respiratory distress syndrome–*cont.*
pulmonary blood pressure control and, 27
relation to asphyxia, 52
renal function and, 218, 219
respiratory depression and, 29
surfactant deficiency and, 23, 25
trauma and, 29
treatment
surfactant, 65
ventilation therapy, 23
Respiratory failure, 23
Respiratory problems, prevention of, 32
Respiratory syncytial virus, 89
Resuscitation, 50–64
drug therapy, 60
evaluation of, 57
failure to respond, 61
intubation in, 57, 58
poor response to, 60
techniques of, 58
temperature control in, 58
Retinopathy of prematurity, 145, 169, 297
Rickets, 147, 156
aetiology, 157
complications, 159
incidence and diagnosis, 156
prevention, 160
treatment, 160

Seizures, 259
Selenium levels, 144
Sensors, multiple, 116
Sensory responses, 313
Septicaemia, 146, 209, 231
Shock, thrombosis and, 185
Shunt surgery, 280
Skin
care during monitoring, 310
drug effects on, 300
immature, 94–105
barrier properties, 95
drug absorption and, 102
trauma to, 103
injury from strapping, 291
maturation, 94
structure of, 94
transepidermal water loss through, 95
Skull
birth injury, 289
fractures, 289
ultrasonography, 261–273
Sleep, 254, 321
Social class, birth weight and, 11
Social interaction, 322
Social needs of parents and baby, 325
Sodium
excretion, 218
intake, 221
reabsorption, 216
role of kidney in metabolism, 213, 215
Sodium pump, 215, 219
Splenic vein thrombosis, 186
Staff–parent interaction, 327
Steroids
crossing placenta, 32
in bronchopulmonary dysplasia, 89
influencing lung maturation, 31
preventing RDS, 32
Stillbirths, 9
Stress
affecting birth weight, 11
causing preterm labour, 3
reduction of, 313
Stridor, 295
Sucking
assessment of, 241
development of, 244
Surfactant
affected by patent ductus, 44
artificial, 37
biochemical maturation, 25
composition of, 25
deficiency, 23, 25
glucocorticoids stimulating, 31
overventilation, 54
pH and, 53
release of, 54
stimulation of, 31
substrate deficiency, 25
synthesis, 53
therapy for RDS, 37, 65
Survival rates, 21
Syndrome of inappropriate antidiuretic hormone secretion, 217

Teeth, abnormalities of, 292
Temperature
control of, 59
water loss and, 101
transepidermal water loss and, 98
Theophylline in ventilation, 70
Thrombocytopenia, 148, 179, 182–184
Thrombocytosis, 148
Thrombosis, 179, 181, 184–187
from aortic cannulation, 297
risk factors, 184
surgery for, 187
treatment of, 186
Thyroid hormones, influencing lung maturation, 36
Tocolysis, 13
in prevention of RDS, 35
Toxaemia of pregnancy, RDS and, 29
Tracheal lavage, 70, 74
Tracheal ulceration, 295
Transfer of patient *in utero*, 13
Transposition of great vessels, 202
Trauma
to immature skin, 103
respiratory distress syndrome and, 29
Tricuspid atresia, 208
Twins, 5, 329

Ultrasonic scanning, 1
calculating fetal size, 12, 233
cranial, 261–273
diagnosis with, 262
purpose of, 262
technique of, 261
value of, 273
importance of, 20, 273
Umbilical artery
blood gas measurement in, 51, 110
catheters, thrombosis and, 185–186
pressure measurement in, 109
Umbilical cord, complications affecting delivery, 16
Umbilical vein
catheters
complications, 299
thrombosis and, 186
Urine, 216
Urokinase in thrombosis, 187
Uterine contractions, manipulation of, 13, 35

Venous stasis, 185
Ventilation
blood gas values during, 68
bronchopulmonary dysplasia complicating, 296
carbon dioxide tension during, 69
complications of, 291
apparatus, 291
continuous positive airway pressure, 67
effect on surfactant, 54
gas composition, 59, 296
humidification in, 70, 74
indications for, 50, 67
inflation pressures, 59
intermittent positive pressure, 67
justification for, 50
management of, 67
oxygenation during, 69
pneumothorax complicating, 296
positive pressure, 50
pressure of gases, 295
in pulmonary air leak, 80, 81
Ventilation–*cont.*
pulmonary perfusion and, 54
synchronous, 69
tracheal lavage in, 70, 74
weaning from, 70
Ventilation–perfusion imbalance, 54
Ventilator
care of infant on, 65–77
equipment, 66
Ventricular septal defect, 202
Vertex presentations, 17, 18, 19, 21
head compression in, 20
mortality rates, 20
Visceral injuries at birth, 291
Vision, assessment of, 234, 241
Visual tracking, 244
Vitamins, 144
bronchopulmonary dysplasia and, 89
Vitamin B_{12}, 170, 171
Vitamin D, 160
Vitamin E, 168
deficiency, 168
periventricular haemorrhage and, 169, 230
Vocal cords, damage to, 295

Water
excretion, 218
metabolism in kidney, 212, 216
reabsorption, 216
transepidermal loss, 95
effect of gestational age on, 96
factors affecting, 98
in incubators, 101
radiation and, 99
temperature and, 101
Weighing, electric scales, 311
White cell antigens, allo-immunization, 174
Wilson–Mikity syndrome, 89–90

X-rays in heart disease, 201

Zinc, 167
deficiency, 144, 167